T0260260

Practical Artificial Intelligence for Internet of Medical Things

This book covers the fundamentals, applications, algorithms, protocols, emerging trends, problems, and research findings in the field of artificial intelligence (AI) and Internet of Things (IoT) in smart healthcare. It includes case studies, implementation, and management of smart healthcare systems using AI. The chapters focus on AI applications in Internet of Healthcare Things, provide working examples on how different types of healthcare data can be used to develop models and predict diseases using machine learning and AI, with the real-world examples.

Features:

- Focuses on the Internet of Healthcare Things and innovative solutions developed for use in the application of healthcare services
- Discusses artificial intelligence applications, experiments, core concepts, and cutting-edge themes
- Demonstrates new approaches to analyzing medical data and identifying ailments using AI to improve overall quality of life
- Introduces fundamental concepts for designing the Internet of Healthcare Things solutions
- Includes pertinent case studies and applications

This book is aimed at researchers and graduate students in Computer Engineering, Artificial Intelligence and Machine Learning, Biomedical Engineering, and Bioinformatics.

Advances in Smart Healthcare Technologies

Editors: *Chinmay Chakraborty and Joel J. P. C. Rodrigues*

This book series focus on recent advances and different research areas in smart healthcare technologies including Internet of Medical Things (IoMedT), e-Health, personalized medicine, sensing, Big data, telemedicine, etc. under the healthcare informatics umbrella. Overall focus is on bringing together the latest industrial and academic progress, research, and development efforts within the rapidly maturing health informatics ecosystem. It aims to offer valuable perceptions to researchers and engineers on how to design and develop novel healthcare systems and how to improve patient's information delivery care remotely. The potential for making faster advances in many scientific disciplines and improving the profitability and success of different enterprises is to be investigated.

Blockchain Technology in Healthcare Applications
Social, Economic and Technological Implications
Bharat Bhushan, Nitin Rakesh, Yousef Farhaoui, Parma Nand Astya and Bhuvan Unhelkar

Digital Health Transformation with Blockchain and Artificial Intelligence
Chinmay Chakraborty

Smart and Secure Internet of Healthcare Things
Nitin Gupta, Jagdeep Singh, Chinmay Chakraborty, Mamoun Alazab and Dinh-Thuan Do

Practical Artificial Intelligence for Internet of Medical Things
Emerging Trends, Issues, and Challenges
Edited by Ben Othman Soufiene, Chinmay Chakraborty, and Faris A. Almalki

Intelligent Internet of Things for Smart Healthcare Systems
Edited by Durgesh Srivastava, Neha Sharma, Deepak Sinwar, Jabar H. Yousif, and Hari Prabhat Gupta

For more information about this series, please visit: www.routledge.com/Advances-in-Smart-Healthcare-Technologies/book-series/CRCASHT

Practical Artificial Intelligence for Internet of Medical Things

Emerging Trends, Issues, and Challenges

Edited by Ben Othman Soufiene,
Chinmay Chakraborty, and Faris A. Almalki

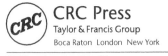

CRC Press
Taylor & Francis Group
Boca Raton London New York

CRC Press is an imprint of the
Taylor & Francis Group, an **informa** business

Designed cover image: © Shutterstock

First edition published 2023
by CRC Press
6000 Broken Sound Parkway NW, Suite 300, Boca Raton, FL 33487–2742

and by CRC Press
4 Park Square, Milton Park, Abingdon, Oxon, OX14 4RN

CRC Press is an imprint of Taylor & Francis Group, LLC

ISBN: 978-1-032-32527-9 (hbk)
ISBN: 978-1-032-32528-6 (pbk)
ISBN: 978-1-003-31547-6 (ebk)

DOI: 10.1201/9781003315476

Typeset in Times
by Apex CoVantage, LLC

Contents

About the Editors

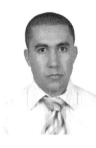

Ben Othman Soufiene is Assistant Professor of Computer Science at the University of Gabes, Tunisia, from 2016 to 2021. He received his Ph.D. in Computer Science from Manouba University in 2016 for his dissertation "Secure data aggregation in wireless sensor networks." He also received M.S. degree from the Monastir University in 2012. His research interests focus on the Internet of Medical Things, Wireless Body Sensor Networks, Wireless Networks, Artificial Intelligence, Machine Learning, and Big Data.

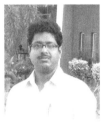

Chinmay Chakraborty is Assistant Professor in the Department of Electronics and Communication Engineering, BIT Mesra, India, and Postdoctoral Fellow of Federal University of Piauí, Brazil. His primary areas of research include wireless body area network, Internet of Medical Things, point-of-care diagnosis, mHealth/e-Health, and medical imaging. Dr. Chakraborty is co-editing many books on Smart IoMT, Healthcare Technology and Sensor Data Analytics with CRC Press, IET, Pan Stanford, and Springer. Dr. Chakraborty has published more than 150 papers in reputed international journals, conferences, book chapters, more than 30 books, and more than 20 special issues. He received Young Research Excellence Award, Global Peer Review Award, Young Faculty Award, and Outstanding Researcher Award.

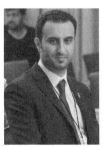

Faris A. Almalki is Assistant Professor of Wireless Communications and Drones in Computer Engineering Department at Taif University and Research Fellow in the Department of Electronic and Computer Engineering at Brunel University, London. He holds a B.Sc. in Computer Engineering from Taif University, an M.Sc. in Broadband and Mobile Communication Networks from Kent University, and a Ph.D. in Wireless Communication Networks from Brunel University London. He is a member of the IEEE Communication Society.

Contributors

Mohammed H. Abdalla
University of Raparin
Ranya, Iraq

Souid Abdelbaki
National Engineering School of Gabes
Gabes University
Tunisia

Jaza M. Abdullah
Erbil Polytechnic University
Erbil, KRG, Iraq

Enes Açıkgözoğlu
Isparta University of Applied Sciences
Isparta, Turkey

Aram M. Ahmed
University of Human Development
Sulaymaniyah, KRG, Iraq

D. Ajitha
Vellore Institute of Technology
Vellore, Tamil Nadu, India

Aso M. Aladdin
Charmo University
Sulaymaniyah, KRG, Iraq

Abeer Alsaddon
Asia Pacific International College
(APIC)
Sydney, Australia

Merve Varol Arisoy
Department of Informatics
Burdur Mehmet Akif Ersoy University
Turkey

Ganesh Babu
International University-Erbil
Erbil, KRG, Iraq

Nebojsa Bacanin
Singidunum University
Belgrade, Serbia

Chokri Baccouch
El Manar University
Tunis, Tunisia

Indradip Banerjee
The University of Burdwan
Burdwan, West Bengal, India

Anirban Bhattacharyya
Techno India University
Kolkata, West Bengal, India

Chinmay Chakraborty
Electronics and Communication
    Engineering
Birla Institute of Technology, Mesra
Ranchi, Jharkhand, India

Pratik Chatterjee
Vellore Institute of Technology
Vellore, Tamil Nadu, India

Amit Chhabra
Guru Nanak Dev University
Amritsar, Punjab, India

Amarendranath Choudhury
Department of Zoology
Patharkandi College
Karimganj, Assam, India

Ziya Dirlik
Isparta University of Applied Sciences
Isparta, Turkey

Leila Ennaceur
National Engineering School of Gabes
Gabes University
Tunisia

Sathish Eswaramoorthy
School of Electronics Engineering
Vellore Institute of Technology
Vellore, Tamil Nadu, India

Bryar A. Hassan
Kurdistan Institution for Strategic
   Studies and Scientific Research
Sulaymaniyah, KRG, Iraq

Nehru Kandasamy
National University of Singapore
Singapore

Ashish Kumar
Aryabhatta Knowledge University
Patna, Bihar, India

Jafar Majidpour
University of Raparin
Ranya, Iraq

Arun Anoop M
Royal College of Engineering &
   Technology
Thrissur, Kerala, India

Mustapha Najjari
National Engineering School of Gabes
Gabes University
Tunisia

Ben Othman Soufiene
PRINCE Laboratory Research
ISITcom
University of Sousse
Hammam Sousse, Tunisia

P. Rajesh
Annamalai University
Annamalai Nagar, Tamil Nadu, India

Karthikeyan P
Velammal College of Engineering and
   Technology
Madurai, Tamil Nadu, India

Shko M. Qader
University College of Goizha
Sulaymaniyah City, KRG, Iraq

Namita Rajput
Sri Aurobindo College
University of Delhi
New Delhi, India

Tarik A. Rashid
University of Sulaimani
Sulaymaniyah, KRG, Iraq

Sukanya Roy
Indian Institute of Technology Ropar
Rupnagar, Punjab, India

Rafid Sagban
University of Babylon
Hillah, Iraq

Hedi Sakli
EITA Consulting
Montesson, France

Nizar Sakli
National Engineering School of Gabes
Gabes University
Tunisia

Kazhan Othman Mohammed Salih
University of Sulaimani
Sulaymaniyah, KRG, Iraq

S. Vimal
Ramco Institute of Technology
Rajapalayam, Tamil Nadu, India

Anurag Shrivastava
Department of ECE
Bansal Group of Institutes
Indore, Madhya Pradesh, India

S.R. Swarnalatha
Patel Institute of Science and Management
Bengaluru, Karnataka, India

Noor B. Tayfor
Qaiwan International University
Sulaymaniyah, KRG, Iraq

Rabiaa Tbibe
National Engineering School
    of Gabes
Gabes University
Tunisia

Nagarjuna Telagam
GITAM University
Bengaluru, Karnataka, India

Abhinay Thakur
Lovely Professional University
Phagwara, Punjab, India

Dhilleshwara Rao Vana
Bharathidasan University
Tiruchirappalli, Tamil Nadu, India

Preface

The Internet of Things (IoT) is one of the most prominent technologies that emerged in recent years. The integration of IoT in the healthcare sector is giving rise to a new paradigm called the Internet of Medical Things (IoMT). IoMT enables collection, transmission, and storage of patients' physiological information. The remote patient monitoring can be performed via wearable sensors. These collected information can be stored, processed, and made available to doctors to give a consultation at any time and from any devices connected to the Internet.

In IoMT, the structure of data is important for accurate predictive analytics due to heterogeneity of data such as ECG data, X-ray data, and image data. So, the Internet of Medical Things requires new methods and technologies to evaluate information objectively. Artificial Intelligence (AI), which is being propelled forward by exponential advances in computer processing and the digitalization of things, has the potential to provide unimaginable benefits to the healthcare industry.

Thus, the integration of AI into IoT healthcare systems creates tremendous opportunities for new research and necessitates interdisciplinary efforts to address these challenges. AI combined with Internet of Healthcare Things can assist doctors in almost every area of their proficiencies such as clinical decision-making using the data generated by the health worker/professionals and the patient feedbacks.

This book covers the fundamental ideas, applications, algorithms, protocols, emerging trends, problems, and research findings in the field of AI and IoT in smart healthcare. It also demonstrates new approaches to analyzing medical data and identifying ailments to improve overall quality of life. The goal of this book is to bring together a diverse group of researchers, academics, and professionals from various communities to share and exchange new ideas, approaches, theories, and practices for resolving the difficult issues associated with the Internet of Healthcare Things by artificial intelligence.

Book Organization

The book consists of 16 chapters in the field of artificial intelligence for Internet of Medical Things.

A summary of each chapter is presented herein.

CHAPTER 1: IOT-BASED TELEMEDICINE NETWORK DESIGN: IMPLEMENTATION OF A SMART HEALTH MONITORING SYSTEM IN COVID-19

The role of telemedicine and big data analysis in the COVID-19 pandemic is highlighted in this chapter along with some real-life applications. The IoT and modern healthcare background exhibit the improvement of technology in the health sector with continuous research and innovation. The primary objectives of this discussion are to portray the impacts of telemedicine in the continuation of advanced healthcare approaches and help individuals to become familiar with modern healthcare. Along with expanding new research opportunities and extending telemedicine principles throughout the future medical sector, health services will become stronger and more easily accessible to everyone.

CHAPTER 2: DETECTION AND EVALUATION OF OPERATIONAL LIMITATIONS OF INTERNET INFRASTRUCTURE OF CRITICAL SYSTEMS BASED ON THE INTERNET OF MEDICAL THINGS IN SMART HOMES

In this study, the technical working principles of health-based IoT objects integrated into smart home systems and the previously measured network traffic and bandwidth consumption will be examined. The current problem situation will be a smart home system equipped with IoT systems, network traffic, and bandwidth usage will be measured through sample scenarios and the working performance of critical IoT systems will be discussed quantitatively based on Internet infrastructures. With this study, it will be easier to accurately plan the Internet infrastructure requirements of IoT-based health objects integrated into smart home environments.

CHAPTER 3: FITNESS-DEPENDENT OPTIMIZER FOR IOT HEALTHCARE USING ADAPTED PARAMETERS: A CASE STUDY IMPLEMENTATION

There are two primary goals for this chapter: first, the implementation of fitness-dependent optimizer (FDO) will be shown step-by-step so that readers can better comprehend the algorithm method and apply FDO to solve real-world applications quickly. The second issue deals with how to tweak the FDO settings to make the meta-heuristic evolutionary algorithm better in the IoT health service system at evaluating big quantities of information. Ultimately, the target of this chapter's enhancement is to adapt the IoT healthcare framework based on FDO to spawn effective IoT healthcare applications for reasoning out real-world optimization, aggregation, prediction, segmentation, and other technological problems.

CHAPTER 4: DIGITAL DISRUPTION IN THE INDIAN HEALTHCARE SYSTEM

The chapter begins with an introduction of the healthcare system in India, its challenges, and solutions to overcome the problems in the healthcare system. The second section of the chapter discusses the story and root cause of the coronavirus pandemic, which devastated the entire health ecosystem in India. Health crisis leads to an opportunity in the third section of the chapter; it throws light on the amalgamation of digital technology in the healthcare system, which brought a radical transformation. The rise in digital technologies in the healthcare domain increases efficiency, accessibility, and affordability. Integrating technologies like artificial intelligence, big data, and virtual reality solves institutional medical problems. The fourth section of the chapter discusses the health-tech start-up landscape in India and throws light on how the government bodies provide schemes and grants to encourage the start-up's ecosystem in the health domain.

CHAPTER 5: SMART HEALTHCARE MONITORING SYSTEM USING LORAWAN IOT AND MACHINE LEARNING METHODS

This chapter aims to study the LoRaWAN architecture involved in the health monitoring system and compare the GPRS-based system and show that LoRaWAN IoT devices provide accurate data. This chapter compares smart healthcare monitoring system using LoRaWAN IoT and Machine Learning Methods using medical data. The sensor medical data uploaded on the cloud are analyzed, and data predictions are explained briefly with the machine learning algorithm–based decision tree and random forest algorithm. The decision tree feature selection and random forest classifiers are used in this chapter. The proposed model shows an accuracy of about 4% for training data and a 5% improvement in accuracy for testing data.

CHAPTER 6: LIGHT DEEP CNN APPROACH FOR MULTI-LABEL PATHOLOGY CLASSIFICATION USING FRONTAL CHEST X-RAY

This chapter propounds custom deep convolutional neural network architecture for classifying COVID-19 CXR images. The method makes use of conglomeration of state-of-the-art CNNs by applying transfer learning. To solve the problem of the data imbalance, we used oversampling. The proposed methods with the MobileNet V3 implementation achieved 95.91% of the test accuracy of four class predictions and 96% recall. According to the obtained results, the model also achieved 97% precision and a 98% F1 score in coronavirus detection task; the other implementations also show good results, with an F1 score of 93–96%. These obtained findings reveal that the suggested techniques exceed the comparison models in classification accuracy, recall, precision, and F1 score, which illustrates their promise in computer-aided diagnosis and smart healthcare.

CHAPTER 7: TRENDS IN MALWARE DETECTION IN IOHT USING DEEP LEARNING: A REVIEW

The aim of the study is to inform about current malware attacks that threaten Internet of Healthcare Things (IoHT) environments, and to provide comprehensive research on the latest developments in the field of deep learning to prevent and detect these attacks. In this context, various malware attacks and the effects of these attacks were examined. A discussion on IoT environment architectures, IoHT-enabling technologies, security requirements of IoT/IoHT environments, and applications of IoT systems in healthcare is also presented. Moreover, an analogy-based study on various DL-based available methods for malware detection and prevention in IoT/IoHT environment is conducted.

CHAPTER 8: IOT-BASED WRIST ATTITUDE SENSOR DATA FOR PARKINSON'S DISEASE ASSESSMENT FOR HEALTHCARE SYSTEM

A detection approach for Parkinson's disease on-off period based on wrist posture is proposed to address the problem of high-precision drug on-off period detection for Parkinson's disease patients in a universal medical scenario. To categorize the condition of Parkinson's disease on-off phase, the motion IoT-based sensor data on the wrist is utilized to compute the attitude, get the information aspects of the wrist posture, and use it as the input of the convolutional neural network. Comparative experiments on clinical patient test data in the hospital show that using attitude information improves detection accuracy by 20.3% compared to the optimal results using motion sensor raw data; compared to the current optimal network structure, the convolutional neural network used in this method maintains a similar detection accuracy (88.7%) but is reduced by 90.4%. Furthermore, investigations on free movement data of clinical patients in the hospital reveal that this system can accurately forecast the patient's on-off state under unconstrained actions, with a 91.5% on-phase and 94.4% off-phase accuracy rate.

CHAPTER 9: ROBOTICS AND THE INTERNET OF HEALTH THINGS TO IMPROVE HEALTHCARE: ESPECIALLY DURING THE COVID-19 PANDEMIC

At the same time, the pandemic has highlighted the need to use new IoT, AI, and robotics technologies to cope. This chapter describes the influence of COVID-19 on the world of work, particularly in the health sector. We aim to highlight the role of new technologies in the improvement of healthcare as well as the advantages of an intelligent care platform that involves robotics coupled with the IoT to fight against the spread of the disease.

CHAPTER 10: ARTIFICIAL INTELLIGENCE AT THE SERVICE OF THE DETECTION OF COVID-19

Toward the end of December 2019, the COVID-19 epidemic appeared in the Chinese city of Wuhan, and due to its rapid spread, the World Health Organization designated it a global pandemic on March 11, 2020. Recently, many researchers from around the world have proposed new ways to detect COVID-19 making use of medical pictures like chest X-rays and CT scans combined with artificial intelligence. In this chapter, we study, analyze, discuss, and compare some of these proposed solutions.

CHAPTER 11: MONITORING ECG SIGNALS USING E-HEALTH SENSORS AND FILTERING METHODS FOR NOISES

In this chapter, we will present the different stages of denoising based on a real ECG and a development in Matlab of the techniques proposed after its reception and before sending it to the doctor. The treatments are carried out on the complete ECG, however, for the sake of readability; only extracts of the ECG relevant to the phenomenon illustrated will be presented. As a result, the available ECG signals are generally contaminated by random noises, and it is in this context that our contribution will intervene in order to minimize the influence of these noises on the ECG signals. As a result, in this study, we used a variety of strategies to eliminate noise from the ECG signal as a denoising technique. The simulation's results are given and then discussed.

CHAPTER 12: ARTIFICIAL INTELLIGENCE–ENABLED WEARABLE ECG FOR ELDERLY PATIENTS

In this chapter, we propose ResNet50, a deep learning model that uses a pooled dataset of 42 511 ECG 12-Lead records to categorize 26 CVD and normal sinus rhythm. When compared to the values obtained in the literature, our proposed model reaches 99.99% accuracy and precision. This result demonstrates the efficacy of the proposed model. ResNet50 will be used as a platform for diagnosing ECG signals and assisting cardiologists in their work in the future.

CHAPTER 13: DIAGNOSING OF DISEASE USING MACHINE LEARNING IN INTERNET OF HEALTHCARE THINGS

This chapter represents an efficient and effective machine learning, including systems such as computer-aided diagnosis (CAD) systems relied on boosting algorithm, principal component analysis (PCA), artificial neural network (ANN), and support vector machine (SVM), to explore an accurate model of predicting numerous diseases such as hepatitis, heart, thyroid, and Alzheimer. In research, it was also demonstrated that using a resilient and adaptable ML approach allows for the creation of well-proportioned organizational models that are rather more precise (86%) than the familiar synchrony metrics (83%) for the Alzheimer's diseases. Through this chapter, the readers and researchers working in the domain will have a quick update about the significance and utilization of ML-based approaches to diagnose and cure several fatal diseases.

CHAPTER 14: HEART ATTACK RISK PREDICTOR USING MACHINE LEARNING AND PROPOSED IOT-BASED SMART WATCH DRONE HEALTHCARE SYSTEM

This research expects to pinpoint the most applicable heart assault hazard factors just as it anticipates the general danger utilizing distinctive AI strategies lastly distinguish the best neural network methods with the "heart disease-UCI" dataset. Furthermore, we performed this performance evaluation using Google research Colab. In addition, we analyzed different optimization algorithms and test functions finally added to its survey. Furthermore, we utilized machine learning to choose the best calculation for foreseeing heart diseases. Different measures, for example, accuracy, recall, F1-measure, and precision, were utilized to test our proposed framework, assessing that the proposed procedure outperforms different models. Finally, IoT-based smart watch drone healthcare framework was likewise created utilizing Arduino.

CHAPTER 15: THERMAL FACE IMAGE REIDENTIFICATION BASED ON VARIATIONAL AUTOENCODER, CASCADE OBJECT DETECTOR USING LIGHTWEIGHT ARCHITECTURES

This chapter proposes a new framework in this regard, which is based on variational autoencoder (VAE) method, cascade object detector method, and three lightweight convolutional neural network (CNN) architectures. The variational autoencoder technique is employed to create the noticeable images out of their corresponding thermal images. Then, the cascade object detector method is used to crop the region of interest in these generated images. Finally, three lightweight CNN methods, namely, MobileNet, SqueezeNet, and ShuffleNet, are used for identification purposes. Carl dataset was used in the simulation experiments of this work and the results confirm that the suggested framework is capable. When an original image is used for testing, the SqueezeNet model returns an accuracy of more than 87%. Moreover, when the generated images are used for testing, the MobileNetV2 returns an accuracy of 94%.

CHAPTER 16: IOT-BASED LABEL DISTRIBUTION LEARNING MECHANISM FOR AUTISM SPECTRUM DISORDER FOR HEALTHCARE APPLICATION

This chapter proposes an IoT-based auxiliary diagnosis method for ASD that addresses the issue of label noise using label distribution learning (LDL), addresses the issue of sample imbalance using a cost-sensitive mechanism, and utilizes a support vector regression (SVR)–based method. By mapping the samples to the feature space, the label distribution learning approach overcomes the classification challenges imposed by high-dimensional features and eventually enables the IoT-based auxiliary diagnosis of multi-class ASD. The experimental findings demonstrate that, in comparison to existing approaches, the suggested method eliminates the imbalance between the majority and minority classes' effects on the results. It successfully addresses the issue of unbalanced data in ASD diagnosis, provides more accurate and consistent classification performance, and aids in ASD diagnosis.

1 IoT-Based Telemedicine Network Design

Implementation of a Smart Health Monitoring System in COVID-19

Anirban Bhattacharyya and Pratik Chatterjee

CONTENTS

1.1 INTRODUCTION

The term "tele," which means transferring over a distance, combines with the word "medicine" to enable a smart and digital approach in the field of medical science, stepping one step forward toward the "world of digitalization." Medical devices, smart health networks, AI-based disease prevention systems, and other equipment development have made significant contributions to global health improvement. Telemedicine has been introduced to intensify modern healthcare using communication networks for providing medical services, consultation, treatment, health advice, and also medical education [1]. However, the use of IoT has not been improved in the health sector throughout the years and the adoption of smart technology has been slower in this industry than in most other industries. The problems started occurring when people couldn't get proper medical treatments due to the unavailability and inaccessibility of the services, suffered from serious illnesses, and became helpless. Much research has been done to overcome this problem and new innovations have been implemented to make a better and more advanced health sector. In the continuation of the healthcare innovations, this chapter concentrates on developing an awareness of telemedicine and modern healthcare by describing all the relevant aspects of the entire architecture. Besides improving people's health and safety, the Internet of Medical Things (IoMT) also ensures that it will decrease healthcare expenses in the coming years [2]. Telemedicine is a modern concept that has recently gained popularity. Various types of telemedicine have been developed to monitor patients smartly (Figure 1.1). Some telemedicine systems are simply used to obtain remote medical advice from a doctor via some means, some are used to book appointments with the doctors and get medical services from the nearest hospitals, while others are used to identify any irregularities in the patient's body through the biometric sensors and give attention immediately to avoid any accidents [3]. Telemedicine allows patients to receive medical care when it is suitable for both the doctor and him while remaining safe. After COVID-19 hit the entire world, going to a doctor's chamber or hospital for general treatment enhances the risk of

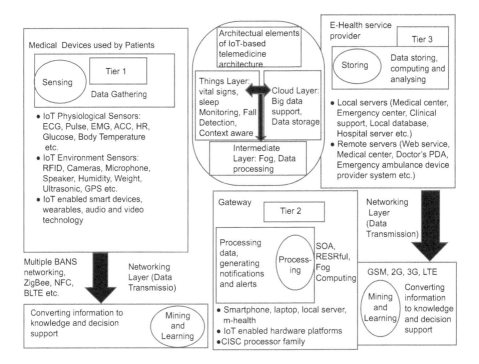

FIGURE 1.1   A theoretical flow diagram involving IoT-based telemedicine network and disease diagnosis solutions.

getting infected by other patients. This is especially harmful to people with weak immune systems or chronic health issues. Also, telehealth service professionals may be able to reduce the overhead costs and supplement their income by providing care to more patients. The patient may be pleased with their doctors if they do not have to travel to the office, wait in the outpatient department (OPD) for the consultation, or become infected while in the hospital [4]. Considering all the advantages, telemedicine has the potential to play a key part in this dangerous COVID-19 epidemic by minimizing viral propagation, making better use of healthcare workers' time, and alleviating depression or anxiety [5]. Coronavirus infection, caused by the severe acute respiratory syndrome coronavirus 2 (SARS-CoV-2), is a highly contagious disease that has been declared a pandemic by the World Health Organization (WHO). This virus has infected approximately 240 million people, resulting in more than 49 lakh deaths worldwide [6]. Social distancing has been used to reduce the frequency of human-to-human disease transmission as well as morbidity and death [7, 8]. However, in larger population densities, maintaining more than a 1-m distance between people, as recommended by the WHO, is challenging. As a result, densely populated developing countries are particularly vulnerable to COVID-19 outbreaks [9]. This chapter highlights the need for telemedicine networks and demonstrates an overall picture of the utilization of IoT-based healthcare systems in this current situation (Figure 1.1). Healthcare systems in low-resource countries face capacity and accessibility challenges. Hospitals are ill-equipped to deal with such a pandemic because they lack ventilators, ICU beds, and staff [5]. Because of the COVID-19 pandemic, telemedicine has become an essential entry point into the process of diagnosis, evaluation, and medication, with the goal of limiting patient displacement to hospitals, allocating hospital capacity, and slowing the spread of the illness. While healthcare innovations such as telemedicine hold great promise, their implementation has the potential to cause significant disparities due to the "generational difference," also known as the "digital divide," which refers to the disparity in the use of digital technology among individuals and communities of various ethnicity or religion and socioeconomic demographics due to cultural, social, language, financial, and other barriers [10]. Apparently, IoT opens new possibilities for telemedicine and makes healthcare more accessible to people. It is intended to be a continuous source of information, a real-time data analytics platform using big data mechanisms, and an end-to-end interface between a patient and a doctor. Application interconnectivity and a thorough clinical history allow physicians to use prudent treatment methods. Considering all the supremacy, it can be predicted that most of the patients and doctors will opt for remote healthcare monitoring and telemedicine systems in the upcoming years [11]. The IoT incorporates concepts of prevalent, versatile, and encompassing computing, which has been progressing for the last two decades and has now matured to the point where it can be used to supplement an experienced human for mass health and well-being. The IoT healthcare market is expected to be worth $188.0 billion by 2024, according to market estimates. The long-anticipated IoT evolution in healthcare provides the ability to adapt effectively, react quickly, and operate on a large scale that influences an entire community, state, city, or nation. The utilization of artificial intelligence (AI) comes up with some more advanced models for disease prediction, as well as prevention. This chapter also deals with some of the biometric sensors that can relate to the smartphones to make daily routine checkups and store the data for analysis by the doctors virtually with the help of a telemedicine network, allowing a healthy body fitness which is the first and foremost priority in this COVID-19 pandemic. This descriptive study incorporates the need for a modern healthcare society where patients will get efficient treatments and timely services from the comfort of their homes, get familiar with the advanced technologies, and the entire world will move one step forward toward digitalization.

1.2 TELEMEDICINE NETWORK FOR DISEASE PREVENTION

Image and video-based patient education, transmission of medical data such as X-rays, computed tomography scans (CT-Scans), and real-time audio or video consultations have all become a reality as wireless broadband technology has evolved and cell phones and Internet use have become dominant over the last several decades to make the best use of technology [12]. Improvement of the telecommunication network, which transmits various types of information over wire, radio, optical, or other electromagnetic systems, has made the people connected throughout the world. Various networking industries are continuously trying to link every sector that provides essential services to the masses and has kept their promises over the past decades. Internet infrastructures have been developed immensely with the introduction of fourth-generation technology. Because of advancements in bandwidth rates, the maximum capacity of a wired or wireless communication link to transmit data over a network has grown. Web service backups and information storage databases have also contributed to the advancement of telecommunication-based systems, making telehealth and telemedicine cost-effective. According to a 2017 American Telemedicine Association survey of 184 healthcare executives, 88% believed that they would invest in telemedicine in the coming future, and 98% believed that it offered a strategic advantage that would help it to become competitive in the market. But 71% believed that lack of representation and reimbursements were barriers to implementation on a larger scale. Recent studies have indicated that telehealth treatments are effective at improving medical outcomes and lowering hospital use in the fields of mental health and chronic illness management, with excellent patient satisfaction [13]. Table 1.1 elaborates the information of various types of disease datasets used in multiple works of literature, including the telemedicine network.

1.2.1 DEVELOPMENT OF TELEMEDICINE NETWORK

Several scientists and researchers have designed various models of telemedicine networks and proposed solutions to prevent diseases. Along with IoT-based healthcare systems, some personnel have studied and executed telemedicine models to combat this COVID-19 pandemic. This section describes some of the implementation and research that had been done before in this sector. Dr. Elisabeth Medeiros de Bustos et al. (2018) investigated the use and effect of a regional rural French telehealth network focusing on surgical and medical or neurological catastrophes [26]. They observed that telemedicine consultation was used by 23,710 patients in that region.

TABLE 1.1

A Theoretical Flow Diagram Involving IoT-based Telemedicine Network and Disease Diagnosis Solutions

S. No.	Name of Disease	Resource Material	Dataset	Algorithms	Techniques	Reference
1.	Cardiovascular	Electrocardiogram (ECG) data from telehealth	250 telehealth data from ECG	Support vector machine (SVM)	–	Liu et al. (2018) [14]
2.	Diabetes	Patients are fitted with sensors to help anticipate their diabetic condition, as well as medical data from the patients' healthcare records	N/A	–	Neural classifier (Fuzzy rule)	Kumar et al. (2018) [15]
3.	Neurodegenerative disease	Unlabeled dataset of patients' vital signs obtained by nanosensor	531 files	Multivariant linear/ logistic regression	–	Bagula et al. (2018) [16]
4.	Dermatology disease	Include photographs of either a visible and clear lesion or a nonvisible lesion; skin swabs, scrapings, nail clippings, and blood samples are collected	43 clear lesions and 48 nonclear lesions	Deep convolution neural network	–	Guo et al. (2018) [17]
5.	Respiratory disease	For sleep analysis, polygraphic signals for the patient with technical aspects of the recorded signals, cough swabs, antral, chest drain fluids, sputum, nasopharyngeal aspirates, etc. samples are tested	30 volunteered patients	–	–	Puthal et al. (2017) [18]
6.	Congestive heart failure	ECG readings from 15 patients with severe cardiomyopathy.	The individual recordings of 15 patients took around 20 hours to complete	Naive Bayes	Rank correlation coefficient (RCC)	Abawajy et al. (2017) [19]
7.	Chronic kidney disease	Benchmark source	In the presence of 24 characteristics, there were 400 cases	Logistic regression	–	Arulanthu et al. (2020) [20]

(Continued)

TABLE 1.1 (*Continued*)
A Theoretical Flow Diagram Involving IoT-based Telemedicine Network and Disease Diagnosis Solutions

S. No.	Name of Disease	Resource Material	Dataset	Algorithms	Techniques	Reference
8.	Disease at the time of pregnancy	Pregnant women, their medical histories, and sociodemographic data were analyzed	205 pregnant ladies were diagnosed with pregnancy-related issues	Nearest neighbor and ensemble classifier (NN)	–	Field et al. (2019) [21]
9.	Lack of balance	Data on a fall occurrence received from sensors on a smartphone	–	Artificial neural network (ANN)	–	Mrozek et al. (2020) [22]
10.	Infectious disease	Deploying the SocioPatterns framework 2016 to assess a genuine dataset of students' contact information	There are 188.508 entries in all, and each one depicts a proximity contact (CPI)	J48 decision tree	–	Sareen et al. (2018) [23]
11.	Alzheimer's syndrome	From 2010 to 2013, information was analyzed at the KFUPM clinic and the University laboratory	30 ECG samples were collected from young and aged individuals	–	–	Raad et al. (2015) [24]
12.	Ophthalmological disease	Capturing photos for normal retinal atlas using the iExaminer system	100 images	Binary decision tree (BDT) and extended nearest neighbor (ENN)	Multikernel	Jebadurai and Peter (2018) [25]

Most of these consultations were 30% for strokes and 36% for brain or spinal injuries. Cerebral tumors were responsible for 9% of the total teleconsultations. They also found that the number of patients examined and treated by telemedicine had increased over 13 years and interhospital transfers had halved for both pathologies. After the detailed 14-year research, they concluded that telemedicine networks make severe neurological assessments easier and reduce the need for additional interhospital transfers.

A study reported that Tamiru et al. (2020) developed a simple telemedicine system that was used to integrate with network design [27]. The system could exchange medical data and information in the hospital networks as well as outside networks. They designed the proposed system in such a way that health professionals could share, access, and retrieve patients' vital biometrics and relevant medical information easily with the help of networks. This telemedicine system was also used to give medical advice and education to the patients, take medical consultations from seniors, and seek guidance from experienced specialists. They described telemedicine architecture, its applications, advantages, and scope that help to make a better understanding of their implementation.

Another research by Nobre et al. (2012) recommended the creation of a state-wide telemedicine corporate network for the Santa Catarina State Department of Health in tropical America to investigate the advantages of telehealth and its future aspects [28]. Based on open-source technology, researchers from the Federal University of Santa Catarina created a web-based system that offers solutions for store-and-forward asynchronous and real-time medical applications, online and videoconferencing, continuous education, and a second constructive viewpoint. Case-based evaluations and evidence-based medical consulting were also incorporated into this application with library support. The primary focus was to decrease the costs of the system and make telemedicine available to everyone by improving the healthcare services in remote areas. They took a great initiative for the advancement of the Brazilian Healthcare system and made the telemedicine networks more demanding in the state of Santa Catarina. The number of doctors and health professionals enrolled and using the telemedicine network has exceeded 5,500 after five years of continuous implementation. The system had performed more than 1,200,000 processes. This service is now available throughout the state, making healthcare more inexpensive for patients.

In Paraguay, Pedro Galván et al. [29] studied the potential of telemedicine as an electrocardiographic (EKG) mapping tool for the interpretation, monitoring, and prevention of cardiac surgery problems. From 2014 to 2018, descriptive research was carried out at 60 tele diagnostic facilities throughout Paraguay to explore the usefulness of telemedicine as an EKG mapping system for the diagnosis and prevention of cardiological problems. The Health Sciences Research Institute Scientific and Ethics Committee accepted this study throughout the observation period, which comprised 246,217 patients with medical requests for an EKG test who were referred to one of 60 rural hospitals. These findings show that in low-resource nations, telemedicine might be used as an EKG mapping tool to identify and prevent cardiovascular disorders, while also improving cardiovascular disease monitoring and employing appropriate resources.

It has been reported that Bokolo Anthony Jnr (2020) researched and published an article on the importance of telemedicine in the COVID-19 pandemic [30]. His study offered a step-by-step tutorial on how to employ telemedicine and enhance the existing technologies to combine with medical science and provide telecare during the COVID-19 pandemic. To contribute to the integration of digital technology into healthcare, this article offered a framework for the possibilities of integrating virtual care solutions shortly.

A study governed by Ohannessian et al. (2020) promoted and scaled up telemedicine networks in the United Kingdom and the United States through their article [31]. Their objective was to propose and define an updated telemedicine framework in the COVID-19 pandemic to reduce the risk of disease transmission in hospitals and health clinics. Because of technology breakthroughs and cost reductions in telemedicine technologies, as well as the ubiquitous availability of high-speed Internet and cell phones, they believed this framework might be applied in the medical sector. They also discussed and reviewed some of the telemedicine systems used in different countries for disease prevention and monitoring.

1.2.2　Different Health Monitoring Systems

Telemedicine is a new concept that emerged as a modern health solution to monitor patients, provide online consultation, prescribe medicines, and give medical advice and health education. As communication and IoT have taken the recent market, telemedicine is becoming a necessity for people and health personnel day by day. The fundamental of introducing a telemedicine network is the advancement of health monitoring systems. This section describes different types of health monitoring systems that enable a digital approach to medical science.

- **Remote Patient Monitoring and Telemedicine:** With the development of telemedicine, patients are allowed to be treated utilizing telecommunications, lowering expenses, and reducing in-facility congestion [32]. Remote patient monitoring, sometimes known as homecare telehealth, enables a patient to do a standard test using smart body sensors and comprehend real-time health records on their smartphones. The data can be sent to the doctors to detect anomalies and provide specific recommendations [33].
- **Electronic Healthcare Records (EHR) Systems:** The primary objective of this type of healthcare system is to monitor a patient and send his/her medical records to the doctor or health professional for analysis [34]. Various health monitoring devices have been introduced to collect the vital biometrics of a patient through smart sensors and send it to the server using the Internet. Thanks to IoT for enabling a modern approach of connecting hardware devices with software technologies to adopt centralization of healthcare records which can be made available from various EHR systems used to monitor the patients. The health records can be accessed by the doctors, lab assistants, nurses, general physicians, and other associated entities for analysis, making predictions, taking preventive measures, and providing immediate medical support in case of an emergency. The users

can also visualize his/her medical records in the interactive UI application created by prominent software developers to keep a track of daily routine checkups [35].

- **Preventive Healthcare:** The healthcare industry's move to embrace IoT technology for preventive healthcare has had a huge influence on how suitable therapies are supplied for unanticipated chronic illnesses and medical problems utilizing IoT's predictive analytics capacity. There is an increasing demand and necessity in the modern period for the healthcare business to provide individualized, collaborative, and preventative treatment [36].

- **Medical Alert System:** Medical alert systems are generally based on IoT and artificial intelligence which help to make the existing system more advanced. Combining both the technology, some interactive and user-friendly medical systems have been designed to monitor a patient through body sensors, take the input data, and make predictions about whether any abnormalities are present or not [37]. A machine learning model analyzes the records coming from the hardware devices and raises alerts in case of any anomalies to make the health providers attentive so that they can take necessary medical action immediately and prevent serious diseases.

1.3   IoT-BASED TELEMEDICINE NETWORK

The IoT is a concept referring to any device, located anywhere on the planet, that can send and receive data across a network unaccompanied by associated computer architecture or an automated mainframe. It also consists of cloud-enabled intelligent technologies that gather, send, and analyze data in connection with the present environment using embedded technologies such as CPUs, trackers, and communications equipment. The sensor detects data from a variety of sources and samples, collects it, and delivers it to an IoT-based cloud database for processing [38]. The IoT offers various advantages to businesses. Some benefits are exclusive to manufacturing, while others are widespread in other industries. IoT is predominantly used to track whole operational procedures to improve the consumer experience, save time and costs, implement smart and advanced systems, increase production efficiency and feasibility, boost staff productivity, and integrate and alter business models. The Internet of Things allows businesses to reconsider how they govern their markets and provides them with the tools they need to establish a market strategy [39]. IoT is extensively employed in the automotive, shipping, and service industries, but it has also found uses in agricultural, telecommunication, and automation, forcing some corporations to go with data-driven technology. Job simplification might benefit IoT farmers. Sensors might collect data on moisture, humidity, temperature, and relative humidity, among other things, to help with the digitalization of agricultural operations with the help of robotics. One of the aspects that may aid IoT is the observation of functionality activities surrounding the foundation. Sensors can be used to identify issues or upgrades in existing buildings, bridges, and other infrastructure, for example [40].

Healthcare industries are no longer deprived of the benefits of IoT with the introduction of the Internet of Medical Things (IoMT) to enable real-time monitoring, knowledge gathering, data collection, and decision-making. Medical professionals and healthcare experts are smart enough to incorporate mobile platforms and applications that help to smoothen customer communication and track vital stats for providing better services. The introduction of patient portals, telemedicine applications, and various medical devices assist consumers to take a telemedicine approach for the betterment of society [41]. Advancement of health monitoring systems leads to a telemedicine-based network where patients not only monitor and test their vital biometrics through different sensors but also connect with the doctors through video- and audioconferencing to get better treatment, online diagnosis, health advice, prescriptions, and all other services that they require to keep themselves healthy [42].

1.3.1 System Design and Topology

Telemedicine follows a hierarchical structure to make the whole network traffic-free. It includes health monitoring devices, local/primary telemedicine centers, city/district hospitals, and specialty centers. Health monitoring devices are used to test the vital biometrics of a patient from the comfort of their home. These devices consist of smart sensors, i.e., pulse sensor, temperature sensor, ECG sensor, blood pressure monitor, etc. Readings are automatically sent to the server through the Internet as these devices relate to some software applications where all the analysis can be done by the doctors [43]. Local/primary telemedicine centers are the primary healthcare units established in rural and isolated locations to address the patients for primary health checkups and collect the data [44]. A patient who needs medical attention and does not have any medical device goes to the nearest telemedicine center where a local expert or health professional reports him/her and does all the preliminaries to gather all the vital statistics, i.e., blood, urines, pressure, pulse, temperature, X-rays and whichever applicable. These centers are connected to the city hospital through the PCs and Internet and all the data are transferred for analysis. City/district hospitals receive the records and checks thoroughly to discover any abnormalities that could cause serious diseases. City hospitals are connected to state hospitals. If they are unable to provide proper infrastructure and analyze the data, then records are transferred to state hospitals for further processing. After carefully examining the data by the city/state hospitals, an online appointment is booked with the patient for teleconsultation. A specialized doctor is appointed to take care of the patient and provide a proper recommendation. To connect with the patient in real time, the doctor employs an audio or videoconference system as well as automates live feeds. E-prescription and further analysis are given to the patient as needed [45]. Specialty centers are connected to the city hospitals for disease-specific assistance. In case of an emergency, these units are responsible to take immediate necessary steps and arrange hospital beds and doctors for faster treatment. A centralized database is used to store all of the patient's data and other medical reports so that these documents can be monitored by the doctors in the future if needed. Teleconference videos and audios are also recorded and sent to the patients for future reference. The recorded data may be accessed via a mobile application or web-based interface [46]. Here, Figure 1.2 demonstrates a general system design of a telemedicine network.

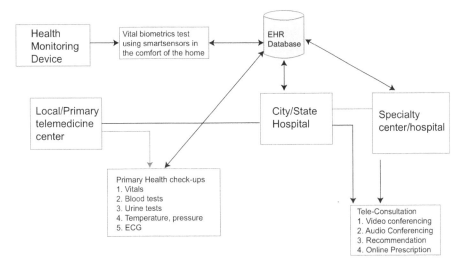

FIGURE 1.2 System design of a telemedicine network.

1.3.2 State-of-the-Art

The major components of a telemedicine system are telemedicine architecture, block diagrams, peripherals, software architecture, and databases. Data storing and forwarding, videoconferencing, and teleconferencing are the three key aspects of a telemedicine network [47]. This section briefly describes the architecture of the same.

- **Data Storing and Forwarding:** This method is responsible for storing patients' medical history, vital tests' readings, prescriptions, diagnostic images, X-ray scans, reports, and other relevant medical documents which are transferred to the diagnostic centers and city hospitals so that associated doctors can analyze and recommend proper treatment. The ability to save and forward solves the challenge of arranging several physicians' consultation schedules. Any consultant can access the patient file (called Electronic Medical Record) and review the details of the condition at his or her leisure to offer his or her professional opinion. This is ineffective in the case of an emergency medical intervention [47, 48].
- **Teleconferencing:** Teleconferencing is a commonly used term in recent days. It connects two or more individuals electronically to share information. Instead of meeting physically, teleconferencing helps different companies and businesses to arrange virtual telephonic meetings, customer interaction, training, and workshops via electronic devices such as laptops, mobile, etc. Participants can exchange relevant information and share individual opinions through teleconference from the comfort of their homes. A telemedicine network uses this virtual conference concept in the healthcare industry and connects the doctors with the patients over the phone or any teleconferencing device [49].

- **Videoconferencing:** Videoconferencing is like teleconferencing, but the only difference is that it is video-based teleconsultation and the most appropriate and effective mechanism [50]. The only thing which is needed for a smooth videoconference is a strong Internet connection and an active laptop webcam or mobile camera. Physicians use this method to diagnose virtually and provide proper treatment to the patients.

A simple block diagram of a telemedicine network is shown in Figure 1.3. The medical records are transferred as a bio signal through a telecommunication channel and received at the doctor's end for further processing. Both the doctor and the patient communicate with each other through a web-based application which includes live chat, audio call, and video call.

1.4   NETWORK ARCHITECTURE

An effective telemedicine network has three major platforms which consist of both the hardware and software. As we discussed the general system design of a whole telemedicine network before, this section deals with an in-depth analysis of each of the platforms which have different user controls and components.

- **Patient Application**

The fundamental aspect of a telemedicine system is the software application that a patient needs to communicate with doctors. Table 1.2 provides the key components of a patient-side telemedicine application.

It can be done with a data collecting device, a PC, a phone, and a scanner, but it will need to be scaled up as the demands grow. Telemedicine applications (to capture

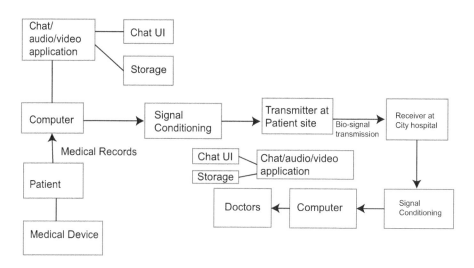

FIGURE 1.3   Block diagram of a telemedicine network.

TABLE 1.2

Patient-side Telemedicine Application Components

Components	Description
Authentication and authorization	The patient needs to register for the application and sign in by providing proper credentials to authenticate himself/herself
Patient profile	The patient can store his/her basic personal details
Storage system	Smart sensor–based medical devices need to be connected to the application through a unique pairing code, allowing the patient to test their vitals and submit information to the server utilizing IoT
Appointment scheduling	Patients can schedule his/her appointment by himself/herself with the respective doctor. City/state hospitals can also book an appointment between the doctor and the patient from their end
Tele and video consultation	Live chat, 24 × 7 support, audio call, and video call allow a patient to get their diagnosis easily from the specialized doctors
Medical education and medicines	Patients can get medical education as well as e-pharmacy services from the comfort of their homes

TABLE 1.3

Doctor-side Telemedicine Application Components

Components	Description
Doctor's profile	It includes the doctor's basic details, education, specialization, etc.
Appointment manager	Doctors can see their appointments and manage the application according to the requirement. They can also schedule their appointments with the patients
EHR	Doctors have access to each patient's electronic health records (EHR), which they may review before meeting with them
Real-time communication	Tele- and videoconference with the patients to provide proper medical care
Prescriptions	When needed, they can write online prescriptions because of the integration with local pharmacies and prescription software

patient data or images), a simple product containing a Pentium PC, a webcam, and some software and a dial-up Internet connection would suffice the same outcomes as sophisticated real-time software [51].

- **Healthcare Provider Application**

The most common type of telemedicine app used by doctors and healthcare providers is a web app. In an office context, a mobile app would be more difficult to utilize. The major components of this application are provided in Table 1.3.

The two different sides of a telemedicine application are controlled and monitored by the admin panel which consists of all the accesses and features to gather the information and arrange necessary steps [52]. City and state hospitals generally control the overall flow to make the system smooth and efficient.

1.5   CONTEXT DIAGRAM

Context diagrams define the boundary between different layers of a software application. Figure 1.3 shows a basic context diagram of a telemedicine network [53]. As a large amount of data has to be processed over the network, big data and cloud computing come into the picture. The system's progress is aided by machine learning and artificial intelligence.

The term "cloud" in cloud computing refers to a collection of networks, like how actual clouds are made up of water molecules. The user always has free access to cloud computing modalities. Instead of constructing their physical infrastructure, cloud computing users often choose to employ an intermediary provider for Internet connectivity. Cloud computing services are classified into three types: platform as a service (PaaS), infrastructure as a service (IaaS), and software as a service (SaaS). People utilize cloud computing regularly, for example, through YouTube, Facebook, Gmail, and Dropboxto, to mention but a few. Because of its scalability, adaptability, flexibility, and accessibility, its business applications are rapidly growing [54].

Web Services are a new type of web application that allows organizations to use a commercial method to put distinct services at multiple network locations by leveraging fundamental Internet infrastructure. The most significant property of Web Services is that they can communicate with each other regardless of the platform on which they were built (operating system and programming language). It offers a global platform for data sharing and dissemination. Web Services are gaining popularity as a structured and extendable framework for application-to-application interaction, based on current web protocols and the open XML Standard [55].

The term "Big Data" refers to datasets that have become so large that working with them using traditional database management systems has become challenging. They are datasets that are too enormous for typical software and storage systems to obtain, store, manage, and analyze in a timely manner [56]. Various data analysis software and platforms are introduced to process huge amounts of data generated every minute from various resources over the Internet.

Machine learning is a sort of artificial intelligence that enables software programs to learn from given datasets and anticipate future events to uncover hidden patterns, identify client experiences, detect anomalies, etc.

For every patient, a massive number of medical records are stored in a telemedicine system. The records include readings of the vital biometrics, test reports, images, meeting recordings, etc. A cloud computing platform, i.e., AWS, Azure is used to maintaining this large amount of data as the database is not enough to process the same [57, 58]. The information is stored in the cloud and can be accessed by the desired recipients. Firewalls, software security, protocols, and other security measures are followed for security purposes. To process real-time data, some of the big data analytics platforms are used. Apache spark is one of the most popular open-source frameworks which is needed to process and analyze real-time streaming data [59]. A machine learning model is trained with the normal human data and asked to predict future data. Based on the readings it finds in the system, it predicts an output and identifies the abnormalities present in that record. Machine learning and AI is used to predict serious diseases in advance and take immediate necessary action

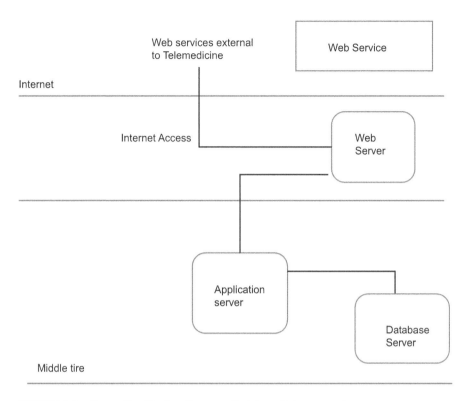

FIGURE 1.4   Context/application diagram of a telemedicine network.

so that any medical accidents can be prevented. Figure 1.4 comprehends the whole context diagram of a telemedicine system as discussed. The three-layer software architecture is shown in this figure. The application server is a server on which the application is created to host business layers, schedule jobs, client UI, etc. The database server has one or more databases hosted which are used to store the data and retrieve it as per the requirements. A web server is a software- or hardware-based appliance that is used to store the contents and data of any website. Web service provides the platform or software to store the modules of a website.

1.6   SERVICE-ORIENTED ARCHITECTURE

This section portrays a detailed service-level architecture of a telemedicine network. To address the issue of consistency, the design incorporates an application and architecture that is readily expandable and interchangeable with other telemedicine networks [60]. The presentation layer, business logic layer, and data layer are the three levels that comprise the software architecture. Figure 1.5 illustrates all the layers and their components in detail.

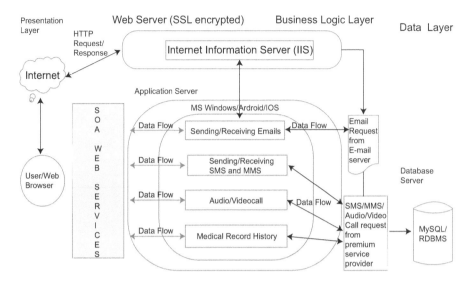

FIGURE 1.5   Service-oriented architecture diagram of a telemedicine network.

- **Presentation Layer**

The presentation layer deals with the presentation or the user interface of the soft-ware application. It consists of client-side rendering of a web browser and Internet. The information is exchanged between doctors and patients in this layer itself. The patient can see his/her medical records, vital statistics, and other relevant details which can be accessed by the doctors as well as healthcare providers to make the diagnosis. The doctor is responsible for writing online prescriptions, checking pre-vious medical history, and recommending medicines through this interactive and impressive UI application [61,62]. Audio and video calling features are included inside the application for the live conference.

- **Business Logic Layer**

The business logic layer manages communication between modules, databases, and external web services such as 3G connection providers, email servers, MMS, and SMS service providers [60]. MySQL (RDBMS) is utilized as a database in this design, while Internet Information Server (IIS) is used as a web server using SSL encryption to safeguard the data. The user sends an HTTP request to the web server, after that the request is transferred to the application server where module-specific configurations and relevant data keep fetching the required information and send it back to the web browser as an HTTP response [63]. The premium service provider's MMS and video calls are accepted by the 3G call module, which isolates photos, videos, and other data and stores it in the Windows file system. It also captures the patient's description as a text and saves all the data in databases. Receiving email is identical to receiving MMS and 3G, except it receives an email from an external email server and stores all of the information in databases. Doctors and experts can access the patient's data based on their most recent prescription history when such MMS, videos, and emails are received by the application server and recorded in the database. The patient videos must be displayed in such a manner that allows them to be easily compared on a computer screen. Doctors can also use a patient's broad description and phone number to seek up their medical history.

- **Data Layer**

Data layer is used to store all the information in the database. When a patient inserts any medical record, it is stored in the database. The doctor can get the data from the data layer with some restrictions. Audio and video calls are also recorded to the database for further use. Big data and machine learning are used in this layer for data analysis.

1.7   COVID-19 AND TELEMEDICINE

The COVID-19 pandemic has been declared a public health emergency of worldwide concern by the WHO [64]. This outbreak is producing a massive number of infections, putting a strain on healthcare systems, and having a negative impact on healthcare personnel, including the danger of infection [65]. The White House Coronavirus Task Force and health authorities have recommended hospitals increase their use of telemedicine for patient assessment [66, 67]. Telehealth promotes enhanced self-monitoring, weight loss, and behavioral changes by allowing children and adolescents to participate in online nutritional help and physical training activities that produce positive outcomes and diminish unproductive attitudes. Many of the basic obstacles in providing healthcare to fat persons during the COVID-19 epidemic can be solved through telemedicine. The present worldwide COVID-19 pandemic emphasizes the critical importance of utilizing digital techniques to improve healthcare delivery during this pandemic period. As limits and constraints on in-person or face-to-face encounters continue, more patients, families, and therapists are becoming more aware of the value of telemedicine [68]. In the era of the COVID-19 epidemic, telemedicine is essential for diagnosis. As we discussed all the advantages of using a telemedicine system to make healthcare systems more modern and effective, doctors and physicians recommend everyone to use telehealth in this recent situation. Telemedicine allows for the continuation of medical therapy while also lowering viral transmission. Even before COVID-19, scientific bodies throughout the world advised the use of telehealth, tailored to patients, their families, healthcare providers, and organizations. According to research, even in very complex medical circumstances, online consultation with a physician can be beneficial [69]. For example, research done some years ago discovered a variety of benefits of using telemedicine to treat chronic congestive heart failure, including shorter inpatient duration and fewer incidences of death. This included reduced infectious disease transmission for both patients and employees, as well as time and expense savings for the elderly, those living in physically inaccessible places, and those with disabilities [70].

The COVID-19 pandemic encouraged the development of several innovative techniques, including telemedicine. Clinician–patient encounters via the Internet were unavoidable because of the necessity for social distance. People who do not have access to the Internet, in general, or lack the necessary technical abilities are likely to have difficulties in seeking medical attention. The current study intends to investigate the relationship between age, eHealth literacy, and telemedicine satisfaction in the context of its use in remote locations during the COVID-19 outbreak. There would be unfavorable associations between age and eHealth literacy, as well as satisfaction with telemedicine. It is also predicted that there would be a positive correlation.

Telemedicine combines the ease of use, relatively inexpensive, and immediate availability of well-being communication and information via the Internet and associated platforms. Telemedicine has evolved from telephone consultations to encompass various virtual communication technologies in order to give healthcare information and services to customers in several places, which is especially crucial in pandemics since it allows the mitigation phase to develop [71]. Table 1.4 depicts an overall view of how telemedicine can play a critical role in the COVID-19 pandemic.

1.7.1 BIG DATA AND DISEASE PREVENTION IN COVID-19 TELEMEDICINE

Massive amounts of data that cannot be handled routinely and require advanced technological algorithms for analysis and pattern identification are referred to as big data. The technology behind big data allows for pattern identification, analysis, and exploration [79]. In this COVID-19 pandemic, health information and data become very crucial things that need to be shared and analyzed thoroughly to prevent serious diseases and reduce the risk of getting infected as human health conditions and reports start varying over a while. Consumers are scanned at airports and seaports, bus terminals, marketplaces, and medical centers, and the scan findings are communicated via smart city networks to process the information. This information is transferred for research and analysis to identify new strains, symptoms, the presence of molecules, etc. Scientists and researchers suggest that data may be provided effectively and timely by using sensors put in various locations to keep people informed about the COVID-19 state [80]. Existing sensors for health monitoring can be modified for the COVID-19 monitoring purpose to keep an eye on the infected patients at a regular interval.

Wearables, which have sensors built in them, are one solution for real-time remote diagnostics that are gaining traction in the IoT domain [81]. The sensors collect data on physiological parameters such as body temperature, blood pressure, and perspiration and send it to remote medical workers through a communications device such as a radio frequency identification tag. Medical officials may send the patient to a specialist or prescribe medication for the ailment. Wearable gadgets for remote patient monitoring are commercially available. Telemedicine holds immense promise for illuminating epidemiological investigation, infection prevention, and therapeutic patient care during a virus outbreak [79,81].

The role of big data in this COVID-19 pandemic is tremendously important to prevent serious diseases and monitor each patient in real time. When IoT real-time tools and techniques are deployed properly, they can not only monitor the spread of infectious illnesses but also provide immediate assistance to the emergency response team [89]. If public health experts can properly combine this universe of data to map and

TABLE 1.4

Role of Telemedicine in COVID-19 Pandemic

S. No.	Functionalities/ Use Cases	Description	References
1.	Time management	Telemedicine reduces the time for diagnosis and initiates faster treatment for quarantined and stabilized patients	Liu et al. (2020) [72]
2.	Reducing inter-hospital infection	It allows a patient to be monitored in the comfort of his/her home, reducing the rate of inter-hospital disease transmission	Rossi et al. (2020) [73]
3.	Medical resources	Telemedicine systems enable an approach to coordinate the required medical services and facilities in distant locations for the people who need necessary medical care every day	Bhat et al. (2021) [74]
4.	Risk prevention for the weak people	Preventing the spread of infection, especially among workers who are essential assets that must be safeguarded in this situation, eliminating direct physical contact, and lowering the chance of nasal secretion exposure	Liang (2020) [75]
5.	Decreasing cost	Lowering the costs of medical facilities and saving costs on antiseptic material	Haleem et al. (2021) [76]
6.	Health education	Arranging different pieces of training and workshops for the health professionals as well as general humans to make everyone aware of the current scenario	Chunara et al. (2021) [77]
7.	Medical records	Telemedicine introduces a platform for storing all the medical records and history of a patient efficiently for analysis	Balasubramanian et al. (2021) [78]

track epidemics in real time, it has the potential to save lives. They can readily foresee the amount of demand for resources and medical personnel if they use the technologies to predict where the sickness will migrate next. Handling health technology is incredibly complicated and taking into consideration all elements is quite difficult. When measuring and implementing technology, we tend to focus on precise structures while missing other and more important qualities. We tend to prioritize accuracy numbers (such as test specificity and sensitivity) above what matters to patients, such as diagnostic effect and subsequent treatment results when examining diagnostic technologies [88]. The primary clinic can administer a telehealth network that connects numerous medical organizations into a single virtual network. This network can encompass a range of physical places, such as hospitals, clinics, and physician offices in both central and outlying areas, as well as all registered patients in their respective areas [89]. Teleconferencing, secure messaging, electronic scheduling, analytics, and laboratory results are all accessible, as are pricing and e-payment, radiological file uploads, integration with electronic health record systems, and e-prescribing.

1.7.2 Artificial Intelligence in COVID-19 Telemedicine

Artificial intelligence has been utilized in therapy in addition to disease diagnosis, and as such it might be applied against COVID-19. It has already been used in Japan, where AI was used to recommend the best treatment for patients with hematological malignancies [82].

It is investigated if AI can be utilized as a prediction tool against COVID-19. The study was observed with two separate commercial AI sites that predicted COVID-19 properly. Bluedot and Metabiota are the names given to these locations. Bluedot is reported to search over 10,000 distinct sources for information in 60 diverse languages [83]. Bluedot looks at places that may be of significant concern based on the search results using clustering methods. Clients are then given the newly found information, which includes the most likely areas to be affected hard by the disease, as well as any other pertinent information such as how the disease spreads, best practices for combating it, and so on. The 2009 H1N1 influenza pandemic, the 2014 Ebola outbreak, the 2016 Zika virus, and the COVID-19 pandemics are all said to have been predicted by Bluedot before they were officially declared worldwide pandemics. Metabiota, similar to Bluedot, is a prediction tool that collects and interprets huge volumes of data from several sources using AI, big data, natural language processing, and neuro-linguistic programming. Official and illicit sources, as well as social media, can be used to obtain information. Insurance firms, nonprofit groups, and government agencies are claimed to gain from metabiota since it helps them make better judgments. Both the 2014 Ebola epidemic and the current COVID-19 outbreak were alleged to have been anticipated by metabiota before they were declared crises.

Artificial intelligence deals with learnings from a given input and making predictions based on future data [87]. Telemedicine integrated with artificial intelligence can become a boon to the future health industries to predict and prevent serious diseases in advance and monitor patients regularly. Figure 1.6 shows a simple diagram of how artificial intelligence is connected with telemedicine to provide better services.

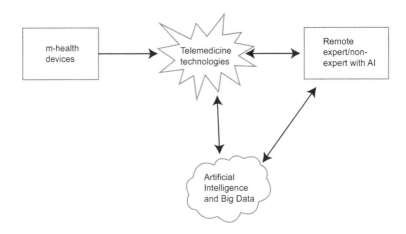

FIGURE 1.6   Artificial intelligence and telemedicine.

1.8　APPLICATION AND CHALLENGES

Despite its many benefits, telemedicine does have certain drawbacks and restrictions. The use of extensive Global Positioning System (GPS) tracking during quarantine in China and Singapore has raised worries about invasions of individual freedoms and the usage of personal data which couldn't be applied in other civilizations or regions of the world [78]. Furthermore, given the exceptional circumstances, the General Data Protection Regulation (GDPR) allowed for a lot of flexibility during the outbreak [84]. Personal data may be used in the public interest or for public health purposes, and personal information may be collected without the data subject's agreement. Under typical circumstances, telemedicine services must ensure and provide access and security, which presents a unique issue for the telemedicine being used. The benefits of greater accessibility, quality, and efficacy of medical diagnosis, however, remove the hazards, thanks to more extensive regulations and legislation providing solid privacy and data protection. Even though telemedicine has numerous advantages of establishing healthy, disease control, and enabling patients to maintain chronic health problems at home, it necessitates the asynchronous, digital collection and interactions of susceptible healthcare data between healthcare professionals and patients, which may pose some vulnerabilities due to the absence of control mechanisms or constraints on the collection and breaches of confidentiality of personal information. A mobile-based healthcare app, for example, maybe sponsored by sharing critically confidential material with third-party advertisers that display advertisements to patients based on app use or go over and above what patients may expect from using a certain application [85]. It is indeed essential to consider concerns about privacy and security risks, such as data breach during collection or transmission to the provider's system; unauthorized access to the functionality of supporting devices, including data stored on them; and untrustworthy distribution of software and hardware to patients [85,86]. It is critical at this time to create rules and procedures for enforcing proper data access, usage, and disclosure limits. Data encryption, face-to-face patient identification, and authenticating the patient's equipment, as well as laws such as the Health Insurance Portability and Accountability Act (HIPAA) and the European GDPR, can all assist to build and sustain public confidence in telemedicine [78,80]. As we discussed, telemedicine has various applications in the health sector. It comprises dealing with real-time patient monitoring, audio- and video-based teleconsultation, online diagnosis, prescriptions, recommendations, and health education. The modern era of the healthcare system has started to rely on telemedicine-based treatment to equip advanced features and hassle-free medical facilities.

1.9　SUMMARY AND FUTURE PERSPECTIVES

IoT-based health monitoring systems have been modified with the introduction of telemedicine networks. Doctors and health professionals are trying to convince patients to make their diagnoses through the telemedicine system to promise a safe and modern treatment. During the coronavirus outbreak, telemedicine became an important aspect for both the doctors and the patients to provide distinctive medical attention while avoiding mass gatherings. Many technologies and healthcare providers are there to monitor patients, but telemedicine becomes extremely relevant to do daily routine checkups, avoid infections from the health clinics and hospitals, store medical records and diagnoses, and arrange audio- and videoconferences with the doctors to get better treatment, etc. During these pandemics, simple and readily available technologies such as phone calls enabled continuity of care and patient–doctor communication; it is expected that if new channels of communication between patients and doctors can be established, communication will become more fluent, easier, and efficient. Telemedicine enables smart health monitoring of the patients at home with more modern technological help. Verifying and educating patients about test findings and minimizing the time it takes to visit a specialist doctor are all examples of what we do in our everyday clinical practice. It demonstrates that telemedicine is a valuable tool in physically isolated places and that it plays a critical role in correcting existing healthcare system inadequacies. Young people and adults with a greater level of education utilized more online search tactics and were more distrustful of the information they found online. The majority of these two groups were enthusiastic about telemedicine and intended to utilize it when the pandemic ended. This group, which is well-versed in eHealth, stands to gain the most from Internet use and digital age medicine technologies.

Under the restrictions of the pandemic, the activity of people with chronic conditions, as well as the healthcare system and healthcare institutions, suggests that a substantial number of service model components, such as a doctor's appointment or conversation with the professionals, may be amended. It is vital to design instructional programs for community people who find it difficult to engage in telemedicine, as well as activities to improve general e-literacy and e-Health literacy in specific. Both patients and physicians should examine their attitudes and sentiments of alienation concerning telemedicine. It would also be useful to look at the extent to which telemedicine is used by people with limited mobility, as well as if telemedicine improves their living standards. Throughout this chapter, we have discussed how the telemedicine network can be beneficial in this pandemic and how a telemedicine system architecture is designed to provide better care to patients. It is easier to establish doctor–patient communication due to the improvement of network channels. Not only during the COVID-19 pandemic but this form of health pipeline should also be integrated with every clinic and hospital in the upcoming future to make the healthcare industry more advanced and provide better care to the patients without having any sorts of risks.

REFERENCES

1. Craig, J., & Petterson, V. (2005). Introduction to the practice of telemedicine. *Journal of Telemedicine and Telecare*, 11(1), 3–9. https://doi.org/10.1177/1357633X0501100102
2. Abdellatif, M. M., & Mohamed, W. (2020). Telemedicine: An IoT based remote healthcare system. *International Journal of Online & Biomedical Engineering*, 16(6). https://doi.org/10.3991/ijoe.v16i06.13651
3. Fong, B., Fong, A. C. M., & Li, C. K. (2011). *Telemedicine technologies: Information technologies in medicine and telehealth*. Chichester: John Wiley & Sons. http://doi.org/10.1002/9780470972151

4. Haleem, A., Javaid, M., Singh, R. P., & Suman, R. (2021). Telemedicine for healthcare: Capabilities, features, barriers, and applications. *Sensors International*, 100117. https://doi.org/10.1016/j.sintl.2021.100117

5. Kadir, M. A. (2020). Role of telemedicine in healthcare during COVID-19 pandemic in developing countries. *Telehealth and Medicine Today*, 4(2), 78–96. https://doi.org/10.30953/tmt.v5.187

6. World Health Organization. (2020). *COVID-19 weekly epidemiological update*, 3 November 2020. www.who.int/publications/m/item/weekly-epidemiological-update-3-november-2020

7. Chen, S., Yang, J., Yang, W., Wang, C., & Bärnighausen, T. (2020). COVID-19 control in China during mass population movements at New Year. *The Lancet*, 395(10226), 764–766. https://doi.org/10.1016/S0140-6736(20)30421-9

8. Wilder-Smith, A., & Freedman, D. O. (2020). Isolation, quarantine, social distancing and community containment: Pivotal role for old-style public health measures in the novel coronavirus (2019-nCoV) outbreak. *Journal of Travel Medicine*, 27(2), 1–4. https://doi.org/10.1093/jtm/taaa020

9. Rocklöv, J., & Sjödin, H. (2020). High population densities catalyse the spread of COVID-19. *Journal of Travel Medicine*, 27(3), taaa038. https://doi.org/10.1093/jtm/taaa038

10. Chunara, R., Zhao, Y., Chen, J., Lawrence, K., Testa, P. A., Nov, O., & Mann, D. M. (2021). Telemedicine and healthcare disparities: A cohort study in a large healthcare system in New York City during COVID-19. *Journal of the American Medical Informatics Association*, 28(1), 33–41. https://doi.org/10.1093/jamia/ocaa217

11. Albahri, A. S., Alwan, J. K., Taha, Z. K., Ismail, S. F., Hamid, R. A., Zaidan, A. A., ... & Alsalem, M. A. (2021). IoT-based telemedicine for disease prevention and health promotion: State-of-the-art. *Journal of Network and Computer Applications*, 173, 102873. https://doi.org/10.1016/j.jnca.2020.102873

12. Chellaiyan, V. G., Nirupama, A. Y., & Taneja, N. (2019). Telemedicine in India: Where do we stand? *Journal of Family Medicine and Primary Care*, 8(6), 1872. https://doi.org/10.4103/jfmpc.jfmpc_264_19

13. Serper, M., & Volk, M. L. (2018). Current and future applications of telemedicine to optimize the delivery of care in chronic liver disease. *Clinical Gastroenterology and Hepatology*, 16(2), 157–161. https://doi.org/10.1016/j.cgh.2017.10.004

14. Liu, C., Zhang, X., Zhao, L., Liu, F., Chen, X., Yao, Y., & Li, J. (2018). Signal quality assessment and lightweight QRS detection for wearable ECG SmartVest system. *IEEE Internet of Things Journal*, 6(2), 1363–1374. https://doi.org/10.1109/JIOT.2018.2844090

15. Kumar, P. M., Lokesh, S., Varatharajan, R., Babu, G. C., & Parthasarathy, P. (2018). Cloud and IoT based disease prediction and diagnosis system for healthcare using Fuzzy neural classifier. *Future Generation Computer Systems*, 86, 527–534. https://doi.org/10.1016/j.future.2018.04.036

16. Bagula, A., Mandava, M., & Bagula, H. (2018). A framework for healthcare support in the rural and low-income areas of the developing world. *Journal of Network and Computer Applications*, 120, 17–29. https://doi.org/10.1016/j.jnca.2018.06.010

17. Guo, K., Li, T., Huang, R., Kang, J., & Chi, T. (2018). DDA: A deep neural network-based cognitive system for IoT-aided dermatosis discrimination. *Ad Hoc Networks*, 80, 95–103. https://doi.org/10.1016/j.adhoc.2018.07.014

18. Puthal, D., El-Sayed, H. E. S. H. A. M., Sankar, S., Wang, Y., Singh, J., & Sangaiah, A. K. (2017). IoT-based wireless polysomnography intelligent system for sleep monitoring. *IEEE Access*, 99, 1. https://doi.org/10.1109/ACCESS.2017.2765702

19. Abawajy, J. H., & Hassan, M. M. (2017). Federated Internet of Things and cloud computing pervasive patient health monitoring system. *IEEE Communications Magazine*, 55(1), 48–53. https://doi.org/10.1109/MCOM.2017.1600374CM

20. Arulanthu, P., & Perumal, E. (2020). An intelligent IoT with cloud centric medical decision support system for chronic kidney disease prediction. *International Journal of Imaging Systems and Technology*, 30(3), 815–827. https://doi.org/10.1002/ima.22424

21. Field, T., Diego, M., & Hernandez-Reif, M. (2010). Preterm infant massage therapy research: A review. *Infant Behavior and Development*, 33(2), 115–124. https://doi.org/10.1016/j.infbeh.2009.12.004

22. Mrozek, D., Koczur, A., & Małysiak-Mrozek, B. (2020). Fall detection in older adults with mobile IoT devices and machine learning in the cloud and on the edge. *Information Sciences*, 537, 132–147. https://doi.org/10.1016/j.ins.2020.05.070

23. Sareen, S., Sood, S. K., & Gupta, S. K. (2018). IoT-based cloud framework to control Ebola virus outbreak. *Journal of Ambient Intelligence and Humanized Computing*, 9(3), 459–476. https://doi.org/10.1007/s12652-016-0427-7

24. Raad, M. W., Sheltami, T., & Shakshuki, E. (2015). Ubiquitous tele-health system for elderly patients with Alzheimer's. *Procedia Computer Science*, 52, 685–689. https://doi.org/10.1016/j.procs.2015.05.075

25. Jebadurai, J., & Peter, J. D. (2018). Super-resolution of retinal images using multi-kernel SVR for IoT healthcare applications. *Future Generation Computer Systems*, 83, 338–346. https://doi.org/10.1016/j.future.2018.01.058

26. Medeiros de Bustos, E., Berthier, E., Chavot, D., Bouamra, B., & Moulin, T. (2018). Evaluation of a French regional telemedicine network dedicated to neurological emergencies: A 14-year study. *Telemedicine and e-Health*, 24(2), 155–160. https://doi.org/10.1089/tmj.2017.0035

27. Munandar, D., Rozie, A. F., & Arisal, A. (2021). A multi domains short message sentiment classification using hybrid neural network architecture. *Bulletin of Electrical Engineering and Informatics*, 10(4), 2181–2191. https://doi.org/10.11591/eei.v10i4.2790

28. Lanzarin, C. M. D. V., von Wangenheim, A., Rejane-Heim, T. C., Nascimento, F. D. S., Wagner, H. M., Abel, H. S., . . . & Xikota, J. C. (2021). Teleconsultations at a pediatrics outpatient service in COVID-19 pandemic: First results. *Telemedicine and e-Health*, 27(11), 1311–1316. https://doi.org/10.1089/tmj.2020.0471

29. Galván, P., Rivas, R., Portillo, J., Mazzoleni, J., Hilario, E., & Ortellado, J. (2019). National electrocardiographic mapping by telemedicine for diagnosis and prevention of cardiological pathologies in Paraguay. *The Journal of Medicine Access*, 3, 12–31. https://doi.org/10.1177/2399202619840627

30. Jnr, B. A. (2020). Use of telemedicine and virtual care for remote treatment in response to COVID-19 pandemic. *Journal of Medical Systems*, 44(7), 132. https://doi.org/10.1007/s10916-020-01596-5

31. Ohannessian, R., Duong, T. A., & Odone, A. (2020). Global telemedicine implementation and integration within health systems to fight the COVID-19 pandemic: A call to action. *JMIR Public Health Surveill*, 6(2), e18810. https://doi.org/10.2196/18810

32. Wang, X., Zhang, Z., Zhao, J., & Shi, Y. (2019). Impact of telemedicine on healthcare service system considering patients' choice. *Discrete Dynamics in Nature and Society*, 2019. https://doi.org/10.1155/2019/7642176

33. Nesbitt, T. S. (2012). The evolution of telehealth: Where have we been and where are we going. In Board on Health Care Services; Institute of Medicine, eds. *The role of telehealth in an evolving health care environment: Workshop summary*. Washington, DC: National Academies Press. https://doi.org/10.17226/13466

34. Jan, S. U., Ali, S., Abbasi, I. A., Mosleh, M. A., Alsanad, A., & Khattak, H. (2021). Secure patient authentication framework in the healthcare system using wireless medical sensor networks. *Journal of Healthcare Engineering*, 2021. https://doi.org/10.1155/2021/9954089

35. Evans, R. S. (2016). Electronic health records: Then, now, and in the future. *Yearbook of Medical Informatics* (Suppl 1), S48–S61. https://doi.org/10.15265/IYS-2016-s006

36. Chakraborty, C., Roy, S., Sharma, S., Tran, T., Dwivedi, P., & Singha, M. (2021). IoT based wearable healthcare system: Post COVID-19. In *The impact of the COVID-19 pandemic on green societies environmental sustainability* (pp. 305–321). Cham: Springer. https://doi.org/10.1007/978-3-030-66490-9_13

37. Hameed, K., Bajwa, I. S., Ramzan, S., Anwar, W., & Khan, A. (2020). An intelligent IoT based healthcare system using fuzzy neural networks. *Scientific Programming*, Article ID 8836927, 15 pages. https://doi.org/10.1155/2020/8836927

38. Riley, A., & Nica, E. (2021). Internet of things-based smart healthcare systems and wireless biomedical sensing devices in monitoring, detection, and prevention of COVID-19. *American Journal of Medical Research*, 8(2), 51–64. link.gale.com/apps/doc/A682130793/AONE?u=anon~cc5666be&sid=googleScholar&xid=106a90f0

39. Aghdam, Z. N., Rahmani, A. M., & Hosseinzadeh, M. (2021). The role of the Internet of Things in healthcare: Future trends and challenges. *Computer Methods and Programs in Biomedicine*, 199, 105903. https://doi.org/10.1016/j.cmpb.2020.105903

40. Nalinipriya, G., & Aswin Kumar, R. (2013). Extensive medical data storage with prominent symmetric algorithms on cloud—A protected framework. *International Conference on Smart Structures and Systems—ICSSS'13*, 171–177. https://doi.org/10.1109/ICSSS.2013.6623021

41. Malasinghe, L. P., Ramzan, N., & Dahal, K. (2019). Remote patient monitoring: A comprehensive study. *Journal of Ambient Intelligence and Humanized Computing*, 10, 57–76. https://doi.org/10.1007/s12652-017-0598-x

42. Albahri, O. S., Albahri, A. S., Mohammed, K. I., et al. (2018). Systematic review of real-time remote health monitoring system in triage and priority-based sensor technology: Taxonomy, open challenges, motivation and recommendations. *Journal of Medical Systems*, 42, 80. https://doi.org/10.1007/s10916-018-0943-4

43. Angelov, G. V., Nikolakov, D. P., Ruskova, I. N., Gieva, E. E., & Spasova, M. L. (2019). Healthcare sensing and monitoring. In Ganchev, I., Garcia, N., Dobre, C., Mavromoustakis, C., & Goleva, R., eds. *Enhanced living environments*. *Lecture notes in computer science*, vol. 11369. Cham: Springer. https://doi.org/10.1007/978-3-030-10752-9_10

44. Yu, S., Hill, C., Ricks, M. L., Bennet, J., & Oriol, N. E. (2017). The scope and impact of mobile health clinics in the United States: A literature review. *International Journal for Equity in Health*, 16(1), 178. https://doi.org/10.1186/s12939-017-0671-2

45. Keshta, I., & Odeh, A. (2021). Security and privacy of electronic health records: Concerns and challenges. *Egyptian Informatics Journal*, 22(2), 177–183. https://doi.org/10.1016/j.eij.2020.07.003

46. Newaz, A. I., Sikder, A. K., Rahman, M. A., & Uluagac, A. S. (2021). A survey on security and privacy issues in modern healthcare systems: Attacks and defenses. *ACM Transactions on Computing for Healthcare*, 2(3), 1–44. https://doi.org/10.1145/3453176

47. Chowdhury, M. S., Kabir, H., Ashrafuzzaman, K., & Kwak, K. S. (2009). A Telecommunication network architecture for telemedicine in Bangladesh and its applicability. *International Journal of Digital Content Technology and its Applications*, 3, 156–166. https://doi.org/10.4156/JDCTA.VOL3.ISSUE3.20

48. Jahan, S., & Ali, F. (2021, October). Advancing health information system with system thinking: Learning challenges of e-health in Bangladesh during COVID-19. In *International conference on health information science* (pp. 15–23). Cham: Springer. https://doi.org/10.1007/978-3-030-90885-0_2

49. Tomlin, E. B. (2021). *The lived experiences of counselors-in-training transitioning to clinical video teleconferencing (CVT) during COVID-19: An interpretive phenomenological analysis* (Doctoral dissertation, Adams State University).

50. Bennett, A. A., Campion, E. D., Keeler, K. R., & Keener, S. K. (2021). Videoconference fatigue? Exploring changes in fatigue after videoconference meetings during COVID-19. *Journal of Applied Psychology*, 106(3), 330. https://doi.org/10.1037/apl0000906

51. Haleem, A., Javaid, M., Singh, R. P., & Suman, R. (2021). Telemedicine for healthcare: Capabilities, features, barriers, and applications. *Sensors International*, 100117. https://doi.org/10.1016/j.sintl.2021.100117

52. Filchev, R., Pavlova, D., Dimova, R., & Dovramadjiev, T. (2021, August). Healthcare system sustainability by application of advanced technologies in telemedicine and eHealth. In *International conference on human interaction and emerging technologies* (pp. 1011–1017). Cham: Springer. https://doi.org/10.1007/978-3-030-85540-6_129

53. Shaikh, A., Memon, M., Memon, N., & Misbahuddin, M. (2009). The role of service oriented architecture in telemedicine healthcare system. *2009 International Conference on Complex, Intelligent and Software Intensive Systems*, 2009, 208–214. https://doi.org/10.1109/CISIS.2009.181

54. Priyanka, E. B., Thangavel, S., & Gao, X. Z. (2021). Review analysis on cloud computing based smart grid technology in the oil pipeline sensor network system. *Petroleum Research*, 6(1), 77–90. https://doi.org/10.1016/j.ptlrs.2020.10.001

55. Haque, M. A., Haque, S., Kumar, K., & Singh, N. K. (2021). A comprehensive study of cyber security attacks, classification, and countermeasures in the Internet of Things. In *Handbook of research on digital transformation and challenges to data security and privacy* (pp. 63–90). Hershey, PA: IGI Global. https://doi.org/10.4018/978-1-7998-4201-9.ch004

56. Elgendy, N., & Elragal, A. (2014, July). Big data analytics: A literature review paper. In *Industrial conference on data mining* (pp. 214–227). Cham: Springer. https://doi.org/10.1007/978-3-319-08976-8_16

57. Jephte, I. F. (2021). *Extract, transform, and load data from legacy systems to Azure cloud* (Doctoral dissertation). https://run.unl.pt/bitstream/10362/118629/1/TGI0408.pdf

58. Kwilinski, A., Litvin, V., Kamchatova, E., Polusmiak, J., & Mironova, D. (2021). Information support of the entrepreneurship model complex with the application of cloud technologies. *International Journal of Entrepreneurship*, 25(1), 1–8.

59. Mareeswari, V., Patil, S. S., & Ramanan, G. (2021). Real time sentiment analysis of Tweets using Apache Spark and Scala. *ACS Journal for Science and Engineering*, 1(2), 9–15. https://doi.org/10.34293/acsjse.v1i2.9

60. Adarsh, A., Pathak, S., & Kumar, B. (2021). Design and analysis of a reliable, prioritized and cognitive radio-controlled telemedicine network architecture for Internet of Healthcare Things. *International Journal of Computer Networks and Applications*, 8(1), 54–66. https://doi.org/10.22247/ijcna/2021/207982

61. Gorelov, V. A., Linskaya, E. Y., Tatarkanov, A. A., Alexandrov, I. A., & Sheptunov, S. A. (2020, September). Complex methodological approach to introduction of modern telemedicine technologies into the healthcare system on federal, regional and municipal levels. In *2020 international conference quality management, transport and information security, information technologies (IT&QM&IS)* (pp. 468–473). Piscataway, NJ: IEEE. https://doi.org/10.1109/ITQMIS51053.2020.9322864

62. Soufiene, Ben Othman, Bahattab, Abdullah Ali, Trad, Abdelbasset, & Youssef, Habib. (2020). PEERP: A priority-based energy-efficient routing protocol for reliable data transmission in healthcare using the IoT. *The 15th international conference on future networks and communications (FNC)*, August 9–12, 2020, Leuven, Belgium.

63. Soufiene, Ben Othman, Bahattab, Abdullah Ali, Trad, Abdelbasset, & Youssef, Habib. (2020). LSDA: Lightweight secure data aggregation scheme in healthcare using IoT. *ACM — 10th international conference on information systems and technologies*, June 2020, Lecce, Italy.

64. Othman, Soufiene Ben, Bahattab, Abdullah Ali, Trad, Abdelbasset, & Youssef, Habib. (2019). RESDA: Robust and efficient secure data aggregation scheme in healthcare using the IoT. *The international conference on Internet of Things, embedded systems and communications (IINTEC 2019)*, HAMMAMET, Tunisia from 20–22 December 2019.

65. Banerjee, A., Chakraborty, C., Kumar, A., & Biswas, D. (2020). Emerging trends in IoT and big data analytics for biomedical and health care technologies. In *Handbook of data science approaches for biomedical engineering* (pp. 121–152). Amsterdam: Elsevier . https://doi.org/10.1016/B978-0-12-818318-2.00005-2

66. Banerjee, S., Chakraborty, C., & Chatterjee, S. (2019). A survey on IoT based traffic control and prediction mechanism. In Balas, V., Solanki, V., Kumar, R., & Khari, M., eds. *Internet of Things and big data analytics for smart generation. Intelligent systems reference library*, vol. 154. Cham: Springer. https://doi.org/10.1007/978-3-030-04203-5_4

67. Covid, C. D. C., Team, R., Covid, C., Team, R., Covid, C., Team, R., . . . & Walters, M. (2020). Characteristics of health care personnel with COVID-19—United States, February 12—April 9, 2020. *Morbidity and Mortality Weekly Report*, 69(15), 477. http://doi.org/10.15585/mmwr.mm6938a3externalicon

68. Chatterjee, P. Comparative study of drug analysis via spike protein binding site recognition and vaccine development of novel Corona virus. https://doi.org/10.22214/ijraset.2021.33145

69. Chou, E., Hsieh, Y. L., Wolfshohl, J., Green, F., & Bhakta, T. (2020). Onsite telemedicine strategy for coronavirus (COVID-19) screening to limit exposure in ED. *Emergency Medicine Journal*, 37(6), 335–337. http://doi.org/10.1136/emermed-2020-209645

70. Garg, L., Chukwu, E., Nasser, N., Chakraborty, C., & Garg, G. (2020). Anonymity preserving IoT-based COVID-19 and other infectious disease contact tracing model. *IEEE Access*, 8, 159402–159414. https://doi.org/10.1109/ACCESS.2020.3020513

71. Calcaterra, V., Verduci, E., Vandoni, M., Rossi, V., Di Profio, E., Carnevale Pellino, V., . . . & Zuccotti, G. (2021). Telehealth: A useful tool for the management of nutrition and exercise programs in pediatric obesity in the COVID-19 era. *Nutrients*, 13(11), 3689. https://doi.org/10.3390/nu13113689

72. Othman, Soufiene Ben, Almalki, Faris A., Chakraborty, Chinmay, & Sakli, Hedi (2022). Privacy-preserving aware data aggregation for IoT-based healthcare with green computing technologies. *Computers and Electrical Engineering*, 101, 108025. https://doi.org/10.1016/j.compeleceng.2022.108025

73. Dopelt, K., Avni, N., Haimov-Sadikov, Y., Golan, I., & Davidovitch, N. (2021). Telemedicine and eHealth literacy in the era of COVID-19: A cross-sectional study in a peripheral clinic in Israel. *International Journal of Environmental Research and Public Health*, 18(18), 9556. https://doi.org/10.3390/ijerph18189556

74. Vidal-Aaball, J., Acosta-Roja, R., Hernández, N. P., Luque, U. S., Morrison, D., Pérez, S. N., . . . & Seguí, F. L. (2020). Telemedicine in the face of the COVID-19 pandemic. *Atencion Primaria*, 52(6), 418–422. https://doi.org/10.1016/j.aprim.2020.04.003

75. Liu, L., Gu, J., Shao, F., Liang, X., Yue, L., Cheng, Q., & Zhang, L. (2020). Application and preliminary outcomes of remote diagnosis and treatment during the COVID-19 outbreak: Retrospective cohort study. *JMIR mHealth and uHealth*, 8(7), e19417. https://doi.org/10.2196/19417

76. Rossi, B., Zoccali, C., Baldi, J., Scotto di Uccio, A., Biagini, R., De Luca, A., . . . & Ferraresi, V. (2020). Reorganization tips from a sarcoma unit at time of the COVID-19 pandemic in Italy: Early experience from a regional referral oncologic center. *Journal of Clinical Medicine*, 9(6), 1868. https://doi.org/10.3390/jcm9061868

77. Bhat, K. S., Jain, M., & Kumar, N. (2021). Infrastructuring telehealth in (In) formal patient-doctor contexts. *Proceedings of the ACM on Human-Computer Interaction*, 5(CSCW2), 1–28. https://doi.org/10.1145/3476064

78. Haleem, A., Javaid, M., Singh, R. P., & Suman, R. (2021). Telemedicine for healthcare: Capabilities, features, barriers, and applications. *Sensors International*, 100117. https://doi.org/10.1016/j.sintl.2021.100117

79. Chunara, R., Zhao, Y., Chen, J., Lawrence, K., Testa, P. A., Nov, O., & Mann, D. M. (2021). Telemedicine and healthcare disparities: A cohort study in a large healthcare system in New York City during COVID-19. *Journal of the American Medical Informatics Association*, 28(1), 33–41. https://doi.org/10.1093/jamia/ocaa217

80. Balasubramanian, V., Vivekanandhan, S., & Mahadevan, V. (2021). Pandemic tele-smart: A contactless tele-health system for efficient monitoring of remotely located COVID-19 quarantine wards in India using near-field communication and natural language processing system. *Medical & Biological Engineering & Computing*, 1–19. https://doi.org/10.1007/s11517-021-02456-1

81. Ullah, W., Yahya, A., Samikannu, R., & Tlale, T. (2021). Robust and secured tele-health system for COVID-19 patients. In *Data science for COVID-19* (pp. 337–349). Amsterdam: Elsevier. https://doi.org/10.1016/B978-0-12-824536-1.00022-8. Epub 2021 May 21. PMCID: PMC8138116.

82. Allam, Z., & Jones, D. S. (2020). On the coronavirus (COVID-19) outbreak and the smart city network: Universal data sharing standards coupled with artificial intelligence (AI) to benefit urban health monitoring and management. *Healthcare*, 8(1), 46. https://doi.org/10.3390/healthcare8010046

83. Elavarasan, R. M., & Pugazhendhi, R. (2020). Restructured society and environment: A review on potential technological strategies to control the COVID-19 pandemic. *Science of the Total Environment*, 725, 138858. https://doi.org/10.1016/j.scitotenv.2020.138858

84. Allam, Z., Dey, G., & Jones, D. (2020). Artificial intelligence (AI) provided early detection of the coronavirus (COVID-19) in China and will influence future urban health policy internationally. *AI*, 1(2), 156–165. https://doi.org/10.3390/ai1020009

85. Hutchinson, A. *US government looking to use cell phone location data to halt the spread of COVID-19*. www.socialmediatoday.com/news/us-government-looking-to-use-cell-phone-location-data-to-halt-the-spread-of/574420/.

86. Aashima, Nanda, M., & Sharma, R. (2021). A review of patient satisfaction and experience with telemedicine: A Virtual solution during and beyond COVID-19 pandemic. *Telemedicine and e-Health*, 21(12), 1325–1331. https://doi.org/10.1089/tmj.2020.0570

87. Hemanta, K. B., & Chinmay, C. (2022). Explainable machine learning for data extraction across computational social system. *IEEE Transactions on Computational Social Systems*, 9, 1–15. http://doi.org/10.1109/TCSS.2022.3164993

88. Kumar, A., Kumar, A., Chinmay, C., & Joel, J. P. C. R. (2022). Real geo-time based secured access computation model for e-Health systems. *Computational Intelligence*, 2022. https://doi.org/10.1111/coin.12523

89. Neha, S., Chinmay, C., & Rajeev, K. (2022). Optimized multimedia data through computationally intelligent algorithms. *Springer Multimedia Systems*, 1–17. https://doi.org/10.1007/s00530-022-00918-6

2 Detection and Evaluation of Operational Limitations of Internet Infrastructure of Critical Systems Based on the Internet of Medical Things in Smart Homes

Enes Açıkgözoğlu and Ziya Dirlik

CONTENTS

2.1 INTRODUCTION

Internet of Things (IoT) defines the hardware that can communicate among themselves and share information with different communication protocols and form an intelligent network. Every object we use in our daily life can connect to the Internet and have a MAC and IP address. The more these objects are connected to each other, the more they can provide us with real-time solutions for our daily needs and resolve potential problems before they arise [1]. IoT will change our lives and make everything much easier and more convenient. IoT refers to the large number of interconnected devices that are connected to the Internet and whose data is

DOI: 10.1201/9781003315476-2

shared worldwide, such as smartphones, tablets, computers, and many other devices. In addition to vehicles, many machines and even objects that we use in our daily life will be connected to each other and form a large network over the Internet [2]. The ever-increasing trend of IoT devices is expected to exceed 100 billion by 2050 [3]. In Figure 2.1, the amount of increase and future forecast of Internet-connected IoT devices by years are given.

Intelligent sensor hardware, which forms the basis of IoT technology, can store and analyze data. In this way, they can create networks and synchronize the information they collect with cloud technology. Therefore, it is necessary to develop an identification protocol that can be used for communication between different types of sensors, especially when these sensors need to exchange data securely without using any third-party software [4]. In addition, it is important that this protocol can provide authentication, integrity, and confidentiality mechanisms to protect information against malicious attacks from external sources [5].

Internet of Things can be defined as virtual objects that use intelligent interfaces to connect social, environmental, and user environments. IoT is a concept that connects all devices (both man-made and natural) over the Internet to enable data exchange. In this way, it makes it possible to automate and monitor the physical world [6]. Some analysts predict that in the coming years, one billion new IoT devices will come online every year. Some people think that the number of IoT devices on the market has already exceeded the number of people living today [7].

If we list the contributions, we hope to achieve as a result of this study.

- The technical Internet infrastructure and bandwidth required by IoT-based health devices integrated into smart home systems will be determined.
- Before the integration of IoT-based health devices into the smart home, the needs analysis will be carried out correctly and will be useful in preventing possible financial and temporal losses.
- It will contribute to the preparation of the feasibility map of the needs that will appear in the modification processes that the currently in use smart home systems will undergo to make them suitable for IoT-based health systems.

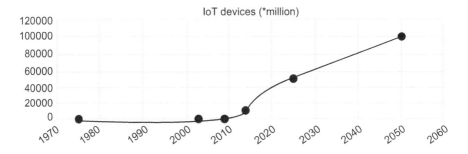

FIGURE 2.1 Uptrend of IoT-connected devices.

In the second part of the study, smart home systems are mentioned. Afterward, a detailed section was prepared by examining medical IoT applications in the third part. In the fourth section, the use of medical IoT applications in smart home systems is examined and current studies are mentioned. The use of artificial intelligence technologies, which is one of the popular areas of recent years, in health-based IoT applications in smart home systems has been examined in the fifth section. In the sixth section, the development of medical IoT infrastructures and the investments made in this field are examined. In the last section, the findings are discussed and interpreted, and the result is presented in a clear language.

2.2 SMART HOME TECHNOLOGY

Smart home is a term used to create a living ecosystem in which air-conditioning technology, lighting systems, heating systems, television, tablet, games, audiovisual systems, and security camera systems can communicate with each other [8]. Smart homes allow remote control of such devices through networking from an operator station (such as web browsers, wireless devices, or smartphones). Components of a smart home can be connected to a local area network (LAN) or wide area network (WAN). This allows communication between devices located in different geographical locations. The basic criterion in designing smart homes or making a building smart is based on the ability to control some equipment in the building regardless of location and time. In order to bring this capability to the devices, a microcontroller that allows us to control the system and communication hardware that allows us to communicate with the microcontroller are needed. In order to control an environment from outside, the priority is to listen to the environment variables in real time. At this point, sensors are the biggest helpers of technology developers. The values obtained from the environment through the sensors are transferred to the controller people via special cards. Objects that qualify as special cards are hardware that uses the Internet infrastructure, which is defined as a special purpose or development card. By examining the data transferred to them, the controllers can carry out monitoring activities or they can manipulate the environment remotely by determining new environment values of the environment. There are studies built on the same basis with different scenarios in the development of smart home technologies. In Table 2.1, sensors, hardware cards, and communication methods used in some studies on smart home systems are given.

Remote-controlled lighting and electrical equipment, automatically changing the settings of heating systems according to regional weather conditions, controlling refrigerators, air conditioners, ovens and more, smart transportation, smart education, people with health problems that need to be constantly monitored living a reliable life with smart medical devices, etc.—the number of IoT-based devices is increasing in many areas [14]. Applications that increase the quality and comfort of our lives are growing exponentially with each passing day. The potential benefits of this new technology are saving energy, making life better for people with disabilities, or providing a safe environment for children [15]. These can be easily realized by using IoT technology without any additional investment by users. The structure of the energy-saving smart heating system offered by Taştan is given in Figure 2.2.

TABLE 2.1

IoT Devices, Sensors, and Communication Techniques Used in Smart Home Systems

Work	The Aim of the Study	Used Sensor and Hardware Card	Communication Method
[9]	Developing flexible, economical, real-time, reliable, and realistic wireless sensors for use in smart homes	Sıcaklık sensor, Pır sensor, ZigBee	Wireless network, RF
[10]	It is aimed to develop a low-cost, expandable, wireless, flexible, smart home system to enable them to control various devices by providing a user-friendly interface	Rf Module, Wi-Fi Module, Pır sensor, gas sensor, Arduino Uno, Arduino Mega	Wireless network, RF
[11]	A communication protocol that is developed for smart home systems is recommended for energy efficiency, security, and privacy	Smoke detector, motion detector, smart meter	Wi-Fi
[12]	A new resource management technique (router) is proposed that utilizes particle swarm algorithm for optimization in fog-enabled cloud computing environments	Light sensor, motion sensor, Pır sensor, temperature sensor, humidty sensor, Esp 8266, Arduino Mega	Wi-Fi
[13]	A full design of an IoT-based detection and monitoring system for smart home automation is proposed	Light sensor, motion sensor, pressure sensor, temperature sensor, humidity sensor, fire sensor, Arduino, Raspberry Pi 3, NodeMCU	Wi-Fi

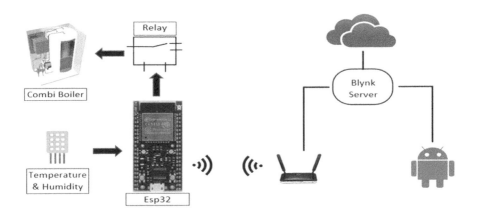

FIGURE 2.2   The general structure of the smart heating system.

2.3   IoT APPLICATIONS IN MEDICAL SYSTEMS

IoT health monitoring systems are systems that collect biological data in the human body and transmit this data via cables to monitoring, processing, or visualization devices. Wired systems have disadvantages such as restricting mobility and not being able to be monitored remotely. This causes a lot of inconvenience to patients and doctors. For example, diabetes and cardiovascular health should be monitored continuously throughout the day. However, traditional healthcare systems often require wired connections between patients' homes and hospitals [16]. This leads to high costs and privacy concerns. Wireless communication technology is promising in overcoming these limitations. It makes communication between users easier and with minimal effort, allowing them to monitor their vital signs anytime and anywhere. In recent years, wireless sensing technologies have been widely used for biomedical applications as they are suitable for wearable, implantable, and noninvasive measurements. Wireless sensors, electrocardiogram, temperature, blood pressure, body acceleration, etc. can follow physiological signals [17]. By integrating IoT applications into healthcare systems, it is considered to have the potential to bring many benefits to human health, including drug prediction, disease prediction, early warning of epidemics, preventive healthcare, and tracking people in need of surveillance [18]. Figure 2.3 shows various classifications made in the past for H-IoT applications.

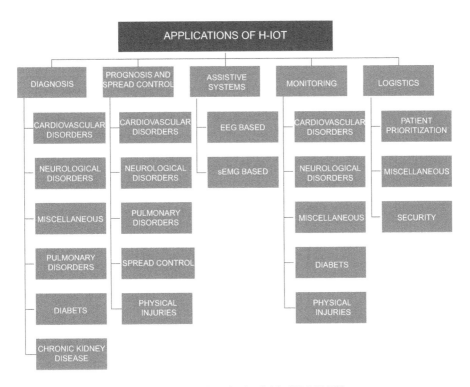

FIGURE 2.3   Classification of applications in the field of H-IoT [19].

Instant follow-up of critically ill patients is of vital importance for the patient. Early intervention can save the life of the patient in adverse developments. For this reason, uninterrupted and instant follow-up of critically ill patients has become a necessity. This situation has become very costly in terms of personnel and time. Thanks to the developing technology, critical patients can be monitored in real time and uninterruptedly, regardless of time and place, via IoT devices and sensors. Elhadad et al. in their study proposed a model in which they can monitor their patients in real time and uninterruptedly by utilizing the temperature sensor, ECG sensor, and blood pressure sensor. The system they recommend can instantly display and store the data received from patients. In extraordinary cases, it is ensured that the necessary interventions are made by warning the interests through notifications [20].

In their study, Lu and Liu proposed a model in which their patients can monitor their ECG values remotely in real time by using RFID and IoT technologies [21]. Drăgulinescu et al. have proposed a new IoT-based architecture that serves home care and hospital services based on a wide area network. Within this architecture, biological values such as heartbeat and body temperature of patients in different locations can be monitored instantly by sending them to the application server with a Lora-based solution [22]. Rathore et al. have developed a real-time emergency alert system in the healthcare field based on IoT technology. In the developed system, values such as glucose level, blood pressure, pulse rate, body temperature, heart rate, and breathing rate were monitored and transferred [23].

For the aged person, home care services are mostly preferred among health amenities for the aged person such as home care services, hospitals, health centers, and aged person care homes [24]. IoT technology is critical for instant tracking of individuals in medically risky groups. The raise in studies in this topic in recent years proves this situation. It is also used as an e-Health application in different subjects such as early diagnosis of diseases, emergency notification and computer-aided rehabilitation, expert systems, and decision support systems [25]. Smartphones have become an indispensable part of people's daily lives, and they can be connected to sensors to monitor people's health. IoT-based health systems provide efficient monitoring. Cloud computing is used to process health data. Cloud computing provides data storage and resource sharing facilities [26].

2.4   USE OF MEDICAL IOT TECHNOLOGY IN MY SMART HOME SYSTEMS

Developing smart home technologies have significantly increased the daily comfort of human beings [27]. Features such as remote control and environment monitoring with IoT technology have led to the creation of a new field that will encompass the concept of smart home. A tremendous benefit has emerged when remote monitoring and control systems are combined with health technologies [28]. Let's expand on this a little bit to understand this situation better. Doctors examine their patients, diagnose, and initiate treatment processes [29]. Treatment processes are carried out sometimes on an outpatient basis and sometimes by staying in the hospital. They want to see their patients' reactions to the treatment so that doctors can monitor the effectiveness of their treatment. In order to observe the patients staying in the hospital, doctors visit their patients in the room at certain times of the day [30].

Some patients may be in critical condition. Intensive care patients and patients who have undergone surgery are examples of this situation [31]. Some patients need to continue their treatment at home, but they should be kept under constant observation. This necessity may sometimes be due to the nature of the disease and sometimes due to the lack of adequate rooms for patients in hospitals. The COVID-19 epidemic disease that we have experienced recently is the warmest and most striking example of this situation. Such patients need to be followed up in real time and continuously. This necessity seriously affects the working hours and working efficiency of doctors [25]. In order to eliminate this limitation, new environments are created by integrating medical IoT technologies into smart home technologies. The provision of medical infrastructures in today's and future smart home systems is now a social need and demand. Even the privacy problems that can be experienced in this regard have lagged the potential health problems to be experienced. Among the conducted studies, the attitudes of users toward video-based monitoring systems were examined for the care of the long-term needs of the elderly in smart home environments or the long-term needs of the physically disabled. As a result of the study, positive results were observed [32].

In his study, Li expressed his ideas on how smart home technologies can be shaped for telemedicine and emergency management. In smart homes, biological data of elderly, disabled, or ordinary individuals can be detected with skilled sensors. These data are instantly transferred to a central monitoring environment. In adverse situations that may occur, the necessary intervention is carried out by specialist physicians without delay [33]. Linkous et al.'s research in the field of remote monitoring of health-based devices and IoT for smart home systems examines the many potential benefits of blending technology and proposes integration with an existing smart home. In the study, many data such as body temperature, blood pressure, pulse, and oxygen in the blood were obtained with wireless body sensors. The obtained data is sent to a Raspberry Pi 3 IoT device that has been converted to an Access point, thanks to Wi-Fi technology. Necessary notification and warning processes are carried out here [34]. In Figure 2.4, the general architecture of medical IoT systems in smart home technologies is shown.

In their study, Mano et al. proposed a model that targets patients' imagery and emotional perception to help patients and older people in the context of home healthcare. In addition, the emotional state of the patient is examined from the facial movements and facial expressions of the patients. It has been determined that this feature is a very important criterion for the patient to recover from a disease [35]. Datta et al. describe an example of personalized health applications in smart homes. In its applications, it has been done to provide a unified approach to discovery, management, and interaction with physical devices, to frame machine measurement to create machine measurement framework, to combine using M3 from cross-domain sensors and to control home automation devices based on health sensor information [36].

The concept of work in this area is expanding. Studies in which smart home technologies and medical IoT technologies are combined have generally focused on

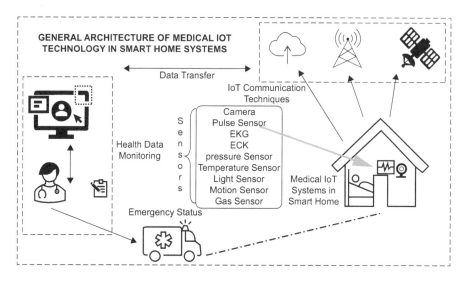

FIGURE 2.4   General architecture of medical IoT applications in smart home systems.

issues such as instant monitoring of patients' biological data, remote monitoring of patients at home, deteriorating instant data of patients, and designing early warning systems. In the expanding concept, it is ensured that home accidents that may occur in the smart home are detected, and cases such as injury and fainting are reported to the emergency response teams and the alarm system is activated [37]. These systems are lifesaving for individuals living alone.

2.5 USE OF HEALTHCARE IOT SYSTEMS WITH ARTIFICIAL INTELLIGENCE TECHNOLOGIES IN SMART HOME DESIGN

Artificial intelligence technologies, which is one of the popular fields of study and pioneering topics of technology in recent years, are frequently used together with other technology fields as well as their own field. Artificial intelligence technology includes machine learning algorithms, deep learning algorithms, and heuristic algorithms. Artificial intelligence technologies, which are very capable in estimating, classification, and optimization problems, have started to be used in the development of expert systems and decision support systems. The accuracy of the model, which will emerge after the operation of artificial intelligence algorithms, is directly dependent on the dataset it is trained on. The quality and heterogeneity of the data in the dataset are important factors that increase the success of the model. Artificial intelligence models trained with accurate data can produce successful results over 90% [38–41].

The use of artificial intelligence technologies in the health field has been frequently encountered in recent days. Algorithms used in both disease diagnosis and data transmission bring together IoT technologies and artificial intelligence technologies [42]. The studies of deep learning algorithms on image classification are very popular fields of study. Many classification studies have been carried out, especially on the images of the lung organ affected by the recent COVID-19 epidemic [43]. It is also used in the diagnosis and classification of other common cough-related lung disorders [44]. Security protocols and secure transmission algorithms as well as diagnostic and classification artificial intelligence algorithms are used in the healthcare field. For example, in the study of Gupta et al., epileptic seizures are detected by EEG signals, and methods for the safe transmission of these signals are described [45].

In smart home technologies, much more effective models are suggested by combining healthcare IoT systems with artificial intelligence technologies. In their study, Javed et al. proposed an improved approach to measure the simple activities of daily life of smart home users using predefined scores assigned by a neuropsychologist. The proposed model also measures the quality of tasks performed by users by making use of supervised classification. The aim of this study is to identify cognitively impaired individuals in their early stages. The ensemble AdaBoost algorithm was preferred to classify individuals into healthy, mildly cognitively impaired, and dementia categories [46]. In their study, Chatrati et al. proposed a smart health monitoring system that helps analyze blood pressure and glucose values for home follow-up of patients and reports abnormal conditions to the health authority board for which they are responsible. The proposed system is structured to predict hypertension values and diabetes status as a mixed use of machine learning algorithms for decision-making. The aim of the study is to predict the hypertension and diabetes status of the patient with high success using glucose values and blood pressure values. The proposed and trained model was trained using different supervised machine learning classification algorithms to predict the patient's diabetes and hypertension status. After many classification algorithm values were measured, it was determined that the support vector machine classification algorithm produced more successful results and therefore it was preferred for the training of the model [47].

Gebrie and Abie proposed a new IoT-based risk-based adaptive authentication model to identify the user's activities and verify the validity of the sensor nodes in their proposed model. The proposed model uses a pure Bayesian machine learning algorithm to classify channel features between the sensor and gateways. Based on the observed variation of channel characteristics, the model selects an appropriate authentication decision for a particular risk score of the model, based on the risk score of the device in question from the assessment. The developed machine learning model classifies the parameter values in user movements and the activities from the user as normal, abnormal, suspicious, and critical [48].

In their proposed study, Manocha et al. proposed a new e-Health framework using the advantages of IoT and fog technology to identify irregularities related to health, behavioral, physical posture, and environmental conditions of the individual. Critical misbehaviors detected in the monitored smart environment are classified by the machine learning model, and the urgent ones are immediately sent to the responsible physician as a notification, while the others are sent to be recorded in the cloud [49]. Lamiae et al. proposed a smart home model in which medical surveillance can be remotely controlled and monitored to contribute to the smart health paradigm. The proposed smart home design and architecture aims to create a comfortable smart home environment for sick individuals, elderly individuals, and individuals with reduced autonomy (convicts). For this reason, various technologies such as wearable sensor technologies, IoT, agent tracking system, and artificial intelligence algorithms have been applied [50].

2.6 INVESTIGATION AND EVALUATION OF INTERNET INFRASTRUCTURES IN MEDICAL IOT SYSTEMS

The architectural structure of a study for electrocardiography follow-up is presented in Figure 2.5. In the same study, the amount of data used to depend on the density situation during the transfer of data on the Wi-Fi network is given in Table 2.2.

Some wireless network standards and features that are frequently used in Internet access of sensors, data collector, and storage devices used in smart home and health automation are given in Figure 2.6 [14].

Bandwidth consumption is an important issue when it comes to Internet connection of IoT devices. Therefore, managing the bandwidth in home networks has also become very important. With an increasing number of IoT devices in the home generating large amounts of data, modern homes have high bandwidth requirements. Especially video streaming is the most bandwidth-consuming phenomenon. There

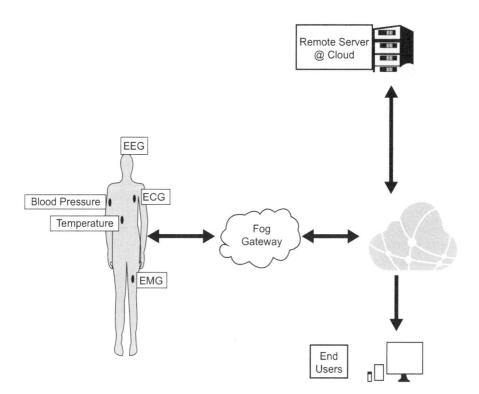

FIGURE 2.5   Electrocardiography tracking system architectural structure.

TABLE 2.2

Density Status Depending on the Amount of Electrocardiography Data [17]

Network State	Data Rate (Mbit/s)	Frequency (GHz)
No busy	18	2.4
Busy	12	2.4
Busiest	9	2.4

		Wireless Protocol				
		ZigBee	**WIFI**	**Thread**	**Z-Wave**	**Bluetooth LE**
Characteristics	**IEEE Standard**	802.15.4	802.11	802.15.4	N/A	802.15.1
	Frequency band	2.4 GHz	2.4 GHz, 5 GHz	2.4 GHz	900 MHz	2.4 GHz
	Nominal range	100 m	150 m	30m	30m	10 m
	Peak current consumption	30 mA	116 mA	12.3mA	17 mA	12.5 mA
	Power consumption per bit	185.9 W/bit	0.00525 W/bit	11.7 W/bit	0.71 W/bit	0.153 W/bit
	Data range	250 Kbps	1Gbps	250 kbps	100 kbps	1 Mbps
	Network topology	Star, Cluster, Mesh	Star, Mesh	Mesh	Mesh	Star-Bus
	Number of nodes per nerwork	65000	250/access point	300	232	one-to-many

FIGURE 2.6 Wireless network standards and features.

was 13.6 zettabyte data flow from IoT devices in 2018, and this data size is estimated to be 79.4 zettabyte in 2025 [3].

The data transfer rate of the devices is called bitrate. The bitrate requirements of some sensors and devices used in smart home and health automation are given in Figure 2.7 [24]. In IoT automations, the importance of upload is greater than download in the process of sending data to remote servers. In addition, bandwidth usage is one of the factors affecting the performance of applications.

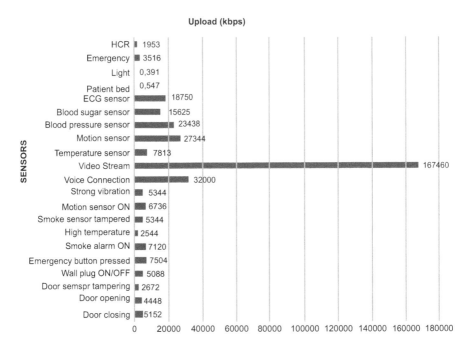

Upload (kbps)

HCR 1953
Emergency 3516
Light 0,391
Patient bed 0,547
ECG sensor 18750
Blood sugar sensor 15625
Blood pressure sensor 23438
Motion sensor 27344
Temperature sensor 7813
Video Stream 167460
Voice Connection 32000
Strong vibration 5344
Motion sensor ON 6736
Smoke sensor tampered 5344
High temperature 2544
Smoke alarm ON 7120
Emergency button pressed 7504
Wall plug ON/OFF 5088
Door semspr tampering 2672
Door opening 4448
Door closing 5152

SENSORS

0   20000   40000   60000   80000   100000 120000 140000 160000 180000

FIGURE 2.7   Bitrate requirements of sensors and devices.

2.7   DISCUSSION AND CONCLUSION

In recent years, IoT systems have developed rapidly. Thanks to IoT devices, systems that make life easier have been proposed. Many devices available with IoT have become smart. Two of the usage areas of the developed devices are health services and smart home systems. Health services should not be considered as services received only in health institutions. Services such as patient follow-up after treatment and the follow-up of the elderly or people in need of care should also be evaluated within the scope of health services. Although patient follow-up is a challenging process, the development of IoT devices has facilitated this process.

In this study, Internet network traffic that may occur with the use of IoT devices used in previous smart home and health services studies in the same environment has been examined. The average performance of countries for mobile Internet is 29.60 Mbps download, 8.44 Mbps upload, and for cable Internet the average performance is 59.86 Mbps download and 25.53 Mbps upload (Speedtest, 2022). In smart home systems, it has been observed that smart home sensors operating in the on/off logic do not create density in Internet traffic. It has been observed that the sensors used in the field of health services cause slightly more Internet traffic density than smart home sensors. In addition, it has been observed that IoT devices with video monitoring feature cause more density to Internet traffic than other IoT devices. In smart home systems, if IoT devices with video monitoring feature used in the field of health services are used in the same Internet network, the number of devices should be determined according to the speed of the Internet. In cases where the number of devices and the bandwidth needs of the devices are not considered, interruptions may occur in critical health services that need to be followed.

According to Speedtest February data on average Internet speeds of countries, it has been concluded that IoT devices used in smart home systems and healthcare services can work without affecting the Internet speed performance.

REFERENCES

1. Madakam, S., Lake, V., Lake, V., & Lake, V. Internet of Things (IoT): A literature review. *Journal of Computer and Communications*, 3(5), 164 (2015).
2. Meydanoğlu, E. S. B., & Klein, M. Nesnelerin İnterneti ve Pazarlama. *V. Tecim, Ç. Tarhan ve C. Aydın, Gülermat Matbaa, İzmir*, 12–19 (2016).
3. EY. *Siber Güvenlik Değerlendirilmesi Raporu, Erişim Tarihi: 15.03.2022, Erişim Linki* (2020). www.ey.com/tr_tr/ey-turkiye-yayinlar-raporlar/ot-ve-iot-siber-guvenlik-degerlendirmesi-raporu
4. Haras, M., & Skotnicki, T. Thermoelectricity for IoT—A review. *Nano Energy*, 54, 461–476 (2018).
5. Ercan, T., & Kutay, M. Endüstride nesnelerin interneti (IoT) uygulamaları. *Afyon Kocatepe Üniversitesi Fen ve Mühendislik Bilimleri Dergisi*, 16(3), 599–607 (2016).
6. Gokhale, P., Bhat, O., & Bhat, S. Introduction to IOT. *International Advanced Research Journal in Science, Engineering and Technology*, 5(1), 41–44 (2018).
7. Dhar, S. K., Bhunia, S. S., & Mukherjee, N. Interference aware scheduling of sensors in IoT enabled health-care monitoring system. In *2014 Fourth International Conference of Emerging Applications of Information Technology* (pp. 152–157). IEEE (2014, December).
8. Taştan, M. Akıllı Ev Uygulamaları için Yeni Nesil IoT Denetleyici ile Gerçek Zamanlı Uzaktan İzleme ve Kontrol Uygulaması. *Süleyman Demirel Üniversitesi Fen Bilimleri Enstitüsü Dergisi*, 23(2), 481–487 (2019).
9. Ghayvat, H., Mukhopadhyay, S., Gui, X., & Suryadevara, N. WSN-and IOT-based smart homes and their extension to smart buildings. *Sensors*, 15(5), 10350–10379 (2015).
10. Govindraj, V., Sathiyanarayanan, M., & Abubakar, B. Customary homes to smart homes using Internet of Things (IoT) and mobile application. In *2017 International Conference on Smart Technologies for Smart Nation (SmartTechCon)* (pp. 1059–1063). IEEE (2017, August).
11. Othman, S. Ben, Bahattab, A. A., Trad, A., & Youssef, H. Lightweight and confidential data aggregation in healthcare wireless sensor networks. *Transactions on Emerging Telecommunications Technologies, Wiley*, 26(11) (2016, November).
12. Gill, S. S., Garraghan, P., & Buyya, R. ROUTER: Fog enabled cloud based intelligent resource management approach for smart home IoT devices. *Journal of Systems and Software*, 154, 125–138 (2019).
13. Al-Kuwari, M., Ramadan, A., Ismael, Y., Al-Sughair, L., Gastli, A., & Benammar, M. Smart-home automation using IoT-based sensing and monitoring platform. In *2018 IEEE 12th International Conference on Compatibility, Power Electronics and Power Engineering (CPE-POWERENG 2018)* (pp. 1–6). IEEE (2018, April).
14. Samuel, S. S. I. A review of connectivity challenges in IoT-smart home. In *2016 3rd MEC International Conference on Big Data and Smart City (ICBDSC)* (pp. 1–4). IEEE (2016, March).

15. Gürfidan, R., & Ersoy, M. A new approach with blockchain based for safe communication in IoT ecosystem. *Journal of Data, Information and Management*, 1–8 (2022).

16. De Michele, R., & Furini, M. IoT healthcare: Benefits, issues and challenges. In *Proceedings of the 5th EAI International Conference on Smart Objects and Technologies for Social Good* (pp. 160–164) (2019, September). https://dl.acm.org/doi/10.1145/3342428.3342693

17. Gia, T. N., Jiang, M., Rahmani, A. M., Westerlund, T., Liljeberg, P., & Tenhunen, H. Fog computing in healthcare internet of things: A case study on ECG feature extraction. In *2015 IEEE International Conference on Computer and Information Technology; Ubiquitous Computing and Communications; Dependable, Autonomic and Secure Computing; Pervasive Intelligence and Computing* (pp. 356–363). IEEE (2015, October).

18. Apthorpe, N., Reisman, D., & Feamster, N. A smart home is no castle: Privacy vulnerabilities of encrypted iot traffic. *arXiv preprint arXiv:1705.06805* (2017).

19. Bharadwaj, H. K., Agarwal, A., Chamola, V., Lakkaniga, N. R., Hassija, V., Guizani, M., & Sikdar, B. A review on the role of machine learning in enabling IoT based healthcare applications. *IEEE Access*, 9, 38859–38890 (2021).

20. Elhadad, A., Alanazi, F., Taloba, A. I., & Abozeid, A. Fog computing service in the healthcare monitoring system for managing the real-time notification. *Journal of Healthcare Engineering*, 2022, Article ID 5337733, 11 pages (2022). https://doi.org/10.1155/2022/5337733

21. Lu, D., & Liu, T. The application of IOT in medical system. In *2011 IEEE International Symposium on IT in Medicine and Education* (Vol. 1, pp. 272–275). IEEE (2011, December).

22. Drăgulinescu, A. M. C., Manea, A. F., Fratu, O., & Drăgulinescu, A. LoRa-based medical IoT system architecture and testbed. *Wireless Personal Communications*, 1–23 (2020).

23. Othman, Soufiene Ben, Bahattab, Abdullah Ali, Trad, Abdelbasset, & Youssef, Habib. PEERP: A priority-based energy-efficient routing protocol for reliable data transmission in healthcare using the IoT. *The 15th International Conference on Future Networks and Communications (FNC) August 9–12, 2020*, Leuven, Belgium, 2020.

24. Khoi, N. M., Saguna, S., Mitra, K., & Åhlund, C. IReHMo: An efficient IoT-based remote health monitoring system for smart regions. In *2015 17th International Conference on E-health Networking, Application & Services (HealthCom)* (pp. 563–568). IEEE (2015, October).

25. Xu, Z., Liu, W., Huang, J., Yang, C., Lu, J., & Tan, H. Artificial intelligence for securing IoT services in edge computing: A survey. *Security and Communication Networks*, 2020, Article ID 8872586, 13 pages (2020). https://doi.org/10.1155/2020/8872586

26. Song, T., Li, R., Mei, B., Yu, J., Xing, X., & Cheng, X. A privacy preserving communication protocol for IoT applications in smart homes. *IEEE Internet of Things Journal*, 4(6), 1844–1852 (2017).

27. Othman, Soufiene Ben, Bahattab, Abdullah Ali, Trad, Abdelbasset, & Youssef, Habib. LSDA: Lightweight secure data aggregation scheme in healthcare using IoT. *ACM — 10th International Conference on Information Systems and Technologies*, Lecce, Italy, June 2020.

28. Othman, Soufiene Ben, Bahattab, Abdullah Ali, Trad, Abdelbasset, & Youssef, Habib. RESDA: Robust and efficient secure data aggregation scheme in healthcare using the IoT. *The International Conference on Internet of Things, Embedded Systems and Communications (IINTEC 2019)*, HAMMAMET, Tunisia from 20–22 December 2019.

29. Hasan, H. M., & Jawad, S. A. IoT protocols for health care systems: A comparative study. *International Journal of Computer Science and Mobile Computing*, 7(11), 38–45 (2018).

30. Selvaraj, S., & Sundaravaradhan, S. Challenges and opportunities in IoT healthcare systems: A systematic review. *SN Applied Sciences*, 2(1), 1–8 (2020).
31. Tyagi, S., Agarwal, A., & Maheshwari, P. A conceptual framework for IoT-based healthcare system using cloud computing. In *2016 6th International Conference-Cloud System and Big Data Engineering (Confluence)* (pp. 503–507). IEEE (2016, January).
32. Almalki, Faris A., Othman, Soufiene Ben, Almalki, Fahad A., & Sakli, Hedi. EERP-DPM: Energy efficient routing protocol using dual prediction model for healthcare using IoT. *Journal of Healthcare Engineering*, 2021(Article ID 9988038), 15 pages (2021).
33. Li, K. F. Smart home technology for telemedicine and emergency management. *Journal of Ambient Intelligence and Humanized Computing*, 4(5), 535–546 (2013).
34. Linkous, L., Zohrabi, N., & Abdelwahed, S. Health monitoring in smart homes utilizing internet of things. In *2019 IEEE/ACM International Conference on Connected Health: Applications, Systems and Engineering Technologies (CHASE)* (pp. 29–34). IEEE (2019, September).
35. Mano, L. Y., Faiçal, B. S., Nakamura, L. H., Gomes, P. H., Libralon, G. L., Meneguete, R. I., . . . & Ueyama, J. Exploiting IoT technologies for enhancing Health Smart Homes through patient identification and emotion recognition. *Computer Communications*, 89, 178–190 (2016).
36. Datta, S. K., Bonnet, C., Gyrard, A., Da Costa, R. P. F., & Boudaoud, K. Applying Internet of Things for personalized healthcare in smart homes. In *2015 24th Wireless and Optical Communication Conference (WOCC)* (pp. 164–169). IEEE (2015, October).
37. Juang, L. H., & Wu, M. N. Fall down detection under smart home system. *Journal of Medical Systems*, 39(10), 1–12 (2015).
38. Kishor, A., & Chakraborty, C. Artificial intelligence and internet of things based healthcare 4.0 monitoring system. *Wireless Personal Communications*, 1–17 (2021).
39. Liu, L., Zhou, B., Zou, Z., Yeh, S. C., & Zheng, L. A smart unstaffed retail shop based on artificial intelligence and IoT. In *2018 IEEE 23rd International Workshop on Computer Aided Modeling and Design of Communication Links and Networks (CAMAD)* (pp. 1–4). IEEE (2018, September).
40. Othman, Soufiene Ben, Almalki, Faris A., Chakraborty, Chinmay, & Sakli, Hedi. Privacy-preserving aware data aggregation for IoT-based healthcare with green computing technologies. *Computers and Electrical Engineering*, 101, 108025 (2022). https://doi.org/10.1016/j.compeleceng.2022.108025.
41. Ziefle, M., Rocker, C., & Holzinger, A. Medical technology in smart homes: Exploring the user's perspective on privacy, intimacy and trust. In *2011 IEEE 35th Annual Computer Software and Applications Conference Workshops* (pp. 410–415). IEEE (2011, July).
42. Chakraborty, C., Banerjee, A., Garg, L., & Rodrigues, J. J. Internet of medical things for smart healthcare. *Studies in Big Data; Springer: Cham, Switzerland*, 80 (2020).
43. Ravi, V., Narasimhan, H., Chakraborty, C., & Pham, T. D. Deep learning-based meta-classifier approach for COVID-19 classification using CT scan and chest X-ray images. *Multimedia Systems*, 1–15 (2021).
44. Kumar, A., Abhishek, K., Chakraborty, C., & Kryvinska, N. Deep learning and internet of things based lung ailment recognition through coughing spectrograms. *IEEE Access*, 9, 95938–95948 (2021).
45. Gupta, A. K., Chakraborty, C., & Gupta, B. Secure transmission of EEG data using watermarking algorithm for the detection of epileptical seizures. *Traitement du Signal*, 38(2), 473–479 (2021).
46. Javed, A. R., Fahad, L. G., Farhan, A. A., Abbas, S., Srivastava, G., Parizi, R. M., & Khan, M. S. Automated cognitive health assessment in smart homes using machine learning. *Sustainable Cities and Society*, 65, 102572 (2021).

47. Chatrati, S. P., Hossain, G., Goyal, A., Bhan, A., Bhattacharya, S., Gaurav, D., & Tiwari, S. M. Smart home health monitoring system for predicting type 2 diabetes and hypertension. *Journal of King Saud University-Computer and Information Sciences*, 34, 862–870 (2020).

48. Gebrie, M. T., & Abie, H. Risk-based adaptive authentication for internet of things in smart home eHealth. In *Proceedings of the 11th European Conference on Software Architecture: Companion Proceedings* (pp. 102–108) (2017, September). https://dl.acm.org/doi/10.1145/3129790.3129801

49. Manocha, A., Kumar, G., Bhatia, M., & Sharma, A. IoT-inspired machine learning-assisted sedentary behavior analysis in smart healthcare industry. *Journal of Ambient Intelligence and Humanized Computing*, 1–14 (2021).

50. Lamiae, E., Fatiha, E., Mohammed, B., & Hicham, G. T. A study on smart home for medical surveillance: Contribution to smart healthcare paradigm. In *Proceedings of the 4th International Conference on Smart City Applications* (pp. 1–6) (2019, October). https://dl.acm.org/doi/10.1145/3368756.3368994

3 Fitness-Dependent Optimizer for IoT Healthcare Using Adapted Parameters
A Case Study Implementation

Aso M. Aladdin, Jaza M. Abdullah,
Kazhan Othman Mohammed Salih,
Tarik A. Rashid, Rafid Sagban,
Abeer Alsaddon, Nebojsa Bacanin,
Amit Chhabra, S. Vimal, and Indradip Banerjee

CONTENTS

3.1   INTRODUCTION

FDO is nothing more than an attempt to emulate the behavior of bees during reproduction. As a scout bee, this algorithm is designed to simulate scout bees using this strategy to choose a new home among the many colonies that are around. A proposed solution to this algorithm is a scout bee that looks for fresh hives; also, selecting the best hive among many good hives is regarded to be approaching optimality [1]. Swarming is an early occurrence that develops when a fresh colony of honeybees is generated. The scout bees leave the previous hive, and the queen bee stays with

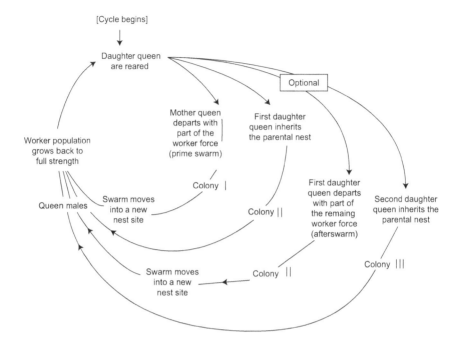

FIGURE 3.1   Bee swarming process cycle.

a group of honeybees; Figure 3.1 illustrates the cycle of bee swarming. A swarm is made up of hundreds to tens of thousands of bees [2]. The scout bees will briefly dwell 20–40 meters outside from the birth beehive for several hours to a few days or weeks.

The colony might contribute attributes to improve this operation. A controlled honeybee colony's health has been reflected in colony characteristics. External factors influencing health and colony production express the production of an organized beehive colony. Bee brand construction and fertilization services are added since they are the driving factors for beekeepers' decision to preserve a honeybee colony [3]. Figure 3.2 includes the diagram to demonstrate the definitions of the elements as well as the interactions between them.

IoT is an area in which massive amounts of data are transferred continuously, and FDO, yet still very new, is very powerful and provides promising results; therefore, the authors of this chapter believe that this algorithm needs step-by-step explanation so that the reader can have a better understanding, the above can be the main motive behind writing this chapter. Consequently, this chapter will also introduce the improved FDO for IoT healthcare using adapted parameters; it is a real case study implementation, which is related to the potential IoT applications. The primary goal of this chapter is to provide a step-by-step implementation guide for the FDO and provide IoT healthcare [4] as a probable application with adapting FDO parameters. The shortened major contributions of this chapter are two crucial points: it illustrates the steps calculation of the novelist swarm intellectual algorithm; besides, it detailed how to use an optimization technique to provide appropriate weights to

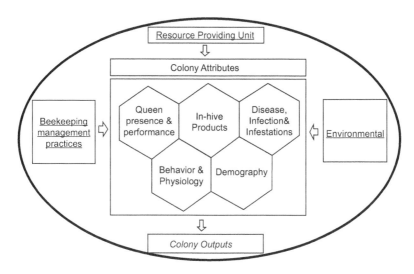

FIGURE 3.2 A comprehensive evaluation of the health.

support the methods in both the explorative and exploitative stages. The second point is concentrated on adapting the parameters of FDO for using IoT healthcare to invent the best accumulation, expectation, and segmentation in the innovative model IoT applications. Another unique aspect of FDO that might be improved for this reason is that it keeps earlier search agent pace for probable reprocess in consequent stages.

This chapter is organized as follows. Section 3.2 is devoted to identifying IoT healthcare technologies. Section 3.3 discusses IoT applications in metaheuristic algorithms and improved FDO parameters in the IoT healthcare system. Section 3.4 examines the mathematical formula, which can be explained for the FDO algorithm, and demonstrates the formulations step-by-step. Section 3.5 is devoted to explaining FDO by simple example as a case study. Section 3.6 concludes the chapter and proposes significant feature works.

3.2   IoT HEALTHCARE TECHNOLOGY

IoT is gradually making its way into a wide range of businesses, from manufacturing to healthcare, communications, and even agriculture [5, 6]. The IoT looks promising in integrating a range of sensors, medical equipment, and healthcare professionals to carry high-value health treatment facilities to those in isolated locations. Using cloud-based IoT in healthcare allows for a smart healthcare system because of its large storage capacity [7]. It has enhanced patient safety, minimized healthcare costs, expanded healthcare service accessibility, and raised operational efficiency in the healthcare business [8]. The technical advancements accumulated over the past have now enabled the detection of various diseases and monitoring systems utilizing tiny technologies, such as smartwatches. Likewise, technological advancements have converted a clinic healthcare system into a physician system [9]. Sensors and IoT-enabled hospital instruments securely transmit sensitive healthcare data to healthcare specialists who might just review and take relevant steps if required without the need for human participation [10]. The technologies employed to construct an IoT of healthcare system are important for this goal. This is because incorporating certain technologies into an IoT system might enhance its capabilities. Hence, a variety of tool technologies have been used to integrate multiple healthcare applications with an IoT structure [11]. IoT is transforming the healthcare industry by changing the way devices and people interact in healthcare service provision. The IoT implementation in healthcare will make life easier for everyone involved, including doctors and patients, while also enhancing the quality of care [12, 13, 14]. IoT sensors collect patient data, which is then analyzed using machine learning techniques [15]. For patients, it is simple to access and use sensors that are built into their health monitoring devices [16, 17]. A doctor, for example, can monitor a patient's heart rate from their office using sensors that periodically collect data [16, 18]; thus, doctors can keep tabs on and communicate with their patients while they are away from the hospital.

Monitoring patients in remote areas, telemedicine, and health technologies are just a few examples of how the IoT might very well support healthcare [19]. In healthcare, IoT has applications that are also beneficial for physicians, patients, hospitals, families, and insurance companies [20]. Accordingly, IoT healthcare technologies are categorized into three parts: identity technology, communication technology, and location technology [21]. The massive amounts of data produced by these associated devices can revolutionize healthcare. Analog data is typically acquired through sensors and other equipment. Next, the data are standardized and preprocessed before they are shipped off to a data center. At the essential level, final data is controlled and evaluated [22]. IoT applications for advanced analytics are revolutionizing healthcare by assuring better care, improving treatment effects, and lowering costs for patients, as well as controlling procedures and operations, improving efficiency, and a bettering patient experience for healthcare professionalization [23]. Using IoT devices and applications in the healthcare industry is shown in Figure 3.3 [16, 24].

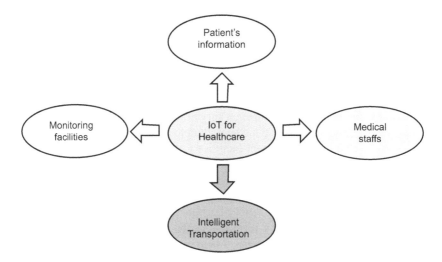

FIGURE 3.3   IoT for healthcare.

3.3   IOT APPLICATIONS IN METAHEURISTIC ALGORITHMS

IoT applications can be adapted in metaheuristic algorithms to simply obtain the behaviors of big data. To make IoT networks last longer, several solutions have been developed; quantum particle swarm optimization (QPSO) is a metaheuristic strategy that researchers have presented earlier as a method for lengthening the lifespan of the IoT network using the cooperative multiple-input multiple-output system, or the so-called MIMO. At the termination of each stage, researchers aim to select dynamically the ideal cooperative MIMO transmitter and receiver equipment that causes a long operational life cycle. Researchers have devised a strategy for finding the best cluster headers in another study [25]. Battery life, storage capacity, and communication range are all significantly reduced in sensor nodes. To transmit data to IoT devices, the author used the suggested communication protocol [26]. Whale optimization algorithm is employed in another metaheuristic study to construct the ideal energy-conscious head collection for the Wireless Sensor Network—Internet of Things (WSN-IoT). The dormancy, workload, energy, length, and thermometer were all taken into description when making the final decision on the best Cluster Head feature to deploy. Algorithms, such as ABC, PSO, GA, and GSA with WOA-based Cluster Head selection methods or adaptive GSA, are compared to the proposed model [27]. The study presented in Augusto et al. investigated ways of controlling the behavior and conditions of nocturnal persons in a healthcare system [28]. It has been suggested by Tomar et al. that data mining algorithms can be used to provide a more accurate forecast, for example, to improve the healthcare system's ability to predict human behavior. Even though typical data mining algorithms might produce significant outcomes for the healthcare system, this research via Tomaret et al., Tsai et al., and Yoo et al. has also advocated that the use of metaheuristics can help improve the outcomes of healthcare system analytics [29, 30, 31]. Because a healthcare system's large data can comprehend a significant collection of potentially useful information, scholars have been interested in learning. Besides, in recent decades, there has been a lot of debate on how to develop a high-performance algorithm for data mining analysis or data science inquiries [32]. As a result, we recommended this parallel metaheuristic algorithm for analyzing the IoT healthcare big data mining methods. IoT and artificial intelligence, on the other hand, are poised to transform most industries, but possibly not any more so than healthcare. Furthermore, both biomedical and computer vision technologies may analyze data collected in public healthcare databases to detect and improve care issues [33, 34]. But, on the other hand, healthcare IoT is concerned with medical equipment connectivity, where recorded data may be saved and evaluated for future diagnostic procedures employing intelligent approaches [35]. Notwithstanding this, this chapter demonstrates that FDO is a swarm technique that provides alternative ideas for analyzing health data and detects abnormalities to increase life quality. According to the above reasoning, it is possible to infer that even though there are various models available, they all have significant power consumption. To solve this issue, a case study of the FDO algorithm can be utilized in IoT healthcare to optimize power consumption by choosing the optimum cluster.

Thus, the FDO algorithm can provide a brief analysis of metaheuristics for the healthcare system as well as a road map for academics working on metaheuristics and healthcare to produce a more proficient and productive health insurance system. This technique offers a learnable data analytics framework that may be collected. Then, the data may be presented with a possible solution by FDO parameters to the incorporation of diverse forms of input data from various devices, sensors, and equipment in addition to a simple evolutionary result to the gigantic data dilemma that a healthcare system would be confronted.

3.4 MATHEMATICAL FORMULATION FOR FDO ALGORITHM

The basis of formulating the FDO problem is mainly concerned with the minimization of real searching for more positions. Scout bees, according to FDO, hunt for better hives by randomly visiting more sites, as seen in Figure 3.1; the previously discovered hive is disregarded once a superior hive is located. As a result, whenever the engine discovers a new candidate, the preceding exposed solution is rejected when FDO discovers the best new solution. Second, if the current motion fails to find a better solution for a main artificial scout bee (hive), it reverts to its former course in the hope of finding a better option. If the prior path fails to yield a better result, it relapses to the earlier solution, which is the premium answer available at the time. Likewise, this FDO framework, which can be utilized in the applications of healthcare, helps to integrate the benefits of cloud computing with IoT into the medical sector. Patients' data from sensors and medical equipment can also be transmitted using the specified methods. IoT also randomizes and calculates the financial benefits and costs of mass implementation of the record systems of electronic health, as well as simulates crucial healthcare and safety benefits depending on the big data [36, 37]. Scout bees, therefore, scout for hives at random in the wild. When adopting this method, artificial scouts initially randomly travel over the landscape to gather information about the terrain's topography. So, when an artificial scout bee speeds up its current location, it expects to find a better option.

First, the procedure begins by generating a random scout colony in the search space X_i (i is the scout bee as inhuman [artificial] and *pace* is the path of the scout bee and the drive rate). Depending on the fitness weight (*fw*), *pace* is indicated. Also, i signifies the presence of the search agent (bee) and t signifies the most recent iteration. The behavior of artificial scout bees is stated in Equation (3.1):

$$X_{i,t+1} = X_{i,t} + pace \tag{3.1}$$

As stated, the direction of *pace* is dependent on an arbitrary mechanism. The *fw* worked on concerning with minimizing problems and it could be formulated in Equation (3.2).

$$fw = \left| \frac{x^*_{i,tfitness}}{x_{i,tfitness}} \right| \tag{3.2}$$

The best global solution for fitness function value is $x^*_{i,t\,fitness}$, which has been exposed from distance. The rate of the current solution for fitness function is specified by

$x_{i,t\ fitness}$ and wf is a weight factor that is predicted either 0 or 1 and is used for adjusting the fw.

Depending on formula (3.2), fw result identified to 0 and 1 can be neglected because it denotes a high and low chance of convergence. Occasionally, as the fitness function cost is reliant on optimization problems, the opposite case occurs. Though the range of fw value ought to be between [0, 1]; particular situations will be $fw = 1$, which is the best global solution. It signifies that the present and best global solutions are indistinguishable, or that they have equivalent fitness values. Furthermore, it is plausible that $fw = 0$, which happens when $x^*_{i,tfitness} = 0$. The rules are illustrated in formulas (3.3)–(3.5):

$$
\left\{
\begin{array}{l}
fw=1 \text{ or } fw = 0 \text{ or } x_{i,t\ fitness} = 0, \quad pace = x_{i,t} * r \qquad (3.3) \\
fw > 0 \text{ and } fw < 1 \left\{
\begin{array}{l}
r < 0, pace = \left(x_{i,t} - x^*_{i,t}\right) * fw * -1 \quad (3.4) \\
r \geq 0, \quad pace = \left(x_{i,t} - x^*_{i,t}\right) * fw \qquad (3.5)
\end{array}
\right.
\end{array}
\right\}
$$

There are other arbitrary pace implementations; however, Levy flight was elected since it gives supplementary steady motions due to its excellent distribution curve [38]. r is a number randomly generated between the range.

If the preceding pace does not lead the scout bee to the best solution, the optimizer will keep the existing solution until the next round. When the answer is accepted in this procedure, the *pace* value is kept for possible reprocess in the subsequent iteration. Two minor deviations are required for implementing this algorithm for maximization problems. Equation (3.2) obliges to be first substituted by Equation (3.6), which is simply the opposite of Equation (3.2):

$$
fw = \left| \frac{x_{i,t\ fitness}}{x^*_{i,t\ fitness}} \right| - wf \qquad \text{(Eq. 3.6)}
$$

The criteria for picking an improved result should be then modified. The condition "if $(X_{t+1,i}\ fitness < X_{t,i}\ fitness)$" required substituting with the condition "if $(X_{t+1,i}\ fitness > X_{t,i}\ fitness)$." In Figure 3.4, the SOFDO pseudocode has displayed both rates.

3.5 CASE STUDY IMPLEMENTATION

Researchers should have acquired numerous lessons about how to formulate models effectively and what sort of algorithm would solve these issues efficiently and reliably after researching various linear or nonlinear optimization problems [39]. While a single example cannot be used to deduce these teachings, it may be used to illustrate them. The train problem for the FDO method is described and summarized for researchers to state succinctly and applied for different aspect models in the future, particularly in the realm of IoT healthcare. As discussed in the previous section, use the FDO algorithm for minimizing real searching positions. Table 3.1 is the random problem, which includes two dimensions and the upper bound ended at (100) with

Initialize scout bee population $X_{t,i}$ (i = 1, 2, ..., n)
while iteration (t) limit not reached
   for each artificial scout bee $X_{t,i}$
     find best artificial scout bee $x^*_{t,i}$
     generate random walk r in [-1, 1] range
     if($X_{t,i}$ fitness ==0) (avoid divide by zero).
       fitness weight = 0
   else
     calculate fitness weight. equation (4.2)
   end if
   if (fitness weight = 1 or fitness weight = 0)
     calculate pace using equation (4.3)
   else
     if (random number>=0)
       calculate pace using equation (4.4)
   end if
   end if
   calculate $X_{t,i+1,i}$ equation (4.1)
   if($X_{t,i+1,i}$ fitness <$X_{t,i}$ fitness)
       move accepted and pace saved
   else
       calcuate $X_{t,i+1,i}$ equation (4.1) with previous pace
       if ($X_{t,i+1,i}$ fitness <$X_{t,i}$ fitness)
          move accepted and pace saved
       else
          maintain current position (don't move)
       end if
     end if
   end for
end while

FIGURE 3.4   Pseudocode of SOFDO.

the lower bound limited at (–100). Consequently, the example problem dimensions equal 2, which means x1 and x2 for every bee in FDO. Three dimensions can be suggested, which means x1, x2, and x3. This example uses two features as a bee pace for IoT healthcare. In several healthcare applications, such as optical, electrochemical, or material physical properties, it might be used as an active sensing element or as providing a substrate [40].

The study selected three bees as suggested by the inquiry, which means the population size equals 3. Conferring to FDO, finding fitness function needs the formula to point out the pace between populations. $F_{(x)} = \sum_{i=1}^{D} X_i^2$ is generated to calculate the fitness function for this case study.

Bee-x1 = r * Upper-bound
Bee-x2 = r * Lower-bound

FDO needs a list of stochastic numbers to evaluate the behaviors. In Table 3.1, use this list of random numbers for generating random numbers respectively, and use each cell only once. The sample of study reaches the algorithm working for two iterations.

TABLE 3.1

Fifteen Random Sequences for Two Parameters

No. of Sequences	Parameter 1	Parameter 2	No. of Sequences	Parameter 1	Parameter 2	No. of Sequences	Parameter 1	Parameter 2	No. of Sequences	Parameter 1	Parameter 2	No. of Sequences	Parameter 1	Parameter 2
1	-0.49	-0.47	11	-0.09	0.92	21	0.34	-0.48	31	0.64	0.41	41	0.77	-0.93
2	0.44	-0.78	12	0.6	-0.45	22	-0.72	0.84	32	-0.19	-0.49	42	0.48	0.31
3	-0.22	-0.52	13	-0.15	0.4	23	0.82	-0.15	33	0.48	0.31	43	-0.19	0.53
4	0.82	-0.22	14	0.36	-0.47	24	-0.4	0.67	34	-0.04	-0.83	44	0.58	0.71
5	-0.81	0.82	15	-0.25	0.61	25	0.77	-0.93	35	0.58	0.31	45	-0.18	0.27
6	-0.94	-0.29	16	0.17	-0.55	26	-0.97	0.62	36	-0.1	0.27	46	0.66	-0.26
7	-0.10	0.95	17	-0.88	-0.64	27	0.8	-0.84	37	0.15	-0.26	47	0.58	0.64
8	0.12	-0.96	18	0.13	0.94	28	-0.28	0.63	38	-0.62	0.38	48	-0.12	0.37
9	-0.89	0.08	19	-0.25	-0.35	29	0.38	-0.55	39	0.42	-0.4	49	0.15	-0.26
10	0.68	-0.06	20	0.08	0.63	30	-0.94	-0.68	40	0.72	0.52	50	-0.98	-0.65

3.5.1 CALCULATING FIRST ITERATION

Regarding FDO, bee one is represented as B1 and the following are the initial stats that may be found:

B1_x1 = −0.49 * Upper-bound = −0.49 *100 = −49
B1_x2 = −0.47 * Lower-bound = −0.47 * −100 = 47

Formerly, it must be finding fitness function optimization according to the given equation $F_{(X)=} \sum_{i=1}^{D} X_i^2$, and it could be obtained this fitness:

$$x_1^2 + x_2^2 = (-49)^2 + (47)^2 = \textbf{4,610}$$

Then, bee two is symbolized as B2 and could be found in initial stat as follows:

B2_x1 = 0.44 * Upper-bound = 0.44 * 100 = 44
B2_x2 = −0.78 * Lower-bound = −0.78 * −100 = 78

Consequently, fitness function optimization must also be found according to the same given equation $F_{(X)=} \sum_{i=1}^{D} X_i^2$, and this fitness could be obtained for the second bee, as follows:

$$x_1^2 + x_2^2 = (44)^2 + (-78)^2 = \textbf{8,020}$$

Finally, bee three is symbolized as B3 and could be found as the initial stat same as B1 and B2:

B3_X1 = −0.22 * Upper-bound = −0.22 *100 = −22
B3_X2 = −0.52 * Lower-bound = −0.52 * −100 = 52

It must also be finding fitness function optimization according to the same given equation $F_{(X)=} \sum_{i=1}^{D} X_i^2$, and this fitness for the third bee is given as follows:

$$x_1^2 + x_2^2 = (-22)^2 + (52)^2 = \textbf{3,188}$$

As a result, the solution of the third bee is defined as the global best solution because it has the lowest fitness value according to the FDO standard and then jumped for the second iteration. To illustrate the calculation results in the first iteration steps following up on Table 3.2 and Figure 3.5:

Global best solution for the first iteration: $x_{i,t \ fitness}^{*}$ = **3,188 [−11, 52]**

3.5.2 CALCULATING SECOND ITERATION

In the second iteration, it should first find the behavior of artificial scout bees by the following clearance steps, although respecting the rules in Equations (3.3)–(3.5) to find fitness weight, as shown at Figure 3.6.

TABLE 3.2

The First Iteration Steps to Find Global Solution

Steps	Pace 1	Pace 2	Fitness Function Solution
1	−49	47	4,610
2	44	−78	8,020
3	−22	52	3,188

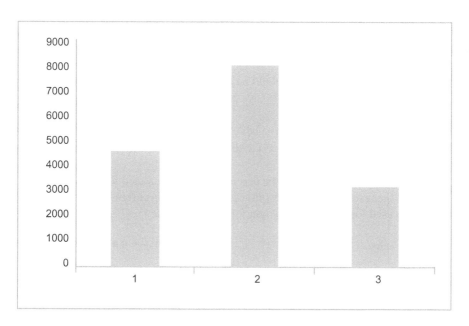

FIGURE 3.5   Prove step 3 is the best global solution for the first iteration.

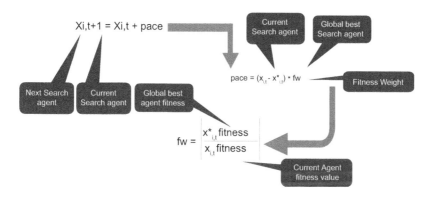

FIGURE 3.6   Implementing FDO sequence rules.

It could be found fitness weight as follows to calculate *pace*:

$$fw = \left| \frac{x^*_{i,t\,fitness}}{x_{i,t\,fitnees}} \right| = \frac{3,188}{4,610} = 0.69$$

After that the pace must be calculated according to the r, which is a number generated randomly between the range [–1, 1] as stated previously and modifying the scout bee location as the simple calculation:

When $r = 0.82$, then $pace = \left(x_{i,t} - x^*_{i,t} \right) * fw$

So, B1_x1_pace = (–49)—(–22)) * 0.69 = –33.82

When $r = -0.22$, then $pace = \left(x_{i,t} - x^*_{i,t} \right) * fw * -1$

So, B1_x2_pace = (47–52) * 0.69 * –1 = 3.45

Then similar previous iterations could be found as a fresh state for bee one; the formula (3.3) is needed as follows:

B1_x1 = $x_{1,1} + pace$ = – 49 + (–33.82) = –82.88
B1_x2 = $x_{1,2} + pace$ = 47 + (3.45) = 50.45

The same given equation used in the first iteration is formulated for the second iteration. Thus, the result shows that new fitness is smaller than current fitness; as a result, it could be used for getting new weight for the second bee:

Fitness value = $x_{i,t\,fitnees}$ = $x_1^2 + x_2^2$ = (–82.88)² + (50.45)² = **9,414**

Since, $x_{i,t\,fitnees}$ = **9,414** > $x^*_{i,t\,fitness}$ = **3,188**

As a result, define Global's best solution: $x^*_{i,t\,fitness}$ = **3,188 [–22, 52]**

For continuity of this iteration and to calculate the fitness function for the second bee, it should find fitness weight as follows to calculate pace for the second bee:

$$fw = \left| \frac{x^*_{i,t\,fitness}}{x_{i,t\,fitness}} \right| = \frac{3,188}{8,020} = 0.397$$

When $r = -0.81$, then $pace = \left(x_{i,t} - x^*_{i,t} \right) * fw * -1$

So, B2_x1_pace = (44– (–22))* 0.397* –1 = – 26.20

When $r = 0.82$, then $pace = \left(x_{i,t} - x^*_{i,t} \right) * fw$

So, B2_x2_pace = (78–52)* 0.397 = 10.32

Also, depending on formula (3.3), we will calculate a new state for bee two as follows:

B2_x1 = $x_{2,1} + pace$ = 44 + (–26.20) = 17.8
B2_x2 = $x_{2,2} + pace$ = 78 + 10.32 = 88.32

Compute the value of fitness via the same fitness function and evaluate it with the current value. The result shows as follows:

$$\text{Fitness value} = x_{i,t\ fitness} = x_1^2 + x_2^2 = (17.8)^2 + (88.32)^2 = \textbf{8,117.26}$$
$$\text{Since, } x_{i,t\ fitnees} = 8,117 > x_{i,t\ fitness}^* = 3,188$$

Hence, the best global value must be defined as the previous step and remain the identical fitness solution: $x_{i,t\ fitness}^* = \textbf{3,188 [–22, 52]}$

In the termination, this iteration ended by computing the fitness function for the third bee. The first step for bee three ought to catch fitness weight:

$$fw = \left| \frac{x_{i,t\ fitness}^*}{x_{i,t\ fitnees}} \right| = \frac{3,188}{3,188} = 1$$

When $r = -0.94$, then $pace = \left(x_{i,t} - x_{i,t}^* \right) * fw * -1$
So, $B3\_x1\_pace = ((-22)—(-22))*(1 * -1) = 0$
When $r = -0.29$, then $pace = \left(x_{i,t} - x_{i,t}^* \right) * fw * -1$
So, $B3\_x2\_pace = (52–52)* (1 * -1) = 0$

Then finding the fitness value and comparing with the current value, the result shows as follows:

$$\text{Fitness value} = x_{i,t\ fitness} = x_1^2 + x_2^2 = (0)^2 + (0)^2 = \textbf{0}$$
$$x_{i,t\ fitnees} = 0 < x_{i,t\ fitness}^* = \textbf{3,188}$$

Here, it should be selected and defined as the global best solution. According to the FDO rules, the novel fitness solution is progressed and should be used in the next iteration. So, the new fitness global best solution is: $x_{i,t\ fitness}^* = 0$ [0, 0]; besides, the steps are explained observably in Table 3.3 and more illustrated in Figure 3.7.

The case study will be continued for the next iterations to pick up the best global solution according to FDO. Thus, the actual problem is about some iterative algorithm. The researcher wants to invent the appropriate parameter (s.t.). As a result, the algorithm terminates in minimal iterations. These parameters, which include scout bee in the FDO algorithm, are similarly approved in physical healthcare in IoT.

TABLE 3.3
Second Iteration Steps to Find Global Solution

Steps	Pace 1	Pace 2	Fitness Function Solution
1	–82.88	50.45	9,414
2	17.8	88.32	8,117
3	0	0	0

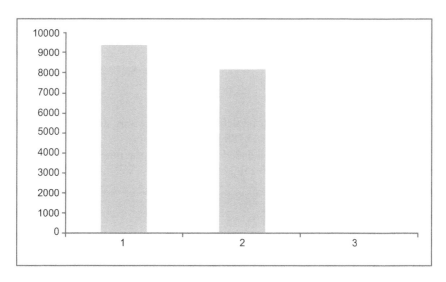

FIGURE 3.7　The output of second iteration.

3.6　CONCLUSION

FDO, a modern meta-heuristic algorithm that simulates the reproduction behavior of the bee swarm in seeking better hives, was presented as one of the most recently formed algorithms. It was a very destructive algorithm when compared to other typical meta-heuristic algorithms since it performed exceptionally well throughout the optimization procedure. Rendering to the original results and outcomes in the FDO paper, the technique of the algorithm is quite powerful and outperforms other standard metaheuristic algorithms. An improvement in this chapter was finished to the FDO from two main viewpoints. First, the case study for calculating FDO mathematical examples accurately explained each step as showing that the fitness global best solution for the second iteration, which is (**0**) is smaller than the first iteration, which is (**3,188**). As a result, readers might just have a greater knowledge of the algorithm, which they could apply to solve real-world problems in the future. The second perspective is on an IoT-based healthcare application system that might be implemented in metaheuristic algorithms to merely collect big data behaviors. Moreover, it has been proposed that FDO parameters be adjusted to enhance the metaheuristic evolutionary algorithm for evaluating large data in the IoT healthcare system. The future scope for this chapter recommends that FDO can be used for a virtualized health IoT architecture and highlighted the best big data system. This scope integrates the health cloud platform for telecommunications to engage and improve user quality and make the health IoT application more intimately related to general human beings.

REFERENCES

1. Abdullah, Jaza Mahmood, and Tarik Ahmed. "Fitness dependent optimizer: inspired by the bee swarming reproductive process." *IEEE Access* 7 (2019): 43473–43486.

2. EFSA Panel on Animal Health and Welfare (AHAW). "Assessing the health status of managed honeybee colonies (HEALTHY-B): a toolbox to facilitate harmonised data collection." *EFSA Journal* 14, no. 10 (2016): e04578.

3. Seeley, Thomas D. *The Five Habits of Highly Effective Honeybees (and What We Can Learn from Them).* Princeton University Press, Princeton, 2010.

4. Farahani, Bahar, Farshad Firouzi, and Krishnendu Chakrabarty. "Healthcare iot." In *Intelligent Internet of Things*, pp. 515–545. Springer, Cham, 2020.

5. Almalki, Faris A., Ben Othman Soufiene, Saeed H. Alsamhi, and Hedi Sakli. "A low-cost platform for environmental smart farming monitoring system based on IoT and UAVs." *Sustainability* 13, no. 11 (2021): 5908.

6. Alsamhi, Saeed H., Ou Ma, Mohammad Samar Ansari, and Faris A. Almalki. "Survey on collaborative smart drones and internet of things for improving smartness of smart cities." *IEEE Access* 7 (2019): 128125–128152.

7. Gupta, Akash Kumar, Chinmay Chakraborty, and Bharat Gupta. "Monitoring of epileptical patients using cloud-enabled health-IoT system." *Traitement du Signal* 36, no. 5 (2019): 425–431.

8. Coetzee, Louis, and Johan Eksteen. "The Internet of Things-promise for the future? An introduction." In *2011 IST-Africa Conference Proceedings*, pp. 1–9. IEEE, 2011.

9. Yang, Geng, Li Xie, Matti Mäntysalo, Xiaolin Zhou, Zhibo Pang, Li Da Xu, Sharon Kao-Walter, Qiang Chen, and Li-Rong Zheng. "A health-IoT platform based on the integration of intelligent packaging, unobtrusive bio-sensor, and intelligent medicine box." *IEEE Transactions on Industrial Informatics* 10, no. 4 (2014): 2180–2191.

10. Othman, S. Ben, A. A. Bahattab, A. Trad, and H. Youssef. "Lightweight and confidential data aggregation in healthcare wireless sensor networks." *Transactions on Emerging Telecommunications Technologies (Impact Factor: 1.354), Wiley* 26, no. 11 (November, 2016).

11. Yuehong, Y. I. N., Yan Zeng, Xing Chen, and Yuanjie Fan. "The internet of things in healthcare: an overview." *Journal of Industrial Information Integration* 1 (2016): 3–13.

12. Karoly, Paul, and Linda S. Ruehlman. "Psychological 'resilience' and its correlates in chronic pain: findings from a national community sample." *Pain* 123, no. 1–2 (2006): 90–97.

13. Čolaković, Alem, and Mesud Hadžialić. "Internet of Things (IoT): a review of enabling technologies, challenges, and open research issues." *Comput Networks* 144 (2018): 17–39. https://doi.org/10.1016/j.comnet.2018.07.017

14. Diène, Bassirou, Joel JPC Rodrigues, Ousmane Diallo, E. L. Hadji Malick Ndoye, and Valery V. Korotaev. "Data management techniques for Internet of Things." *Mechanical Systems and Signal Processing* 138 (2020): 106564.

15. Kishor, Amit, and Chinmay Chakraborty. "Artificial intelligence and internet of things based healthcare 4.0 monitoring system." *Wireless Personal Communications* (2021): 1–17.

16. Salih, Kazhan Othman Mohammed, Tarik A. Rashid, Dalibor Radovanovic, and Nebojsa Bacanin. "A comprehensive survey on the Internet of Things with the industrial marketplace." *Sensors* 22, no. 3 (2022): 730.

17. Atzori, Luigi, Antonio Iera, and Giacomo Morabito. "The internet of things: a survey." *Computer Networks* 54, no. 15 (2010): 2787–2805.

18. Da Xu, Li, Wu He, and Shancang Li. "Internet of things in industries: a survey." *IEEE Transactions on Industrial Informatics* 10, no. 4 (2014): 2233–2243.

19. Gupta, Akash, Chinmay Chakraborty, and Bharat Gupta. "Medical information processing using smartphone under IoT framework." In *Energy Conservation for IoT Devices*, pp. 283–308. Springer, Singapore, 2019.

20. Goyal, Sukriti, Nikhil Sharma, Bharat Bhushan, Achyut Shankar, and Martin Sagayam. "IoT enabled technology in secured healthcare: applications, challenges and future directions." In *Cognitive Internet of Medical Things for Smart Healthcare*, pp. 25–48. Springer, Cham, 2021.

21. Pradhan, Bikash, Saugat Bhattacharyya, and Kunal Pal. "IoT-based applications in healthcare devices." *Journal of Healthcare Engineering* 2021 (2021).

22. Greco, Luca, Pierluigi Ritrovato, Thanassis Tiropanis, and Fatos Xhafa. "IoT and semantic web technologies for event detection in natural disasters." *Concurrency and Computation: Practice and Experience* 30, no. 21 (2018): e4789.

23. Iwendi, Celestine, Praveen Kumar Reddy Maddikunta, Thippa Reddy Gadekallu, Kuruva Lakshmanna, Ali Kashif Bashir, and Md Jalil Piran. "A metaheuristic optimization approach for energy efficiency in the IoT networks." *Software: Practice and Experience* 51, no. 12 (2021): 2558–2571.

24. Horwitz, Lauren. "Patient health data is increasingly democratized—despite data quality." March, 2020, Date of Access (1 March 2022), Available online: www. iotworldtoday.com/2020/03/03/democratization-of-patient-health-data-empowers-despite-data-quality-issues/.

25. Song, L., Kok Keong Chai, Yue Chen, Jonathan Loo, Shihab Jimaa, and Youssef Iraqi. "Energy efficient cooperative coalition selection in cluster-based capillary networks for CMIMO IoT systems." *Computer Networks* 153 (2019): 92–102.

26. Jesudurai, S. Anthony, and A. Senthilkumar. "An improved energy efficient cluster head selection protocol using the double cluster heads and data fusion methods for IoT applications." *Cognitive Systems Research* 57 (2019): 101–106.

27. Reddy, M., and M. R. Babu. "Implementing self adaptiveness in whale optimization for cluster head section in Internet of Things." *Cluster Computing* 22, no. 1 (2019): 1361–1372.

28. Othman, Soufiene Ben, Faris A. Almalki, Chinmay Chakraborty, and Hedi Sakli. "Privacy-preserving aware data aggregation for IoT-based healthcare with green computing technologies." *Computers and Electrical Engineering* 101 (2022): 108025. https://doi.org/10.1016/j.compeleceng.2022.108025.

29. Tsai, Chun-Wei, and Joel J. P. C. Rodrigues. "Metaheuristic scheduling for cloud: a survey." *IEEE Systems Journal* 8, no. 1 (2013): 279–291.

30. Yoo, Illhoi, Patricia Alafaireet, Miroslav Marinov, Keila Pena-Hernandez, Rajitha Gopidi, Jia-Fu Chang, and Lei Hua. "Data mining in healthcare and biomedicine: a survey of the literature." *Journal of Medical Systems* 36, no. 4 (2012): 2431–2448.

31. Tsai, Chun-Wei, Ming-Chao Chiang, Adlen Ksentini, and Min Chen. "Metaheuristic algorithms for healthcare: open issues and challenges." *Computers & Electrical Engineering* 53 (2016): 421–434.

32. Sanjukta, B, and C. Chinmay. "Machine learning for biomedical and health informatics." *CRC: Big data, IoT, and Machine Learning Tools and Applications, Ch. 4* (2020): 353–373, ISBN 9780429322990. https://doi.org/10.1201/9780429322990

33. Chinmay, C., B. Amit, H. K. Mahesh, G. Lalit, and C. Basabi. *Internet of Things for Healthcare Technologies*, Springer—Studies in Big Data, 73, 2020. ISBN 978-981-15-4111-7.

34. Tarik, R., C. Chinmay, and F. Kym. *Advances in Telemedicine for Health Monitoring: Technologies, Design and Applications*, IET, 2020. ISBN 978-1-78561-986-1.

35. Dash, Sabyasachi, Sushil Kumar Shakyawar, Mohit Sharma, and Sandeep Kaushik. "Big data in healthcare: management, analysis and future prospects." *Journal of Big Data* 6, no. 1 (2019): 1–25.

36. Othman, Soufiene Ben, Abdullah Ali Bahattab, Abdelbasset Trad, and Habib Youssef. "RESDA: robust and efficient secure data aggregation scheme in healthcare using the IoT." *The International Conference on Internet of Things, Embedded Systems and Communications (IINTEC 2019)*, HAMMAMET, Tunisia from 20–22 December 2019.

37. Othman, Soufiene Ben, Abdullah Ali Bahattab, Abdelbasset Trad, and Habib Youssef. "PEERP: a priority-based energy-efficient routing protocol for reliable data transmission in healthcare using the IoT." *The 15th International Conference on Future Networks and Communications (FNC) August 9–12, 2020*, Leuven, Belgium, 2020.

38. Kamaruzaman, Anis Farhan, Azlan Mohd Zain, Suhaila Mohamed Yusuf, and Amirmudin Udin. "Levy flight algorithm for optimization problems-a literature review." In *Applied Mechanics and Materials*, vol. 421, pp. 496–501. Trans Tech Publications Ltd, 2013. doi:10.4028/www.scientific.net/amm.421.496

39. Othman, S. Ben, A. A. Bahattab, A. Trad, and H. Youssef. "Secure data transmission protocol for medical wireless sensor networks." In *The 28th IEEE International Conference on Advanced Information Networking and Applications*, IEEE AINA 2014, Victoria, Canada, 13–16 May 2014.

40. Bolotsky, Adam, Derrick Butler, Chengye Dong, Katy Gerace, Nicholas R. Glavin, Christopher Muratore, Joshua A. Robinson, and Aida Ebrahimi. "Two-dimensional materials in biosensing and healthcare: from in vitro diagnostics to optogenetics and beyond." *ACS Nano* 13, no. 9 (2019): 9781–9810. doi:10.1021/acsnano.9b03632

4 Digital Disruption in the Indian Healthcare System

Sukanya Roy

CONTENTS

DOI: 10.1201/9781003315476-4

4.1 INTRODUCTION/BACKGROUND

The pandemic has contributed to the rapid adoption of technology in the healthcare domain and transformed the face of the healthcare system. Digital technology helps to build a sustainable healthcare system. It includes data analytics, artificial intelligence (AI), and the blockchain technology that addresses the problem of accessibility and shortage of human resources. This chapter broadly discusses the challenges of the Indian health system. Also, it explains how the rapid adoption of digital technology in the pandemic era disrupts the healthcare system and transforms primary care services in rural areas. Incorporating digital technology in the healthcare system increases efficiency and reduces cost. The flow of the chapter is arranged as follows. The first section gives a detailed explanation of the Indian healthcare system, the levels and functions of the healthcare system, and the healthcare market in India. The second section explains the challenges and solutions faced by India's health system. The third section explains India's digital health-tech space and attempts to understand the future scope of digital healthcare services in remote areas. And lastly, the study discussed the conclusion, recommendation, and future scope of the study. The World Health Organization (WHO) defined health as a "state of physical, mental and social well-being." Healthy person is free from any diseases and impairment.

4.1.1 HEALTH SYSTEM/HEALTHCARE SYSTEM

A health system comprises all organizations, institutions, and resources committed to providing health actions to the community. The objective of the healthcare system is to protect and facilitate the health of the people. The WHO (World Health Organization, 2000) redefined the health system as "medical activities whose objective is to promote and deliver quality health to the last mile of the community."

4.2 INDIAN HEALTHCARE SYSTEM

Indian healthcare is the largest sector that provides employment and generates revenue [1]. It comprises hospitals, medical tourism, health insurance, medical equipment, and telemedicine. The Indian healthcare industry has been growing fast, and it is broadly categorized into two major components: public and private healthcare services. The government usually provides public healthcare [2] and it mainly comprises primary health centers (PHCs), with a limited number of secondary and tertiary care institutions. In contrast, private healthcare has not been operated by the government, and it is facilitated by secondary and tertiary care institutions in urban areas. India has a mixed healthcare system that includes public and private service providers. Private service providers are situated mainly in urban areas and provide secondary and tertiary healthcare services, whereas public healthcare providers are located in rural areas and provide primary and secondary healthcare services [3]. As per WHO, the healthcare delivery system is divided into three groups based on their services:

Primary Healthcare Services: Primary healthcare services primarily focus on the essential healthcare services that address the health issues. In addition, primary healthcare services spread awareness regarding healthcare practices. A general physician and nurses run the PHC (primary healthcare centers).

Secondary Healthcare Services: Secondary healthcare services are more focused on treating patients suffering from complex health conditions. The secondary healthcare centers are run by doctors and specialists.

Tertiary Healthcare Services: Tertiary healthcare services are specialized medical care that involves advanced and complex diagnostic treatment. Tertiary care is mainly located at the regional and national levels depending on the size and resources.

4.2.1 LEVELS OF HEALTHCARE SYSTEM IN INDIA

- **Primary Level**

Primary healthcare services are the touch points where patients directly connect with healthcare institutions. Primary health level mainly comprises subcenters (SC) and primary healthcare centers (PHC). Subcenters are the most peripheral and first touch point of connection between the primary healthcare system and the community. The tasks allotted to the health workers of subcenters are mainly focused on neonatal and child health, family planning program, vaccination, and contagious disease. The staff size of the SC consists of one auxiliary nurse midwife, female staff, and male health worker. In India, there are 7,821 SC functioning in rural areas. The numbers of subcenters escalated from 43.8% in 2005 to 75.3% in 2019.

Primary healthcare center is the first touch point between the rural people and the medical officers. The objective of PHC is to deliver therapeutic and preventive healthcare to the countryside people. PHC has been functional in the country, including 24,855 rural PHC and 5,190 urban PHC. The primary tasks of PHC include preventive, therapeutic, and promoting family planning programs. Staff size of the PHC consists of 8 medical officers, including 14 paramedical staff. Primary healthcare centers increased significantly from 69% in 2005 to 94.5% in 2019.

- **Secondary Level**

This is the first referral point. The patients are referred based on severe health conditions. The secondary level comprises community health centers (CHC). CHC is maintained and established by state governments. The staff size of the CHC consists of four medical specialists, including surgeon, physician, gynecologist, and pediatrician supported by 21 paramedical and other medical staff. CHC includes in-door beds with one OT, X-ray, labor room, and laboratory facilities. The percentage of community health centers has increased significantly from 91.6% in 2005 to 99.3% in 2019. As per the government record, 5,335 community healthcare centers are in the countryside.

- Tertiary Level

This is the second referral level that includes hospitals and medical colleges.

4.2.2 Challenges of Indian Healthcare System

The Indian healthcare system is paradoxical, and advanced healthcare is accessible only to a small percentage of Indians. In contrast, large populations in rural areas do not access primary and quality healthcare. Secondary and tertiary healthcare infrastructures are concentrated in urban areas where rural people cannot access specialized and complex healthcare facilities.

In 2020, when the pandemic hit the entire nation, COVID-19 has exposed the failure of the Indian healthcare system. Lack of healthcare infrastructure, shortage of well-equipped medical institutes, imbalance doctor–patient ratio, and the expensive treatment [4] were the primary reasons due to which a large number of patients lost their lives in the COVID-19 pandemic. Kasthuri [5] considered five A's challenges:

- **Awareness or Lack of It:** Indian population has a lack of understanding about important issues regarding their health, e.g., adequate knowledge regarding diseases like breast and cervical cancer among the women population. A study showed that one-third of the countryside people were unaware of breast cancer. The prime factors for the low level of health awareness include low education status, low priority of health in the population, poor functional literacy, and lack of health-related education.
- **Accessibility:** Urban people had little difficulty in accessing good quality healthcare services, whereas 70% of the population residing in countryside regions had access to 20% of total hospital beds in the country. The difference in access to healthcare services across rural and urban areas was the prime reason for existing disparities in healthcare outcomes. According to the report published by NHRC (National Rural Health Mission), in rural India, 8% of PHCs did not have adequate medical staff and doctors, 39% did not have a lab technician, and 18% of PHCs did not have a pharmacist. People in rural areas lacked access to even vital primary medical care services. Hence, access to diagnosis and treatment of complex disease conditions such as cancer was nonexistent.
- **Absence of Human Resources:** Lack of quality care, inappropriate/inadequate treatment due to lack of high-quality medical facilities, short supply

of medical staff, and lack of financial resources were the prime factors for delayed treatment in the country.

- **Affordability or Cost of Healthcare:** The private sector is the dominant player in the health system. In private healthcare services, 75% of healthcare expenditures come from the pocket of the household. For example, the treatment of breast cancer depends on the stage of cancer. The treatment includes chemotherapy, radiation, hormone therapy, and surgery. The cost of therapy included doctor's fee, admission fee, hospitalization fee (which depended on the type of hospital), cost of diagnostics testing, etc. Many of these costs depended on the patient's medical condition at treatment. The cost of breast cancer treatment varies from US$1,300 (INR 97,560) to US$23,500 (about INR 1.8 million) in India [6]; comparable costs in the United States were in the range of US$125,000 (INR 95 million). The treatment cost in India was beyond the reach of poor people in the country.

- **Accountability or Lack of It:** In the health system, being accountable is defined "as the processes by which one party justifies and takes responsibilities for its activities" (Kasthuri, A. 2018).

4.3   SOLUTIONS TO OVERCOME HEALTHCARE CHALLENGES

Healthcare providers should focus on building a patient-centric business model: with the power of digitalization in the healthcare sector, patients can receive information with the help of smartphone devices. With the help of technology, it improves the rural healthcare facilities: the rise of digital technology in the medical domain benefits people. An amalgamation of digital technology in the healthcare domain provides standard healthcare facilities to the rural community at a sustainable cost. An outbreak of pandemics led the Indian healthcare system to experience a new wave of opportunities. According to the report released by PwC (Prince Waterhouse Coopers) [7], three emerging trends change the course of the healthcare industry. First, private sector partnerships through health PPPs (public–private partnerships) were gaining acceptance. Second, the role of the government has been transformed, from provider to payer, and has led to expanded financial risk protection coverage to the marginalized. Third, the significant demand–supply mismanagement has led healthcare to emerge as an attractive sector for private equity investment.

4.4   INDIAN HEALTHCARE MARKET

According to the IBEF (Indian Brand Equity Foundation), healthcare has become the second-largest sector in revenues and employment. The following are the factors that drive the rapid growth of the healthcare market in India:

- Lifestyle diseases
- Emergence of digital technology advancements
- Increasing demand for affordable healthcare systems

Statistical figures released by the IBEF reported that the healthcare industry was valued at US$190 billion in 2020 and estimated to reach US$372 billion by 2022. Similarly, the digital healthcare market was valued at US$116.61 billion in 2018 and is estimated to reach US$484.53 billion by 2024 at a CAGR of 27.41%. Likewise, the diagnostics market was valued at US$5 billion in 2012 and estimated to arrive US$32 billion in 2022 at a CAGR of 20.4%. The value of the medical industry was around US$61.79 billion in 2017 and is estimated to reach US$123.84 billion by 2022. India has the world's largest medical insurance scheme known as "Ayushman Bharat," which is supported by the central government of India.

4.5   DIGITAL HEALTHCARE MARKET

India has emerged as a rapid growing digital economy in the past few years; as per the data from the year 2014 to 2017, a 90% growth at digital adopting index has been found [8]. The rapid amalgamation of digital technology in the medical sector has embraced the transformation and improved healthcare services quality, accessibility, and affordability. According to the IBEF (Indian Brand Equity Foundation) [9], the revenue from the digital healthcare market in India was valued at INR 116.21 billion in 2018, and it is estimated that value will increase to INR 485.43 billion by 2024. The digital healthcare market is segmented into telehealth, mHealth, electronic health records (EHR), remote diagnostics, and healthcare analytics. According to IBEF report [10], it is estimated that by 2024 mHealth will dominate the digital healthcare market (40% share) as many people use health and fitness apps to track health activities. The telehealth segment follows this. The telemedicine market is growing in India. The market value of the telemedicine market reached US$32 million. Similarly, the adoption of AI in the healthcare space reached US$6 million in 2021. Furthermore, wearable technology in the health space is growing. In 2021, the value of the wearable medical device market was US$61 billion. It is estimated to reach US$30.1 billion. According to the research by Markets and Markets, the market size of virtual reality technologies in healthcare space is estimated to reach by US$125.2 billion by 2026, at a compound annual growth rate (CAGR) of 30.6% between 2021 and 2026 [11]. The increasing adoption of digital health and technologies has fueled capital investment and many health-tech start-ups have raised during the pandemic.

4.6   THE STORY OF THE CORONAVIRUS PANDEMIC

The COVID-19 pandemic is popularly known as coronavirus pandemic. The novel coronavirus was first identified in Wuhan, China, in December 2019 [12]. The WHO announced COVID-19 a pandemic on 11th March 2020. Since 2021, many variants of the virus have appeared. Delta virus was the most virulent among them. It was first found in India and spread rapidly across the globe. According to a report published in *World Street Journal*, 2020 found that delta variant associated with increased risk for severe disease and hospitalization [13].

4.7 ROOT CAUSE OF THE CORONAVIRUS PANDEMIC

Experts, researchers, and environmentalists considered that human intervention in nature was the prime cause of a pandemic. The researchers claimed that COVID-19 originated from animals, directly impacting the coronavirus health crisis. A study released by UN report 2020 found that 70% of emerging infectious diseases were zoonotic [14] in nature. Zoonotic diseases are those caused by animals to humans. A study by Dr. Michael Greger reported that all the sources of infection diseases like EBOLA, bird flu, and swine flu were originated from the human–animal interface. A study by Professors Rachel et al. at Harvard Chan School of public health has found that the risk of COVID-19 death was high when people live in places with poor air quality [15]. In addition, lack of sanitation facilities, use of manufactured chemicals, and repetitive use of fossils fuel were the factors that increase the risk of infectious diseases, including COVID-19 [16].

4.8 COVID-19 IMPACT ON THE HEALTHCARE SYSTEM

The outbreak of COVID-19 has affected the lives of all sections of society. The delta variant of coronavirus was first detected in India, and it led to a massive number of COVID-19 cases in the country. The second tsunami of coronavirus resulted in thousands of lives lost and the high incremental cost to the healthcare system [17]. According to the government figures, 27 million corona cases were registered during the second wave, and more than 300,000 people lost their lives; India was the worst-hit country affected by the deadly coronavirus [18].

Shortage of essential resources like oxygen cylinders, medicines, and hospitals beds was evident in the supply chain mismanagement. Heart-wrenching stories from every corner of the country showed the failure of the Indian healthcare system. The paper proposed by Roy et al. (2021) suggested that the pandemic led to the panic situation across the globe [19].

Technology played an essential role during the pandemic—millions of individuals leveraged social media platforms by sharing the availability of necessary medical supplies. An amalgamation of technology with healthcare broadens the horizon of healthcare infrastructure. Central and state governments also leveraged technology and developed various healthcare apps. Arogya Setu app, widely used during pandemic outbreaks, helps assist individuals in syndrome mapping, contact tracing, and self-assessment. Similarly, the Co-WIN app has been widely used to access vaccines. The digital healthcare market saw boom during the pandemic. Indian health-tech industry was valued at US$1.9 billion in 2020 [20]. The emergence of telemedicine and teleconsultations is driving the healthcare market in India [21]. The Indian healthcare industry and the public and private sectors took a robust response plan to tackle the pandemic and build the bridge between the demand and supply of essential medical facilities.

The economic disturbance that occurred during the coronavirus pandemic was devastating. Employment opportunities shrunk, and millions of people became unemployed. A report released by WHO showed that 3.3 million global workforces lost their livelihoods [22]. COVID-19 has impacted the people's livelihoods, health, and food systems globally.

4.8.1 Digital Health

Digital health is a new concept with the usage of digital technologies enabling health-care access. Tech revolutionizes eHealth and its whole ecosystem. Digital technology is a new ray of hope in a time of the pandemic. It helps to provide affordable, accessible, and quality healthcare. Digital technologies facilitate clinical support, like teleconsultation, telemedicine, and tracking the supplies of medicines and vaccines [23]. Health information technology (HIT) is a vital tool to enhance the quality of a healthcare services in remote areas. During COVID-19, mobile phone check-in helps to minimize the waiting time and increases efficiency and patient safety. Likewise, in teleconsultation, doctors provide a virtual consultation. Similarly, e-pharmacy imparts a home delivery drug service. It is an effective means in delivering better health services in remote areas.

4.8.2 Scope of Digital Health

The wide scope of digital health comprises the following categories like mHealth (mobile health), wearable devices, telehealth, teleconsultation, health information technology (IT), and personalized medicine [24].

4.8.3 Mobile Health (mHealth)

mHealth is a common term used for mobile phone usage in medical care. The applications of mHealth are used to upskill consumers about preventive healthcare services. It is also used mainly for disease surveillance, treatment support, and tracking records. The utilization of mHealth is becoming popular in emerging nations like India, where there is a large population and widespread penetration of the Internet and smartphones.

4.8.4 Telemedicine

Telemedicine, which is popularly known as telehealth, provides the remote delivery of healthcare services. It broadly deals with medical care–related services.

The following are the benefits of telemedicine [25]:

a. **Comfort and Convenience:** Virtual consultation is easier and more convenient for both patients and doctors.
b. **Control of Infectious Illness:** Rapid adoption of telehealth technology in the healthcare domain was on the rise to protect the spread of deadly coronavirus and other infectious diseases. It saves sick people, pregnant women, and elderly people from the COVID-19 virus.
c. **Better Assessment:** Telemedicine provides a good way to get a mental health assessment and counseling.

4.9   HIT (HEALTH INFORMATION TECHNOLOGY)

HIT involves the work that includes processing, exchanging, and storing health-related data in the electronic environment [26]. Extensive HIT usage in the healthcare space revamp healthcare quality, check medical errors, minimize medical care expense, elevate administrative efficiencies, enhance paperless work, and extend the access to affordable healthcare.

4.9.1   WEARABLE TECHNOLOGY IN HEALTHCARE

Wearables are small electronic devices placed on human bodies to detect or measure the body temperature, blood pressure, oxygen, breathing rate, and the electrical activity of the heart, muscle, and brain. Wearable technology is extensively used in the healthcare space to enable patients to monitor their health records.

4.9.2   PERSONALIZED MEDICINE

Personalized medicine is also known as precision medicine. In the era of digitalization, personalized medicine is an evolving application of medicine, where the medical experts utilize the patient's genetic profile to counsel to make decisions regarding the prevention, diagnosis, and therapy of diseases. A better understanding of a patient's genetic descriptive charts assists medical expert's physicians in choosing the proper medication or therapy. Personalized medicine is upgrading through data from the Human Genome Project [27]. *Applications:* Personalized care medicine is largely used to diagnose certain types of cancer cells.

4.9.3   DIGITAL TECHNOLOGY TRANSFORMING HEALTHCARE SYSTEM

Technology has become an integral part of the healthcare system. Digital technology is a new ray of hope in the pandemic. It provides a standard, accessible, and budgetable healthcare at the PHC center. It helps to facilitate clinical support, like teleconsultation, telemedicine, and tracking the supplies of medicines and vaccines [28]. Health information technology (HIT) is a vital tool to enhance the quality of healthcare services in remote areas.

4.9.4   BLOCKCHAIN

Blockchain is defined as a distributed database that stores information in a digital format [29]. Blockchain differs from the typical database on the basis of how data are structured, and in the blockchain, information is gathered and stored in the form of blocks (WooHyun et al, 2022) [30]. It is an outstanding technology to protect the confidential data in the system, as well as it helps to exchange the critical data and keeps it secure and confidential. In other words, blockchain can be described as a decentralized peer-to-peer (P2P) personal computer network that stores and records historical data. Blockchain is rapidly transforming the ballgame of the healthcare industry. It has a broad range of applications that are used in the healthcare domain [31].

According to the research paper by Gordon W.J. and Catalini C. (2018), blockchain technology transforming institutions has driven interoperability to patient-centric interoperability [32]. Blockchain technology imparts access to patients' medical data and automatically connects to other hospitals. In addition, blockchain technology serves healthcare by resolving drug counterfeit and improving data storage and security [33]. According to the research study by Haleem et al. [34], blockchain is an emerging technology used in the medical care domain to create innovative solutions. The blockchain's primary application in healthcare is to preserve and exchange patients' data through medical institutions like hospitals, diagnostics labs, pharmacies, and physicians. In addition, blockchain provides insights and encourages the better analysis of medical records to the medical institutions (Chakraborty et al., 2022) [35].

4.10　ARTIFICIAL INTELLIGENCE (AI)

John McCarthy defined AI 2004 as "AI helps build an intelligent machine, and it is designed to understand human intelligence" [36]. AI have numerous real-world applications:

- **Speech Recognition**: Speech recognition is also known as ASR (automatic speech recognition). This process can use NLP (natural language processing) to process human speech into a written format. Many smartphones device incorporate ASR in the system to conduct a voice search.
- **Customer Service:** In the present business scenario, online virtual agents are replacing human agents to provide a better customer journey. For example, message chatbots used in e-commerce sites use virtual agents to assist and engage the customers in a meaningful way.
- **Recommendation Engines:** AI algorithms used historical consumption behavior data to discover the data trends and insights to develop effective marketing and selling strategies.

4.10.1　USES OF AI IN HEALTHCARE

The applications of AI transformed the healthcare system radically. The *Harvard Business Review* paper "10 Promising AI application in health care" showed that AI in healthcare assists healthcare providers in many aspects [37]. AI-assisted robotic surgery has increased efficiency. Similarly, AI-enabled technology helps to detect early-stage cancer and generate automated image diagnostic reports. Likewise, AI works like a virtual nursing attendant and resolves the workforce shortage. The increasing adoption of AI helps to cut the drug delivery cost. Furthermore, AI has extensive usage in the field of healthcare. AI systems help physicians provide the latest medical information from medical journals and research papers to notify the proper patient care. Similarly, AI extracts data from the large patient datasets that make an actual inference for health-risk alerts and prediction outcomes. Moreover, AI-related applications help to reduce diagnostic and therapeutic errors (Yirui et al., 2022) [38].

4.10.2 Types of AI Used in the Healthcare Industry

Machine learning is the most common configuration of AI in healthcare. Machine learning is a division of AI and CS (computer science) that concentrate on using data and algorithms to increase accuracy. The large sections of AI technology in healthcare use machine learning, known as supervised learning (Chakraborty et al., 2022) [39]. NLP is a branch of AI within computer science that mainly focuses on assisting computers in understanding the way that humans write and speak. In the healthcare industry, the NLP system analyzes the unstructured clinical notes of the patients and provides an incredible and quality insight that can give better results to patients.

4.10.3 IoT in Healthcare

Internet of Things is defined as a "digitally connected universe of everyday physical devices." IOT has an extensive application in the field of the healthcare system. The convergence of IoT and Cloud has given rise to sensor-clouds, which integrates multisensory services into cloud computing. It enhances the electromedical devices that significantly contribute to the overall decrease of healthcare costs while increasing the health outcomes. In addition, IoT in medical care provides an effective healthcare service delivery with the help of machine-to-machine communication, information exchange, and data movement. Similarly, IoT devices accumulate, report, and analyze real-time information data, and the healthcare organization uses this data to make an error-free decision.

4.10.4 Cloud Computing in Healthcare System

As per NIST, cloud computing is a model supported by computing resources. It requires minimal effort or service to provide valuable interaction. The cloud computing vendor supplies online access to configurable computing resources at very nominal operating costs. The market of cloud computing in the field of medical and health is increasing at a speedy rate, it is estimated that the market of cloud computing in the medical area will reach US$56 billion with average of CAGR of 18% [40]. The merits of cloud computing in healthcare are described in the following points. *Increased security:* Patients personal data and information are protected in online services. *Reduces costs:* In the present scenario, cloud computing services operate based on a subscription model, which saves healthcare providers' money on expensive systems and equipment. With the help of cloud computing in the healthcare industry, it can provide remote access to information and offer a monitoring service to protect the data from unauthorized access.

4.11 VIRTUAL REALITIES (VR)

VR is defined as a 3D computer-generated environment that provides effortless interaction with persons (Virtual Reality, 2009). In healthcare space, virtual reality is the biggest adopters of virtual reality. The applications are described in the following sections.

4.11.1 Uses of Virtual Reality in Healthcare Space

- **VR in Diagnostics:** Virtual reality is an essential and powerful diagnostic tool that helps doctors and physicians diagnose accurately.
- **VR in Medical Education:** Virtual reality simulations are primarily used in medical education and training. Medical professionals use VR technology to provide a risk-free environment to improve basic skills and knowledge.

4.11.2 Virtual Reality in Medical Surgery

In the present situation, virtual reality usage in surgery has gained immense popularity among the medical expert community. With the use of virtual reality techniques in surgery, it eases the surgery operations and reduces both the time and risk associated with surgical complications. Moreover, virtual reality plays a significant role in telesurgery, where the surgeon performs the processes at remote locations. Incorporating technologies like blockchain, AI, virtual reality, and IOT transformed the healthcare domain.

4.12 DIGITAL HEALTHCARE IN INDIA

Internet penetration and rapid digitization in the healthcare system has ameliorated the diagnostics, preventive, and medical care facilities. Digital technology connects patients with the doctors effectively. In the recent year, the advancement in digital technologies includes the following:

(a) Telemedicine, which provides remote delivery of healthcare services
(b) Personalized diagnosis with smart healthcare monitors
(c) Health apps increase health awareness among people
(d) AI-enabled tools to detect genetic diseases

4.12.1 Primary Medical Care System in India

Primary healthcare centers are the first touch point of connection where patients receive a first health-related treatment. In an emerging nation like India, PHC is the functional unit of public health services. Its objectives are to provide affordable and accessible healthcare services to both urban and rural areas. According to the report released by Rural Health Statistics in 2019, 30,045 PHC have been functional [41]. Though the PHC figures look spectacular, the ground reality is different. PHCs are in a dilapidated condition. Sriram's (2018) research paper examined that PHCs severely lack workforce and infrastructure [42]. According to the Ministry of Health, 58% of PHCs in India are located in six states with 54% of the rural population. These data showed that the Indian primary healthcare system lacks PHC in remote areas, and PHC has a shortage of adequate resources and quality of care. The pandemic has severely impacted primary healthcare services. This leads to the disrupted vaccination and neglect of non-communicable diseases. To improve the performance of primary healthcare services, the government should provide financial support to the PHC and recruit more health workers, including doctors, nurses, and lab technicians. Lastly, the government should implement digital technology in the remote healthcare system, including telemedicine e-pharmacy [43]. Primary healthcare is popularly essential healthcare. PHC is the first touch point [44]. Primary healthcare primarily addresses health needs and ensures that people receive quality care. PHC is the backbone of the nation's healthcare system [45], but the sudden outbreak of pandemic has affected the PHCs in remote areas. The impact of COVID-19 badly impacts the primary medical care services, especially in countryside regions. So, there is growing need for access to primary medical care services, government, and medical providers implementing digital technologies (like teleconsultation) to improve the services for the last mile of the community. With the help of digital technology in healthcare services, it bridges the gaps between patients and healthcare providers by providing medical care services regardless of location. In addition, digital health platform enhances the accessibility and availability of quality healthcare at a minimum cost.

Digital technology disrupts the primary healthcare system. A research study by University of Arkansas scholar showed that telemedicine had been an effective health service provider in far-flung areas. Anjan Bose, secretary-general of the Healthcare Federation of India, recommended that medical centers in the rural region restructure and transform from traditional to online providers. Technology helps to provide inexpensive and standard medical care in remote areas. In Ref. [45], the authors proposed that rapid adoption of telemedicine could eradicate the healthcare disparities in far-flung areas.

4.12.2 E-PHARMACY

Internet penetration in urban and rural areas has given rise to diverse technology-driven models to serve consumers efficiently. In the past few years, the rapid adoption of digital technology in the health sector improved healthcare services. Telemedicine has one of the progressive technology models that enabled access to doctors at the click of a bottom. Similarly, e-pharmacy has been an attractive technology model which bridges the gap by providing affordable medicines to consumers. As per the research study by FICCI (Federation of Indian Chambers of Commerce and Industry), the e-pharmacy concept will drive the nation's health sector [46]. The sudden outbreak of coronavirus pandemic has given rise to the adoption of e-pharmacy. E-pharmacy models provide a doorstep drugs delivery service. The establishment of e-pharmacy in the Indian context has improved the supply chain management of medicines. Online pharmacy services are not restricted to urban areas; it also assists in remote areas. For example, online pharmacy 1MG delivers medication in remote areas through common services centers (CSCs) [47]. Similarly, Pharmeasy, an online e-pharmacy platform, partnered with CSC to provide medicines at the last mile of society at an affordable price.

4.12.3 E-PHARMACY MARKET SIZE

Rapid penetration of the Internet across the nation improves the digitalization of healthcare services. According to the report released by Frost and Sullivan, e-pharmacy emerged in 2015 and is at its nascent stage in India. Many e-pharmacy players such as Medlife, Netmeds, 1MG, Sehat Sathi operate in the e-pharmacy segment. Medlife is the leading player in the e-pharmacy segment [48]. The current value of the e-pharmacy market is US$0.5 billion in 2019, and it is expected to increase by 44% to reach US$4.5 billion by 2025 [49].

4.12.4 E-PHARMACY EMPOWERS CUSTOMERS

E-pharmacy addressed the several problems that Indian healthcare consumers [50] suffered:

- **Consumer Convenience:** E-pharmacy helps the consumer to order the medicines conveniently. Deliver medicines at home in one click.
- **Patients' Education:** Online pharmacies provide patients with value-added information such as drugs reminders, drug interactions, and side effects of the medicines. Online pharmacy keeps the consumer more aware of the drugs.
- **Medicine Authenticity:** Online pharmacies can trace counterfeit medicines with complete advancement in technology. It makes a transaction more transparent.
- **Data Analytics**: E-pharmacy stores and analyzes extensive data on consumers; this data can be very beneficial for planning public health policies.
- **Transaction Records:** Organized online players have a systematic description of complete tax-paid transactions—this helps to generate the market size.
- **Industry Experts' Opinion:** Online pharmacy boosts the nation's health sector domain and provides tangible benefits to patients.

4.12.5 E-PHARMACY: LAST-MILE ACCESS TO MEDICINES

India is a nation with a deep geographical spread. According to the statistics released by the Census, 70% of the population inhabit the rural regions. Due to lack of access to healthcare services in the rural areas, a large number of people do not have the facilities to avail the life-saving drugs [51]. However, according to the government data, there is one pharmacy accessible for 1,700 people. In the present context, technology has been changing the healthcare sector in India. The following are the examples of e-pharmacy start-up in India:

- **Sehat Sathi App:** Nikhil Baheti and Saida Dhanavath founded the "Sehat Sathi" health-tech start-up in 2017. The foundation aims to introduce digital transformation in the retail pharmacy segment. The founders started the Sahet Sathi app to empower local pharmacies to organize business, enhance sales, serve customers, and access new services and products. Sehat Sathi App has a vast network of medical stores. It covers more than 30,000 local medical pharma retail across 15 states of India.

- **1MG Online Pharmacy:** Prashant Tandon, Gaurav Agarwal, and Vikas Chauhan founded the 1MG online pharmacy in 2013. The start-up aims to provide accessible and affordable medicines to patients. IMG platform associated with government to expand its services to the last mile of the society. Online pharmacy is a boon to the secluded region. It offers a reasonable cost than brick-and-mortar pharma stores, and medicines are easily accessible through online mode. E-pharmacy provides doorstep delivery within a short period and delivers authentic drugs through a licensed pharmacist. According to the study by A.R Mahesh (2020), customers prefer online pharmacies to obtain medicines in an emergency. Apart from emergency cases, patients who have been prescribed multiple medications also like to use online pharmacies to purchase drugs as online pharmacies give a high discount rate.

4.13 START-UPS IN THE HEALTHCARE DOMAIN

A start-up is a company that works at the initial stages of business. It primarily focuses on a single product or service. Health-tech start-ups are where the companies integrate the technology with the healthcare industry to solve health-related problems.

4.13.1 HEALTHCARE START-UP LANDSCAPE IN INDIA

According to the report Indian Healthtech Landscape in a Post–COVID-19 World released by Inc 43 Plus [5], pandemics severely influence the healthcare system. The crisis leads to an opportunity to opt for innovative healthcare systems. The market size of the Indian health-tech start-up is rapidly growing, and it is estimated to reach US$21 billion by 2025. Indian health-tech start-ups worked with GOI (Government of India) to support the healthcare infrastructure. The digital healthcare landscape predominantly works on technology-based service models, where companies like Netmeds and 1MG play the vital role of the pharmacist and deliver medicines to patients. Digital healthcare start-ups cater to rural areas and provide quality and affordable healthcare to patients. Start-ups like Karma Healthcare provide telemedicine solutions by connecting patients in rural areas to physicians located in urban areas.

4.13.2 HEALTH-TECH START-UPS IN INDIA

HelloLyf is an online platform that provides video consultations with doctors. Dr. Sahabat Azim launched HelloLyf in 2016. The health-tech start-up aims to offer affordable medical care to the last mile of society. HelloLyf offers multispecialty services, including medicine, pediatrics, cardiology, gynecology, sexology, dental, psychology, nutrition, and lifestyle. HelloLyf Digital Dispensary delivers affordable healthcare to remote locations; it provides complete primary healthcare solutions, including consultation, confirmatory tests, and medicine at a single point. In a

digital dispensary, the doctors connect online and examine the patent with an electronic stethoscope [52]. Likewise, nurses feed the patient information and record
the necessary test such as blook pressure, EGC, temperature, oxygen saturate rate,
and upload the investigation reports like MRI and X-rays in the digital dispensary
software.

- **Agile Healthcare:** Dr. Vishal Upadhyaya founded the Agile healthcare
  start-up in 2019. The foundation aims to provide thorough primary and preventive medical care via telemedicine through Medi junction E-clinics [53].
  According to Vishal, Medi junction provides healthcare to the masses in
  remote areas where doctors are unavailable.

Agile Healthcare Work Process: Agile healthcare start-ups provide primary
healthcare services, diagnosis, and treatment in the Medi Junction e-Clinics. The
Agile clinic is also known as a hospital in the bag that caters to three essential
aspects:

- Medical inspection
- Medical history taking via videoconference
- Medical examination (IoT devices and prescription and dispensing of
  medication)

- **Niramai:** This health-tech start-up used AI to detect early-stage breast
  cancer. Dr. Geeta Manjunath founded the Niramai in 2016. It used
  AI-enabled tool that used thermal analytics. The core solution was known
  as Thermalytic, which detects premature stage of breast cancer. In this solution, lab technicians measure the temperature variation in the chest and
  analyze it using the software. The product's core value is no see, no touch,
  no pain, and no radiation.
- **Xaant (TerraBlue):** This health-tech start-up used AI to detect overall mental health. Rajlakshmi Borthakur founded the TerraBlue in 1998.
  AI-enabled Xaant was the world's first medical diagnostic device to identify mental health states automatically.
- **Qure.ai:** This is a health-tech start-up developing deep learning to interpret
  radiology images. Prashant Warier founded it in 2016. The start-up aims
  to use AI to make healthcare services affordable and accessible. Queri.ai
  setup is primarily valuable for remote areas with a shortage of radiologist
  specialists. It leverages deep learning to detect and diagnose disease and
  create an automated diagnostic report. The automated diagnostic reports
  help doctors and radiologists to make faster and more accurate decisions.
  Adoption of AI-driven healthcare improves productivity and efficiency.
  According to the report released by McKinsey, AI impacts healthcare in
  three areas: population health management, improving operations, and
  strengthening innovation [54].

4.14 ROLE OF GOVERNMENT IN BUILDING HEALTH-TECH START-UPS

Start-ups have a significant role in building the nation's economic growth. It creates jobs and provides employment opportunity to the youth of the nation. Start-ups are the centers of innovation. These are the important factors for which government are providing beneficial schemes to start-ups. To build a solid ecosystem to nurture the start-ups in the country, GOI launched the "Start-ups India Action Plan" [55] which provides support to start-ups like legal support, tax exemption, and financial, academia, and industry support. According to the Science and Technology minister, GOI will launch a unique incentive scheme to support the start-ups in telemedicine, digital health, and artificial intelligence. The special incentive program will be launched by BIRAC (Biotechnology Industry Research Assistance Council) [56].

4.15 CONCLUSION

Digital technology radically transformed the healthcare domain. Technology in the medical sector changed the conventional medical care system. The growing demand for telemedicine, teleconsultation, mHealth, and e-pharmacy in the healthcare domain provides affordable medical facilities to the last mile of society.

4.15.1 RECOMMENDATIONS

The pandemic miserably impacted the country's economic and healthcare system. This showed the failure of the government and the healthcare system of India. Pandemics are generally unpredictable. The government should make prior planning and strategy in advance to stop future pandemics. Moreover, the disaster department should depend on transparent data to create a good strategy. In addition, the government should invest in healthcare infrastructure and focus on the primary healthcare system. Generally, the Indian government has been allocating 1.5% of GDP to healthcare, whereas the government should ideally spend 5–6% of GDP on the healthcare system. Pandemic leads to the growth of digital healthcare solutions. Healthcare start-ups in artificial intelligence, machine learning, and decision-support systems completely transform healthcare ecosystems. Digital technology and artificial intelligence have become the mainstream for healthcare access.

4.15.2 FUTURE STUDY

The author of this chapter acknowledges that this chapter has a few limitations. First, the chapter did not discuss the possibilities of balancing the utilization of the latest technology like AI and virtual reality with the traditional healthcare methods and processes. Second, the chapter has adopted the systematic literature review approach. In future, researchers can explore the same study by applying the qualitative and quantitative approaches to get an insightful result.

REFERENCES

1. Health Care Industry in India. (2021, October 12). IBEF. Retrieved from www.ibef.org/industry/healthcare-india.aspx

2. Basu, S., Andrews, J., Kishore, S., Panjabi, R., & Stuckler, D. (2012). Comparative performance of private and public healthcare systems in low-and middle-income countries: a systematic review. *PLoS Medicine*, *9*(6), e1001244. www.ncbi.nlm.nih.gov/pmc/articles/PMC3378609/

3. Sheikh, K., Saligram, P. S., & Hort, K. (2015). What explains regulatory failure? Analysing the architecture of health care regulation in two Indian states. *Health Policy Plan*, *30*(1), 39–55.

4. Danigond Ashvini. (2021, May 28). 5 reasons why Indian healthcare is struggling. *The Hindu Business Line*. Retrieved from www.thehindubusinessline.com/news/national/5-reasons-why-indias-healthcare-system-is-struggling/article34665535.ece

5. Kasthuri, A. (2018). Challenges to healthcare in India-the five A's. *Indian Journal of Community Medicine: Official Publication of Indian Association of Preventive & Social Medicine*, *43*(3), 141.

6. Breast Cancer Treatment in India. (2021, October 13). Practo. Retrieved from www.practo.com/health-wiki/breast-cancer-treatment-india/296/article#:~:text=The%20minimum%20price%20for%20Breast,7%2C00%2C000

7. Digital Healthcare Market. (2019). Retrieved from www.researchandmarkets.com/reports/4988978/digital-healthcare-market-in-india-2019

8. Digital Healthcare in INDIA "Healthcare of the Future." (2020, September). Indian Health. Retrieved from www.indiahealth-exhibition.com/content/dam/Informa/india-health-exhibition/en/downloads/Digital%20health%20report%202020.pdf

9. Digital Healthcare to Witness Exponential Growth in India. (2020, November 30). IBEF. Retrieved from www.ibef.org/blogs/digital-healthcare-to-witness-exponential-growth-in-india

10. Tremosa, L. (2022, January 1). Beyond AR vs RR, what is the difference between AR VS MR VS XR. *Interaction Design*. Retrieved from www.interaction-design.org/literature/article/beyond-ar-vs-vr-what-is-the-difference-between-ar-vs-mr-vs-vr-vs-xr

11. Coronavirus History: Origin and Evolution. (2021, August 14). Webmed. Retrieved from HTTPs://www.webmd.com/lung/coronavirus-history

12. Abbot, Brianna. (2021, June 9). Covid 19 Delta variant. *The Wall Street Journal*. Retrieved from www.wsj.com/articles/covid-19-variant-first-found-in-india-is-quickly-spreading-across-globe-11623257849

13. Fleming Sean. (2020, July 7). It's time to get serious about the cause of the pandemic. *World Economic Forum*. Retrieved from www.weforum.org/agenda/2020/07/it-s-time-to-get-serious-about-the-causes-of-pandemics-un-report/

14. Bernstein, A. (2020). Coronavirus, climate change, and the environment. A conversation on COVID-19 with Dr. Aaron Bernstein, Director of Harvard Chan C-CHANGE. *C-Change*. www.hsph.harvard.edu/c-change/subtopics/coronavirus-and-climate-change/

15. Othman, Soufiene Ben, Bahattab, Abdullah Ali, Trad, Abdelbasset, & Youssef, Habib. (2020). LSDA: Lightweight secure data aggregation scheme in healthcare using IoT. *ACM — 10th International Conference on Information Systems and Technologies*, Lecce, Italy, June 2020.

16. Mistry, Lal. (2021, February 1). *Indian Healthcare Sector Transformation in the Post Covid 19 Era*. Retrieved from https://home.kpmg/in/en/home/insights/2021/02/india-healthcare-sector-transformation-in-the-post-covid-19-era.htm

17. Agarwal, Vibhuti. (2021, June 11). The future of healthcare post covid. *Economic Times*. https://health.economictimes.indiatimes.com/news/industry/the-future-of-healthcare-post-covid/83423336

18. Sukanya, R., & Chinmay, C. (2021). Panic buying situation during COVID-19 global pandemic. *Journal of Information Technology Management*, *13*(2), 231–244. http://doi.org/10.22059/jitm.2021.80625

19. Agarwal, Vibuti. (2021, June 29). The future of healthcare post covid. *Innovaccer Blog*. Retrieved From https://innovaccer.com/blogs/careers/the-future-of-healthcare-post-covid/

20. Bajaj, Akriti. (2021, November 1). Invest India. Retrieved from www.investindia.gov.in/sector/healthcare

21. Chriscaden Kimberly. (2020, October 13). WHO. Retrieved from www.who.int/news/item/13-10-2020-impact-of-covid-19-on-people's-livelihoods-their-health-and-our-food-systems

22. World Health Organization. (2018). *Digital Technologies: Shaping the Future of Primary Health Care* (No. WHO/HIS/SDS/2018.55). World Health Organization. Retrieved from www.who.int/docs/default-source/primary-health-care-conference/digital-technologies.pdf?sfvrsn=3efc47e0_2

23. What is Digital Health. (2022, September 22). FDA. Retrieved from www.fda.gov/medical-devices/digital-health-center-excellence/what-digital-health

24. Hasselfield, W. Benefits of medicine. *Hopkins Medicine*. Retrieved from www.hopkins-medicine.org/health/treatment-tests-and-therapies/benefits-of-telemedicine

25. Health Information Technology. (2020, August 31). HHS. Gov. Retrieved from www.hhs.gov/hipaa/for-professionals/special-topics/health-information-technology/index.html

26. Personalized Medicine. *National Human Genome Research Institute of India*. Retrieved from www.genome.gov/genetics-glossary/Personalized-Medicine#:~:text=Personalized%20medicine%20is%20an%20emerging,diagnosis%2C%20and%20treatment%20of%20disease

27. Digital Technologies: Shaping the Future of Primary Health Care. (2018). World Health Organization. Retrieved (No. WHO/HIS/SDS/2018.55). World Health Organization from www.who.int/docs/default-source/primary-health-care-conference/digital-technologies.pdf?sfvrsn=3efc47e0_2

28. Hayes, A. (2022, March 5). Block chain explained. *Investopedia*. Retrieved from www.investopedia.com/terms/b/blockchain.asp

29. WooHyun, P., Isma, F. S., Chinmay, C., Nawab, M. F. Q., & Dong, R. S. (2022). Scarcity-aware SPAM detection technique for big data ecosystem. *Pattern Recognition Letters*, *57*, 67–75. https://doi.org/10.1016/j.patrec.2022.03.021

30. Daley, S. (2021, July 30). How using blockchain in healthcare is reviving the industry capabilities. *Builtin*. Retrieved from https://builtin.com/blockchain/blockchain-healthcare-applications-companies

31. Gordon, W. J., & Catalini, C. (2018). Blockchain technology for healthcare: Facilitating the transition to patient-driven interoperability. *Computational and Structural Biotechnology Journal*, *16*, 224–230.

32. Othman, Soufiene Ben, Bahattab, Abdullah Ali, Trad, Abdelbasset, & Youssef, Habib. (2019). RESDA: Robust and efficient secure data aggregation scheme in healthcare using the IoT. *The International Conference on Internet of Things, Embedded Systems and Communications (IINTEC 2019)*, HAMMAMET, Tunisia from 20–22 December 2019.

33. Haleem, A., Javaid, M., Singh, R. P., Suman, R., & Rab, S. (2021). Blockchain technology applications in healthcare: An overview. *International Journal of Intelligent Networks, 2*, 130–139.

34. Hemanta, K. B., & Chinmay, C. (2022). Explainable machine learning for data extraction across computational social system. *IEEE Transactions on Computational Social Systems, 9*(4), 1–15. http://doi.org/10.1109/TCSS.2022.3164993

35. McCarthy, J. (2004). *What is Artificial Intelligence*. Retrieved from http://www-formal.stanford.edu/jmc/whatisai.html.

36. Othman, Soufiene Ben, Bahattab, Abdullah Ali, Trad, Abdelbasset, & Youssef, Habib. (2020). PEERP: A priority-based energy-efficient routing protocol for reliable data transmission in healthcare using the IoT. *The 15th International Conference on Future Networks and Communications (FNC) August 9–12*, 2020, Leuven, Belgium, 2020.

37. Agarwal, Y., Jain, M., Sinha, S., & Dhir, S. (2020). Delivering high-tech, AI-based health care at Apollo hospitals. *Global Business and Organizational Excellence, 39*(2), 20–30.

38. Yirui, W., Haifeng, G., Chinmay, C., Mohammad, R. K., Stefano, B., & Shaohua, W. (2022). Edge computing driven low-light image dynamic enhancement for object detection. *IEEE Transactions on Network Science and Engineering*, 1–13. http://doi.org/10.1109/TNSE.2022.3151502

39. Neha, S., Chinmay, C., & Rajeev, K. (2022). Optimized multimedia data through computationally intelligent algorithms. *Springer Multimedia Systems*, 1–17. http://doi.org/10.1007/s00530-022-00918-6

40. IkInk, R. (2021, March 4). 25 cloud trends for 2021 and beyond. *Accenture*. Retrieved from www.accenture.com/nl-en/blogs/insights/cloud-trends

41. Primary Health Centres. (2020, Spetember 18). Pib.gov. Retrieved from https://pib.gov.in/PressReleasePage.aspx?PRID=1656190

42. Sriram, S. (2018). Availability of infrastructure and human resources for primary health centers in a district in Andhra Pradesh, India. *Journal of Family Medicine and Primary Care, 7*(6), 1256

43. Vyas, S., Sharma, N., Archisman, P. R., & Kumar, R. (2021). Repercussions of lockdown on primary health care in India during COVID 19. *Journal of Family Medicine and Primary Care, 10*(7), 2436.

44. What is Primary Healthcare. (n.d). University of Bristol. Retrieved from www.bristol.ac.uk/primaryhealthcare/whatisphc.html

45. American College of Physicians. (2006). Reform of the dysfunctional healthcare payment and delivery system. *Acpoline.com*. Retrieved from www.acponline.org/system/files/documents/advocacy/current_policy_papers/assets/dysfunctional_payment.pdf

46. Mathur, P., Srivastava, S., Lalchandani, A., & Mehta, J. L. (2017). The evolving role of telemedicine in health care delivery in India. *Prime Health Care, 7*(260), 2167–1079.

47. Mehta, Shreyans. (2021, February 25). Empowering local medical stores-the future of medicine. *Business World*. Retrieved from www.businessworld.in/article/Empowering-Local-Medical-Stores-The-Future-Of-Medicine/25-02-2021-381733/

48. Malik, Yuvraj. (2019, August 9). Online pharmacy deliver medicines in rural areas through CSCs. *Business Standard*. Retrieved from www.business-standard.com/article/companies/online-pharmacy-1-mg-to-deliver-medicines-in-rural-areas-through-cscs-119080901272_1.html

49. Sriram, Ganesh. (2021, June 22). E-Pharmacies bridging gap Indian healthcare. *Times of India Blogs*. Retrieved from www.investindia.gov.in/team-india-blogs/e-pharmacies-bridging-gap-indian-healthcare

50. How E-Pharmacy Can Empower Consumers. (n.d). *Economic Time*. Retrieved from https://health.economictimes.indiatimes.com/news/health-it/how-e-pharmacy-can-empower-consumers/47420428

51. How Indian Healthtech Start-ups Are Empowering the Country Healthcare Ecosystem, (2021, June 21). *Inc42Brand Labs*. Retrieved from https://inc42.com/videos/the-dialogue-how-indias-healthtech-startups-are-empowering-the-countrys-healthcare-ecosystem/

52. Narayan, Dinesh. (2017, September 13). Digital dispensaries take affordable healthcare to remote locations. *Economic Times*. Retrieved from https://economictimes.indiatimes.com/industry/healthcare/biotech/healthcare/digital-dispensaries-take-affordable-healthcare-to-remote-locations/articleshow/60503121.cms

53. Varshney, Ravi. (2020, March 5). *Healthtech Start-up Yourstory*. Retrieved from https://yourstory.com/2020/03/doctor-healthtech-startup-agile-healthcare-medi-junction/amp

54. Jenkins, J., Spatharou, A., & Hieronimus, S. (2020, March 10). Transforming healthcare with AI. *Mckinsey.com*. Retrieved from www.mckinsey.com/industries/healthcare-systems-and-services/our-insights/transforming-healthcare-with-ai

55. Startup India. (n.d). *Government of India*. Retrieved from www.startupindia.gov.in/content/sih/en/international/go-to-market-guide/government-initiatives.html

56. Awastha, R. (2021, August, 25). Government to launch incentive schemes to support 75 startups in telemedicine digital healthcare. *Economic Time*. Retrieved from https://economictimes.indiatimes.com/tech/startups/govt-to-launch-incentive-scheme-to-support-75-startups-in-telemedicine-digital-health/articleshow/85626654.cms?utm_source=contentofinterest&utm_medium=text&utm_campaign=cppst

5 Smart Healthcare Monitoring System Using LoRaWAN IoT and Machine Learning Methods

Nagarjuna Telagam, Nehru Kandasamy, and D. Ajitha

CONTENTS

5.1 INTRODUCTION

Healthcare devices and technology have been interrelated for a long time ago. The IoT is advanced in data techniques in multiscale, distributed, homogeneous, and heterogeneous datasets. This has created numerous opportunities in healthcare services. IoT helped analyze the medical research domain and created data accessibility, data availability, patient personal data, and efficient delivery cost.

DOI: 10.1201/9781003315476-5

Today, the latest IoT technologies such as wearable sensors, body area sensors, and smartwatches play an essential role in human life [1]. The authors present the watch-based sensor network, and it describes the platform that works in 868 MHz. the heart rate monitoring and sleep time monitoring are possible with 868 MHz and 2.45 GHz frequency bands. The simulation results are compared with commercial Bluetooth-based watches in the indoor environment [2]. The panoply applications of IoT technology play an essential role in human body monitoring. The network has intelligent sensors and communication cables, making it possible to monitor physical and mental health. The data availability at different scales and temporal longitudes in different processing algorithms can lead to an evolution in the medical field, treating the diseases such as post facto diagnosis [3]. The healthcare solutions have a relevant application to the doctor's respective departments by IoT in the next generation [4]. The IoT devices generate unrivalled data, with which cloud computing algorithms can be processed. The delay between cloud and application of the data is unacceptable in real-time health monitoring applications. The authors have proposed remote monitoring for patients in their smart homes with fog concepts at different gateways. This proposed model uses advanced techniques for distributed storage, embedded data mining, and response time in determining an event's state compared with other classification algorithms [5]. Monitoring patients remotely generates awareness and guides them to proper health [6]. This proposed algorithm or platform has inbuilt Wi-Fi modules, an integrated microprocessor, an analogue to digital converter, a digital to analogue converter, a piezoelectric sensor, etc. The users or patients can check the generated data remotely from any other device [7]. The data routing strategy in IoT environment-based health monitoring is explained [8]. The insecure patient data needs to be stored in the cloud server which consists of primary healthcare parameters. The healthcare monitoring systems can exist with single-mode communications in the global system for mobile communications or data access on the web application. The author proposes that the health monitoring system increases healthcare delivery for multiplexed data over GSM and Wi-Fi [9], [10]. Wearable devices will realize a new electronics class, which will apply to health monitoring and other electrical devices [11]. These lightweight and wearable devices are critical for personal health monitoring systems, and they are not confined by time and space. The wearable sensor devices are based on engineered nanomaterials with unique sensing capabilities to detect diseases [12].

Wrist-worn actigraph devices have been used for the sleep data of human beings for over two decades [13]. Digital health data continuously increases and transforms healthcare and optimizes the patient's experience [14]. The skin-based wearable devices have good potential for health monitoring and heart diagnosing diseases. The innovation and attention to materials used and technologies in fabrication play a crucial role in healthcare device development. The authors of this chapter give insight into the effects of skin-based wearable devices. The parameters that can be monitored in those devices are temperature, strain, biomarker analysis, etc. The advanced materials supporting sensitivity, durability, and biocompatibility are used to design skin-based wearable devices [15]. This approach can also notify critical health data through email reports [16]. The integration of IoT, cloud computing, and big data in the healthcare system leads to innovative health [17] actively. Due to the increasing usage of smartphone applications, the smartphone's edge computation can highly assist network traffic management [18]. A medical system prototype consists of a wireless health monitoring device and a smartphone base station [19]. Table 5.1 shows the traditional machine learning methods.

TABLE 5.1

Conventional Machine Learning Methods for Smart Healthcare Systems

Reference	Aim	Used Dataset	Preprocessing Technique and Feature Extraction	Machine Learning Technique	Accuracy
Chai et al. [41]	Diagnosis of glaucoma	Beijing Hospital provided the data	Normalization and local binary features	Logistic regression	60.84%
Zhang et al. [42]	MMSE values prediction in Alzheimer's disease	ADNI dataset	Five-level brain segmentation and Level 1	Linear regression	AUC = 0.318
Liu et al. [43]	Diagnose the bacterial sepsis	Guangzhou hospital provided the data	Normalization	Procalcitonin	78.4%
Viegas R et al. [44]	ICU readmission patients prediction	MIMIC II	Scope of patients entering and specificity curves	Ensemble decision process	AUC = 0.78
Dong et al. [45]	Detection of cataract	Hospital data	Wavelet	Support vector machine	81.8%
Zheng et al. [46]	Prediction of hospital admission patients	Hospital data	Scope of patient data from admission	Neural network	56.1%
Fialho et al. [47]	Predict ICU readmission	MIMIC II	Deleted data from the database	Sequential forward selection	74%
Ajam et al. [48]	Analyze the medical data	Hospital data	Neural network	Feed forward backpropagation Neural network	88%
Roostaee et al. [49]	Analyze the medical data	Hospital data	Machine learning	Support vector machine	84.4%
Latha et al. [50]	Analyze the medical data	Hospital data	Machine learning	Ensemble classifiers	85.4%

In this chapter, the following contributions are made:

1. The new innovative healthcare techniques for patient monitoring, especially using ECG signals, are identified.
2. Low power wireless area network for health monitoring system–based IoT is briefly reviewed and compared with GPRS technology concerning architecture, range, and cost.
3. The patient path estimator is explained briefly with hospital database controller technologies.
4. The machine learning methods or intelligent system methods that contribute to smart healthcare systems are briefly discussed, and precise heart disease prediction using machine learning algorithms is proposed. We achieved more than 4% of accuracy for training data.

This chapter is classified into four sections. Section 5.1 explains the literature survey of the intelligent healthcare system and related works. Section 5.2 describes the 6LoWPAN health monitoring system model, which combines layered architecture and network architecture, with comparisons to conventional techniques. Section 5.3 describes the Internet of Things–based devices in LoRaWAN architecture and patient data gathering and flow charts in IoT architectures. Section 5.4 discusses the ECG signals–based healthcare monitoring system. Section 5.5 explains the patient data analysis using machine learning methods. The preprocessing of the data and neural network schemes are discussed. Section 5.6 discusses the results obtained and compares it with conventional systems. Finally, Section 5.7 concludes the chapter with machine learning methods analysis and a performance comparison with the traditional methods.

5.2   LoWPAN HEALTH MONITORING SYSTEM

The vision of Internet of Things is that objects will communicate with each other concerning process information. Figure 5.1 shows the layered architecture where the LoRaWPAN adaptation layer receives data from the network and MAC layers. The data packets through radio frequency are communicated between layers. Most

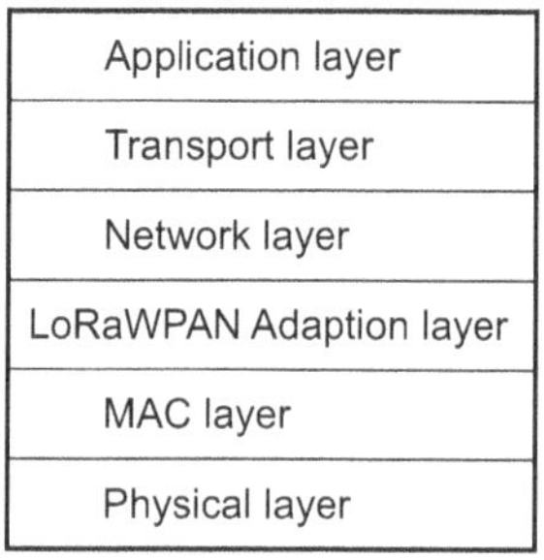

Application layer
Transport layer
Network layer
LoRaWPAN Adaption layer
MAC layer
Physical layer

FIGURE 5.1   LoWPAN-layered architecture.

items or devices are small, have less power constraints, and have small computing and storage resources. The Internet is mandatory for wireless networks to interconnect for information exchange. The 6LoWPAN network architecture is shown in Figure 5.2. Sensor networks have been emerging in recent years because of their self-organized and self-configuration capabilities. Mobility support is needed for the success of the Internet of Things [20].

Devices of all kinds, irrespective of size or shape, have become standard for human beings in their daily lives. These devices are intelligent devices present in buildings, cars, and even public infrastructures such as roads, railway stations, bus stands, and bridges. The authors employed open hardware platforms and emphasized embedded systems' singularities, such as fewer operations, less power consumption, and less bandwidth capability, intending to optimize road structures' maintenance [21].

Internet applications have potential in many domains, such as healthcare, technological, social, and economic. The authors describe the telemedicine architecture for innovative home security solutions, and the classification depends on the layers. The first layer is a comprehensive analysis of the client and server sides. The monitoring of patients remotely benefits security requirements [22]. Critical infrastructure protection is a high priority for every country in the world. It reduces vulnerabilities and has increased the protection of essential infrastructures against vulnerable attacks from terrorists. CIP and structural health monitoring (SHM) gather basic information to detect and quantify vulnerabilities, thereby improving the CI's resilience [23]. The Internet of Things plays a significant role in healthcare systems in today's modern era, monitoring and communicating, storing, and displaying. The authors measure the ECG's monitors, EEG waveforms, temperature, heart rate, pulse rate, etc. These parameters are transmitted with Wi-Fi technology. Additionally, the system can generate a notification for nurses in emergency treatment [24]. Network sniffers are one kind of tool used for testing and designing distributed embedded

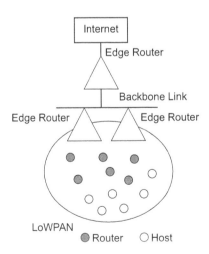

FIGURE 5.2   LoWPAN network architecture.

systems. They have been helpful for LoWPAN networks for quality of service. The Z-monitor is designed with a low-cost, open-source protocol analyzer for 6LoWPAN networks, and here the packet sniffing can be performed by IEEE 802.15.4 complaint nodes with Java coding [25]. Artificial intelligence–based deep neural networks play a crucial role in detecting IoT healthcare systems [26]. Different studies of healthcare systems are classified and discussed [27],[28].

5.3   IoT-BASED HEALTHCARE SYSTEM USING LORAWAN

The medical sensor data is monitored through low-cost, low-power, secure communication. The main parameters such as pulse rate, glucose levels, and body temperature are collected in rural areas where the cell phone coverage area is less or where the data transmission from medical devices is impossible. In addition, the authors conduct experiments concerning the LoRa network and power dissipation. With 30-km radius coverage, the gateway is placed at a 12-meter altitude. As a result, the low power utilization is reduced to at least ten times.

The medical expert executes the developed plans through the fourth component treatment plan. Some of the medical experts' challenges include patient data privacy and the security links for data leakage that must be kept confidential. The second challenge is to expand low-cost and less-power network protocol suitable for comprehensive area communication. The third challenge is to analyze the patient's health data to generate the appropriate treatment plans. Figure 5.3 shows the IoT4HC

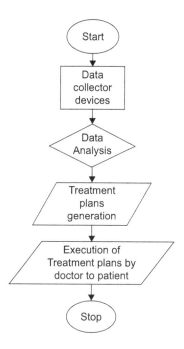

FIGURE 5.3   Flow chart of IoT4HC architecture.

architecture [29]. LoRaWAN is deployed on the gateway, which gathers data packets from the sensor end nodes present in the LoRaWAN transceivers. It also forwards the server data with encryption-based Internet protocol packets through ethernet cables 4G data links, as shown in Figure 5.4.

This architecture is low-cost, corresponding to 4G solutions. The infrastructure cost is ten times less than a conventional GSM network [30]. The most essential for the devices is the duty cycle percentage of 1% for a fair transmission rate. The latency time will be 5 seconds, using the AES algorithm with a 128-bit key. The security encryption depends on frame size and random tokens [31]. The encryption algorithm and message integrity can also be deployed in low-power microcontrollers or Arduino boards. The conventional monitoring approach uses standard different transmission protocols. Table 5.2 shows the differences between LoRaWAN with standard 3G or 4G cellular networks. The coverage area and data rate for these networks will be the same as the conventional networks. The frequency licenses of the network usage, taxes, and cost of the GSM-based networks are very high in nature, but LoRaWAN uses only accessible unlicensed frequencies.

This end node also sends the data to the medical experts or the gateways according to the LoRaWAN specifications. The gateway comprises a concentrator board and an inbuilt processor. This gateway function is to convert the RF packets to IP packets. The concentrator sends radiofrequency packets and then sends them to the hosts. The latter has a packet forwarder installed already, which transforms the radio frequency packets from the concentrator to the UDP packs and configures through the server with the Internet's help. The concentrator will also include a data buffer to avoid the data loss problem and provides privacy. Furthermore, the data can be

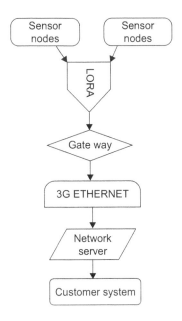

FIGURE 5.4   The general architecture of LoRaWAN.

TABLE 5.2

Comparison of LoRa and Conventional Systems

Technology	Consumption of Energy in Milliampere	The Hardware Cost of Equipment and Distance Covered	Highest Data Rate
LoRaWAN	Idle mode: 2.8 mA Receiving mode: 14.2 mA Transmitting mode: 38.9 mA	The transmitter and receiver cost is US$10, and the gateway cost is US$250. The distance covered is 60 km	The uplink and downlink speed is the same, i.e., 50 kbps
GPRS	Idle mode: 20 mA Receiving mode: 130 mA Transmitting mode: 2,000 mA	The transmitter and receiver cost is US$50, and the gateway cost is US$1,000. The distance covered is 60 km	The downlink speed is 85.6 kbps, and the uplink speed is 14 kbps

plotted for web dashboards graphically to visualize the real-time analysis. The web dashboard is an Internet-based interface for displaying the data in computers and mobiles, allowing doctors or health professionals to track patients remotely [32].

5.4 ECG SIGNALS-BASED SMART HEALTH MONITORING SYSTEM

The body sensor network for healthcare applications and monitoring of patients remotely has brought more attention to the researchers and created a passion for researchers. The sensors are present in the wireless body area network, monitoring any typical patient body changes. This data is given for medical expert analysis. The data changes can happen if the patient has suffered from electrocardiogram (ECG), and the physiological sensors data will change rapidly. The authors present a centralized approach for detecting abnormalities. A simplified Markov model will notice the changes in the ECG signal data. With the help of a sequence pattern, the ECG data forms a feature set. The research results show that the detection rate is almost 5% and 10% abnormalities in the patient data [33]. A signal quality–aware Internet of Things has three modules: the first one is the ECG signal-sensing module, the second one is the signal quality assessment, and the last one is signal quality awareness. The lightweight electrocardiogram method is used to classify, which acquires ECG signals from the sensors automatically. The signal quality-aware method is suitable for assessing ECG signals' clinical acceptability for a high-reliability diagnosis system [34].

The signal quality assessment method is the intermediate step. It plays an essential strategy in the applications such as heart rate analysis, biometric application, and unsupervised health monitoring systems for clinical diagnosis. The ECG signal quality is classified into excellent, good, bad, and unacceptable ranges. The conventional methods have a very high demand for accuracy and reliability for the ECG signals. Still, some ways show less precision and are degraded in the solution-finding

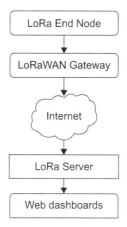

FIGURE 5.5 LoRaWAN-based IoT4HC architecture.

problems. The signal detection and communication nodes will be in sleep mode if the unexpected noise level is detected in the ECG signals and can significantly reduce the ECG signal features [35]. Figure 5.5 shows the IoT architecture with a signal quality awareness program. The hidden Markov model chain is developed for healthcare systems with IoT technology integration. This system helps cardiovascular disease patients to improve their medical services. This IoT-based medical healthcare system makes remote monitoring of patients in rural areas or urban areas possible. This system uses a patient path estimator and alert management scheme to facilitate cardiovascular disease patients' treatment [36]. Architecture is required to ensure the precise nature of administration (QoS) necessities [37].

The proposed engineering is demonstrated in shown Figure 5.6. It is made out of heterogeneous gadgets such as user equipment (UE), inbuilt sensors, the base station (BS), and access points (AP), which interface with the nearest towers and gateways to trade information and yield data in real time. Patients are considered one of the other static or versatile in the IoT climate [38]. As shown in Figure 5.6, the heart data was gathered from the patient's body's clinical sensors to remove the ECG signal [39]. All the information is communicated using Bluetooth to the UE. The UE sends all approaching data and localization to the nearest AP or BS, speaking with the clinic information base. Regulators interact with every quiet sign and store it on the patient's table afterward. The clinical staff manages every one of the refreshed tables, and on account of the crisis, the regulators create an alarm which prompts the clinical team to intercede in an ideal way [40]. The proposed structure appeared in Figure 5.7. It comprises four head parts: patient way assessor, ECG signal sensors, patient table administrator, and medical clinic alert framework/dataset regulator. When an unusual pulse movement is recognized, the regulator creates new principles to produce an alarm/alert to the clinical staff. The segment portions of the framework are depicted which advertise their activity point by point as shown in Figure 5.8.

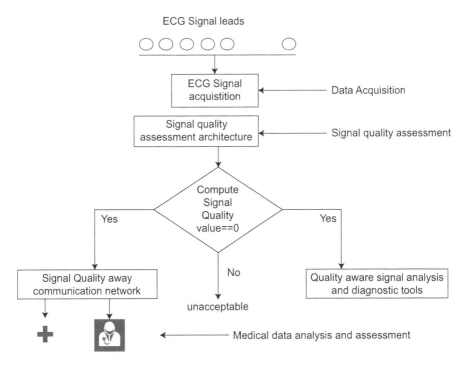

FIGURE 5.6   Signal quality awareness program with IoT framework.

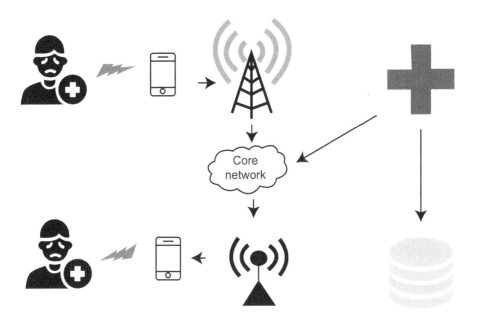

FIGURE 5.7   The architecture of S-health IoT.

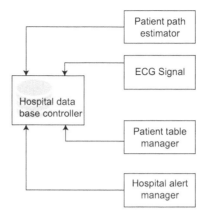

FIGURE 5.8   Patient path estimator framework for patient monitoring.

5.4.1   PATIENT PATH ESTIMATOR

The uplink scenario is considered where the user equipment communicates with base stations and access points with a cellular network or wireless fidelity. The access points will forward the user's location and intimates the hospital's database. The HMM predictor is further used to estimate the patient's future locations or devices.

5.4.2   ECG SIGNAL SENSORS

It is an electrical sign related to the action of the human heart musicality. ECG information securing in the telecardiology medical care administration gives average complex factors expected for analysis. Prompt $\Delta R–R$ span is a component utilized in telecardiology, and it is characterized as the time term between the two nearby R tops. The clinical staff, along these lines, build up a framework utilizing ECG signals misusing $\Delta R–R$ spans to recognize untimely pulses. The authors analyzed that R tops are gathered at periods. The sequence of steps shows the ECG signal securing system identifying unpredictable ventricular cadence for CVD patients shown in Figure 5.8. Figure 5.9 shows the ECG signal generated with signal sensors.

5.4.3   THE PATIENT TABLE MANAGER

The regulator checks the $R–R$ span deviation every 6 seconds and stores the data information in the patient table directory. Thus, every persistent table directory has all the character data, the clinical meeting's historical backdrop for the cardiovascular diagnosed patients, and the progressive $\Delta R–R$ spans.

5.4.4   THE HOSPITAL ALERT SYSTEM

As the ECG signals are identified, the medical clinic information base framework investigates and updates every quiet table. In crisis cases, new standards create and

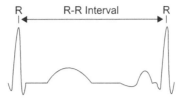

FIGURE 5.9   ECG complex waves showing *R* peak values.

speak over the emergency clinic's organization to a distant information worker, and an alarm message is shipped off to the clinical staff. The above framework gives the more significant development opportunity for patients conceded to the CVD ward as an alarm created in the emergency clinic when an unusual circumstance emerges.

5.5   PATIENT DATA ANALYSIS USING MACHINE LEARNING ALGORITHMS

5.5.1   DEEP LEARNING AND BIG DATA

Big data analytics and deep learning are two high-focal points of information science. Big data has become significant as numerous public and private associations have gathered enormous space in explicit data measures, containing valuable data about public knowledge, digital protection, extortion discovery, advertising, and clinical informatics. Complex reflections are learned at a given level depending on moderately detailed deliberations formed in the progression's former level. A particular kind of figuring equipment called graphics processing units (GPUs) is upgraded to deal with these multifaceted neural networks.

5.5.2   DATA PREPROCESSING

A few stages are associated with preprocessing the information and making it suitable for information examination or AI calculations. The essential things to be dealt with while preparing are missing qualities, categorical information, splitting the informational collection, feature scaling, and feature extraction. The names utilized for this information should reflect clinical reality since they will prepare the AI framework. Any error in naming will seriously restrict the AI calculation precision, paying little mind to the exertion will put resources into improving the calculation. The AI architecture for clinical applications fixates on information curation, an interaction of renaming information into clinically or legitimately important subgroups that may improve the AI device's prescient precision for the expected clinical issue.

5.5.3   NEURAL NETWORKS

The neural network commonly includes a few stages, beginning with utilizing a convolution channel to prehandled data. The track empowers the organization to distinguish a specific shape in a picture or word in a content report by filtering the information and computing a worth that addresses a rundown of the input's highlights. Another significant element of neural networks is backpropagation, which includes preparing the model from a known result through minor, iterative changes [51–54]. Beyond the scope of this review, a thorough evaluation of the iterative cycle of testing various model architectures is not possible. For instance, information researchers should utilize a deliberate and experimental way to deal with engineer neural network structures comparable to the assignment, use a decent number of neural network layers, and change the loads. Table 5.1 shows the conventional methods which used machine learning methods have achieved the highest accuracy of 82%.

5.6   RESULTS AND DISCUSSIONS

Dataset from UCI repository is used to predict the heart disease. Table 5.3 shows the list of input attributes, key attributes, and predictable attributes. The random forest classifier from the sklearn.ensemble module is imported. After importing the libraries, we tuned the hyperparameters using GridSearchCV. The best hyperparameters values are found, such that maximum features = 4, minimum sample leaf = 5, number of estimators = 10, the training accuracy is 87.67%, and the testing accuracy is 89.07%. Figure 5.10 shows the confusion matrix details and how the accuracy is calculated for testing and training dataset.

The disease identification is explained based on the ECG value and Gini index, and the cholesterol value and thalach values are considered for the decision. The age parameter and sample size also classify the disease identification, as shown in Figure 5.10. The calculation of the confusion matrix is explained in Figures 5.11 and 5.12.

The decision tree is a tree-like model to make predictions, and it shows an upside-down tree, i.e., it splits the data into multiple sets of data. Each set is further divided into subsets to arrive at a decision finally. It works on nested if-then-else structure, i.e., each node divides the data into either left or right direction. The top node in the

---

TABLE 5.3
Heart Data Attributes Collected from the UCI Database

Input Attributes	Key Attributes	Predictable Attributes
Age	Patient ID	Target values
Sex (male: 1, female: 0)		0: Patient is suffering from heart disease
Chest pain (1: angina pain, 2: non-angina pain, 3: asymptotic)		1: The patient is not suffering from heart disease
Blood pressure and cholesterol		
Fasting blood sugar		
Resting electrocardiographic results		
Max heart rate achieved and induced angina		
Old peak and slope		
Number of major vessels and thalach value		

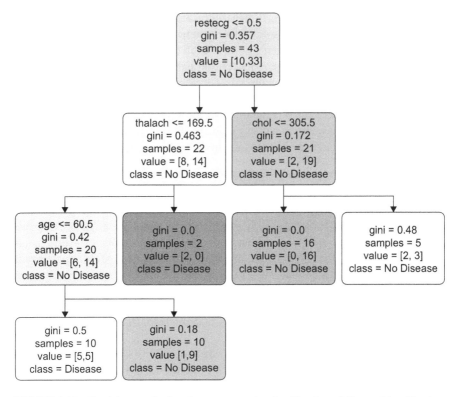

FIGURE 5.10 Decision tree leaf node represents the classification of disease identification.

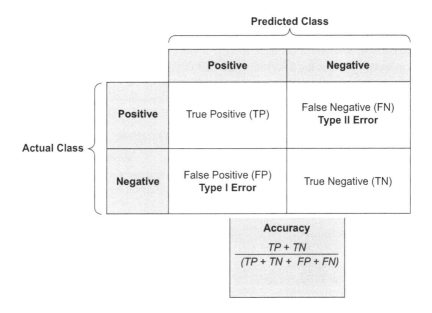

FIGURE 5.11 Confusion matrix values are calculated for the random forest classifier.

decision tree is called the root node. The node can be classified into a leaf node, and the intermediate nodes between the root and the leaf nodes are called internal nodes, as shown in Figure 5.12. Table 5.4 shows that the proposed work has demonstrated improvement in accuracy. The previous models have 79% and 84.4% accuracy with different features selection and classifiers.

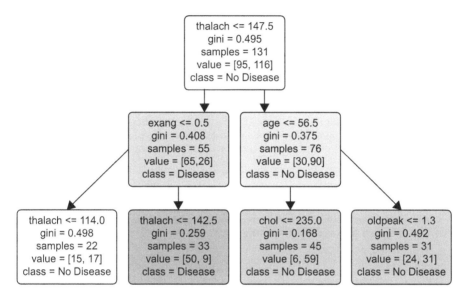

FIGURE 5.12   Decision tree model with nodes and leaf nodes classification using Graphviz library.

TABLE 5.4
Comparison with Conventional Methods

Research Article	Techniques Used	Evaluation Metrics
Khempila et al. [55]	Feature selection: Information gain Classification selection: Multilayer perceptron with backpropagation algorithm	Accuracy: • Training: 89.56% • Testing: 80.99%
Chitra et al. [56]	Classification: Artificial neural network with backpropagation network–cascaded correlation neural network	Accuracy with ANN: • Training: 72.6% • Testing: 79.45% • Accuracy with CNN: • Training: 78.55% • Testing: 85%
Roostaee et al. [57]	Feature selection: Binary Cuckoo optimization Classification: SVM (support vector machine)	Accuracy: 84.4%
Proposed method	Feature selection: Decision tree Classification: Random forest classifier	• Accuracy: • Training: 87% T• esting: 89%

5.7 CONCLUSION

In this chapter, machine learning–based smart health methods are analyzed broadly. This chapter presents medical sensor data with low-power wide area network architecture, ECG signals, and machine learning methods in the smart healthcare field. The sensor data uploaded on the cloud is analyzed, and predictions are explained briefly with the machine learning algorithm–based K-means clustering algorithm. The implementation schemes such as ECG sensors and hidden Markov model chain are used in e-Health. The systems will improve the monitoring of patients, leading to enhanced medical services. The 6LoWPAN is the most energy-efficient communication in smart sensor networks, and it is also used to analyze the operation time of the wireless network for the health monitoring system. Patients' electrocardiogram (ECG) signals for remote real-time monitoring are also analyzed. This chapter concludes the new innovative healthcare techniques for patient monitoring using ECG signals. This chapter also briefly reviewed the low-power wireless area network–based health monitoring system. The patient path estimator is explained briefly with hospital database controller technologies and the machine learning methods that contribute to smart healthcare systems. The dataset is taken from the UCI repository. The decision tree feature selection and random forest classifiers are used in this chapter. The proposed model shows an accuracy of about 4% for training data and 5% improvement in accuracy for testing data.

Heart disease, alternatively known as cardiovascular disease, or any disease that encases various conditions that impact the human body is the primary cause of death worldwide over the past few decades. The numerous datasets are available in the Cleveland database of the UCI repository for analysis. The researchers can use data mining techniques to process numerous complex data to predict diseases. The supervised and unsupervised machine learning algorithms will play a significant role in identifying diseases from huge complex medical data in the future decade.

5.8 FUTURE SCOPE

As the technologies are developing rapidly, this chapter can be extended in numerous ways, and the deep neural network algorithm plays a significant role in the heart disease prediction system. The RNN and CNN architectures also show their capability in the machine learning era. The LoRaWAN IoT medical device data can be integrated into machine learning methods to overcome the certain drawbacks of the conventional method. The ResNet, DNN, and CNN are majorly used in smart health for future generations.

REFERENCES

[1] Farahani, Bahar, Farshad Firouzi, and Krishnendu Chakrabarty. "Healthcare IoT." In *Intelligent Internet of Things*, pp. 515–545. Springer, Cham, 2020.
[2] Kumar, Sanjeev, John L. Buckley, John Barton, Melusine Pigeon, Robert Newberry, Matthew Rodencal, Adhurim Hajzeraj, et al. "A wristwatch-based wireless sensor platform for IoT health monitoring applications." *Sensors* 20, no. 6 (2020): 1675.

[3] Hassanalieragh, Moeen, Alex Page, Tolga Soyata, Gaurav Sharma, Mehmet Aktas, Gonzalo Mateos, Burak Kantarci, and Silvana Andreescu. "Health monitoring and management using Internet-of-Things (IoT) sensing with cloud-based processing: Opportunities and challenges." In *2015 IEEE International Conference on Services Computing*, pp. 285–292. IEEE, 2015.

[4] Zamfir, Mădălina, Vladimir Florian, Alexandru Stanciu, Gabriel Neagu, Ştefan Preda, and Gheorghe Militaru. "Towards a platform for prototyping IoT health monitoring services." In *International Conference on Exploring Services Science*, pp. 522–533. Springer, Cham, 2016.

[5] Verma, Prabal, and Sandeep K. Sood. "Fog assisted-IoT enabled patient health monitoring in smart homes." *IEEE Internet of Things Journal* 5, no. 3 (2018): 1789–1796.

[6] Ghosh, Ananda Mohon, Debashish Halder, and S. K. Alamgir Hossain. "Remote health monitoring system through IoT." In *2016 5th International Conference on Informatics, Electronics and Vision (ICIEV)*, pp. 921–926. IEEE, 2016.

[7] Abdelgawad, Ahmed, and Kumar Yelamarthi. "Internet of things (IoT) platform for structure health monitoring." *Wireless Communications and Mobile Computing* 2017 (2017): Article ID 6560797, 10 pages. https://doi.org/10.1155/2017/6560797

[8] Tokognon, C. Arcadius, Bin Gao, Gui Yun Tian, and Yan. "Structural health monitoring framework based on Internet of Things: A survey." *IEEE Internet of Things Journal* 4, no. 3 (2017): 619–635.

[9] Swaroop, K. Narendra, Kavitha Chandu, Ramesh Gorrepotu, and Subimal Deb. "A health monitoring system for vital signs using IoT." *Internet of Things* 5 (2019): 116–129.

[10] Mdhaffar, Afef, Tarak Chaari, Kaouthar Larbi, Mohamed Jmaiel, and Bernd Freisleben. "IoT-based health monitoring via LoRaWAN." In *IEEE Eurocon 2017–17th International Conference on Smart Technologies*, pp. 519–524. IEEE, 2017.

[11] Takei, K., W. Honda, S. Harada, T. Arie, and S. Akita. "Toward flexible and wearable human-interactive health-monitoring devices." *Advanced Healthcare Materials* 4, no. 4 (2015): 487–500.

[12] Ha, Minjeong, Seongdong Lim, and Hyunhyub Ko. "Wearable and flexible sensors for user-interactive health-monitoring devices." *Journal of Materials Chemistry B* 6, no. 24 (2018): 4043–4064.

[13] Mantua, Janna, Nickolas Gravel, and Rebecca Spencer. "Reliability of sleep measures from four personal health monitoring devices compared to research-based actigraphy and polysomnography." *Sensors* 16, no. 5 (2016): 646.

[14] Kikidis, Dimitrios, Votis Konstantinos, Dimitrios Tzovaras, and Omar S. Usmani. "The digital asthma patient: The history and future of inhaler based health monitoring devices." *Journal of Aerosol Medicine and Pulmonary Drug Delivery* 29, no. 3 (2016): 219–232.

[15] Jin, Han, Yasmin Shibli Abu-Raya, and Hossam Haick. "Advanced materials for health monitoring with skin-based wearable devices." *Advanced Healthcare Materials* 6, no. 11 (2017): 1700024.

[16] Abdullah, Amna, Asma Ismael, Aisha Rashid, Ali Abou-ElNour, and Mohammed Tarique. "Real-time wireless health monitoring application using mobile devices." *International Journal of Computer Networks & Communications (IJCNC)* 7, no. 3 (2015): 13–30.

[17] Tang, Qian, Min-Hsin Yeh, Guanlin Liu, Shengming Li, Jie Chen, Yu Bai, Li Feng, et al. "Whirligig-inspired triboelectric nanogenerator with ultrahigh specific output as the reliable portable instant power supply for personal health monitoring devices." *Nano Energy* 47 (2018): 74–80.

[18] Wcislik, M., M. Pozoga, and P. Smerdzynski. "Wireless health monitoring system." *IFAC-PapersOnLine* 48, no. 4 (2015): 312–317.

[19] Oliveira, L. M., A. F. de Sousa, and J. J. Rodrigues. "Routing and mobility approach in IPv6 over LoWPAN mesh networks." *International Journal of Communication Systems* 24, no. 11 (2011): 1445–1466.

[20] Lazo, C., P. Gallardo, and S. Céspedes. "A bridge structural health monitoring system supported by the Internet of Things." In *IEEE Colombian Conference on Communication and Computing (IEEE COLCOM 2015)*, pp. 1–6. IEEE, 2015, May.

[21] Talal, M., A. A. Zaidan, B. B. Zaidan, A. S. Albahri, A. H. Alamoodi, O. S. Albahri, . . . & K. I. Mohammed. "Smart home-based IoT for real-time and secure remote health monitoring of triage and priority system using body sensors: Multi-driven systematic review." *Journal of Medical Systems* 43, no. 3 (2019): 42.

[22] Alonso, L., J. Barbarán, J. Chen, M. Díaz, L. Llopis, and B. Rubio. "Middleware and communication technologies for structural health monitoring of critical infrastructures: A survey." *Computer Standards & Interfaces* 56 (2018): 83–100.

[23] Fotouhi, H., A. Čaušević, M. Vahabi, and M. Björkman. "Interoperability in heterogeneous low-power wireless networks for health monitoring systems." In *2016 IEEE International Conference on Communications Workshops (ICC)*, pp. 393–398. IEEE, 2016, May.

[24] Tennina, S., O. Gaddour, A. Koubâa, F. Royo, M. Alves, and M. Abid. "Z-monitor: A protocol analyser for IEEE 802.15. 4-based low-power wireless networks." *Computer Networks* 95 (2016): 77–96.

[25] Vimal, S., Y. H. Robinson, S. Kadry, H. V. Long, and Y. Nam. "IoT based smart health monitoring with CNN using edge computing." *Journal of Internet Technology* 22, no. 1 (2021): 173–185.

[26] Telagam, N., S. Lakshmi, and N. Kandasamy. "Performance analysis of parallel concatenation of LDPC coded SISO-GFDM system for distinctive pulse shaping filters using USRP 2901 device and its application to WiMAX." *Wireless Personal Communications* 121, no. 4 (2021): 3085–3123.

[27] Nagarjuna, T., S. Lakshmi, and K. Nehru. "USRP 2901-based SISO-GFDM transceiver design experiment in virtual and remote laboratory." *The International Journal of Electrical Engineering & Education* (June 2019). http://doi.org/10.1177/0020720919857620

[28] Telagam, N., D. Ajitha, and N. Kandasamy. "Review on hardware attacks and security challenges in IoT edge nodes." *Security of Internet of Things Nodes: Challenges, Attacks, and Countermeasures*, p. 211. Chapman and Hall/CRC, Boca Raton, FL, 2021.

[29] Mdhaffar, Afef, Tarak Chaari, Kaouthar Larbi, Mohamed Jmaiel, and Bernd Freisleben. "IoT-based health monitoring via LoRaWAN." In *IEEE EUROCON 2017–17th International Conference on Smart Technologies*, pp. 519–524. IEEE, 2017.

[30] Khan, Farrukh Aslam, Nur Al Hasan Haldar, Aftab Ali, Mohsin Iftikhar, Tanveer A. Zia, and Albert Y. Zomaya. "A continuous change detection mechanism to identify anomalies in ECG signals for WBAN-based healthcare environments." *IEEE Access* 5 (2017): 13531–13544.

[31] Satija, Udit, Barathram Ramkumar, and M. Sabarimalai Manikandan. "Real-time signal quality-aware ECG telemetry system for IoT-based health care monitoring." *IEEE Internet of Things Journal* 4, no. 3 (2017): 815–823.

[32] Neyja, Maryem, Shahid Mumtaz, Kazi Mohammed Saidul Huq, Sherif Adeshina Busari, Jonathan Rodriguez, and Zhenyu Zhou. "An IoT-based e-health monitoring system using ECG signal." In *GLOBECOM 2017–2017 IEEE Global Communications Conference*, pp. 1–6. IEEE, 2017.

[33] Banerjee, Bitan, Amitava Mukherjee, Mrinal Kanti Naskar, and Chintha Tellambura. "BSMAC: A hybrid MAC protocol for IoT systems." In *2016 IEEE Global Communications Conference (GLOBECOM)*, pp. 1–7. IEEE, 2016.

[34] Qi, Nan, Ming Xiao, Theodoros A. Tsiftsis, Mikael Skoglund, Phuong L. Cao, and Lixin Li. "Energy-efficient cooperative network coding with joint relay scheduling and power allocation." *IEEE Transactions on Communications* 64, no. 11 (2016): 4506–4519.

[35] Atat, Rachad, Lingjia Liu, and Yang Yi. "Privacy protection scheme for eHealth systems: A stochastic geometry approach." In *2016 IEEE Global Communications Conference (GLOBECOM)*, pp. 1–6. IEEE, 2016.

[36] Du, Rong, Lazaros Gkatzikis, Carlo Fischione, and Ming Xiao. "Energy efficient sensor activation for water distribution networks based on compressive sensing." *IEEE Journal on Selected Areas in Communications* 33, no. 12 (2015): 2997–3010.

[37] Othman, Soufiene Ben, Abdullah Ali Bahattab, Abdelbasset Trad, and Habib Youssef. "LSDA: Lightweight secure data aggregation scheme in healthcare using IoT." *ACM — 10th International Conference on Information Systems and Technologies*, Lecce, Italy. June 2020.

[38] Lin, Chin-Teng, Kuan-Cheng Chang, Chun-Ling Lin, Chia-Cheng Chiang, Shao-Wei Lu, Shih-Sheng Chang, Bor-Shyh Lin, et al. "An intelligent telecardiology system using a wearable and wireless ECG to detect atrial fibrillation." *IEEE Transactions on Information Technology in Biomedicine* 14, no. 3 (2010): 726–733.

[39] Chinmay, C., and N. A. Arij. "Intelligent Internet of Things and advanced machine learning techniques for COVID-19." *EAI Endorsed Transactions on Pervasive Health and Technology* (2021): 1–14. http://doi.org/10.4108/eai.28-1-2021.168505

[40] Chinmay, C., B. Gupta, and S. K. Ghosh. "Chronic wound characterization using Bayesian classifier under telemedicine framework." *International Journal of E-Health and Medical Communications* 7, no. 1 (2016): 78–96. http://doi.org/10.4018/IJEHMC.2016010105

[41] Chai, Y., L. He, Q. Mei, H. Liu, and L. Xu. "Deep learning through two-branch convolutional neuron network for glaucoma diagnosis." *Proceedings of International Conference on Smart Health*, pp. 191–201. Springer, 2017.

[42] Zhang, J., Y. Luo, Z. Jiang, and X. Tang. "Regression analysis and prediction of mini-mental state examination score in Alzheimer's disease using multi-granularity whole-brain segmentations." *Proceedings of International Conference on Smart Health*, pp. 202–213. Springer, 2017.

[43] Liu, Y., and K. S. Choi. "Using machine learning to diagnose bacterial sepsis in the critically Ill patients." *Proceedings of International Conference on Smart Health*, pp. 223–233. Springer, 2017.

[44] Viegas, R., C. M. Salgado, S. Curto, J. P. Carvalho, S. M. Vieira, and S. N. Finkelstein. "Daily prediction of ICU readmissions using feature engineering and ensemble fuzzy modeling." *Expert Systems with Applications* 79 (2017): 244–253.

[45] Dong, Y., Q. Wang, Q. Zhang, and J. Yang. "Classification of cataract fundus image based on retinal vascular information." *Proceedings of International Conference on Smart Health*, pp. 166–173. Springer, 2016.

[46] Othman, Soufiene Ben, Abdullah Ali Bahattab, Abdelbasset Trad, and Habib Youssef. "RESDA: Robust and efficient secure data aggregation scheme in healthcare using the IoT." *The International Conference on Internet of Things, Embedded Systems and Communications (IINTEC 2019)*, HAMMAMET, Tunisia from 20–22 December 2019.

[47] Fialho, A. S., F. Cismondi, S. M. Vieira, S. R. Reti, J. M. Sousa, and S. N. Finkelstein. "Data mining using clinical physiology at discharge to predict ICU readmissions." *Expert Systems with Applications* 39, no. 18 (2012): 13158–13165.

[48] Ajam, N. "Heart diseases diagnoses using artificial neural network." *IISTE Network and Complex Systems* 5, no. 4 (2015).

[49] Roostaee, S., and H. R. Ghaffary. "Diagnosis of heart disease based on meta heuristic algorithms and clustering methods." *Journal of Electrical and Computer Engineering Innovations (JECEI)* 4, no. 2 (2016): 105–110.

[50] Latha, C. B. C., and S. C. Jeeva. "Improving the accuracy of prediction of heart disease risk based on ensemble classification techniques." *Informatics in Medicine Unlocked* 16 (2019): 100203.

[51] Hemanta, K. B., and C. Chinmay. "Explainable machine learning for data extraction across computational social system." *IEEE Transactions on Computational Social Systems* 9, no. 4 (2022): 1–15. http://doi.org/10.1109/TCSS.2022.3164993

[52] WooHyun, P., F. S. Isma, C. Chinmay, M. F. Q. Nawab, and R. S. Dong. "Scarcity-aware SPAM detection technique for big data ecosystem." *Pattern Recognition Letters* 157 (May 2022): 67–75. https://doi.org/10.1016/j.patrec.2022.03.021

[53] Neha, S., C. Chinmay, and K. Rajeev. "Optimized multimedia data through computationally intelligent algorithms." *Springer Multimedia Systems* 1–17 (2022). https://doi.org/10.1007/s00530-022-00918-6

[54] Yirui, W., G. Haifeng, C. Chinmay, R. K. Mohammad, B. Stefano, and W. Shaohua. "Edge computing driven low-light image dynamic enhancement for object detection." *IEEE Transactions on Network Science and Engineering* 1–13 (2022). http://doi.org/10.1109/TNSE.2022.3151502

[55] Othman, Soufiene Ben, Faris A. Almalki, Chinmay Chakraborty, and Hedi Sakli. "Privacy-preserving aware data aggregation for IoT-based healthcare with green computing technologies." *Computers and Electrical Engineering* 101 (2022). https://doi.org/10.1016/j.compeleceng.2022.108025

[56] Chitra, R., and V. Seenivasagam. "Review of heart disease prediction system using data mining and hybrid intelligent techniques." *ICTACT Journal on Soft Computing* 3, no. 4 (2013): 605–609.

[57] Roostaee, S., and H. R. Ghaffary. "Diagnosis of heart disease based on meta heuristic algorithms and clustering methods." *Journal of Electrical and Computer Engineering Innovations (JECEI)* 4, no. 2 (2016): 105–110.

6 Light Deep CNN Approach for Multi-Label Pathology Classification Using Frontal Chest X-Ray

Souid Abdelbaki, Ben Othman Soufiene,
Chinmay Chakraborty, and Sakli Hedi

CONTENTS

6.1 INTRODUCTION

Today, COVID-19 is considered undoubtedly an invasive malignancy caused by the SARS-CoV-2 [1], and is designated coronavirus owing to its visual similarity to the solar corona (a coronation) [2]. The effort against COVID-19 has encouraged

DOI: 10.1201/9781003315476-6

researchers across the globe to examine, grasp, and develop novel diagnostics and treatment mechanisms that could help eradicating this risk to our generation. In this study, we will investigate on how computer vision scientists encounter this issue by recommending new techniques and boost the efficiency and speed of current projects.

Blood testing, virus tests, and medical imaging are the most routinely utilized diagnostic methods [3]. Blood tests reveal the existence of antibodies to the severe acute respiratory syndrome SARS-CoV-2 within the patient blood. Yet, as reported in Ref. [4], accuracy of this exam in diagnosing COVID-19 is just as low as 5% or less [5]. Using respiratory tract samples, viral tests identify SARS-CoV-2 antibodies. The rapid diagnostic test (RDT) is considered a form of antibody isolation test that delivers results in about half an hour. The rapid diagnostic test kits, on the other hand, are not generally accessible, and their effectiveness is contingent on the sample quality check and the onset of illness. Furthermore, since this test cannot discriminate the coronavirus from other viral infections, it may yield false positive findings; consequently, it is not recommended for coronavirus diagnosis [6]. Another frequent process used is the reverse transcription-polymerase chain reaction (RT-PCR). This exam is a common approach for first-line screening with a large-scale investigation; on the other hand, the result has indicated that the sensitivity of test findings varies somewhere around 50% [7]. This shows that a negative RT-PCR result is possible at first. As a consequence, several tests are done over two weeks in order to guarantee the legitimacy of the provided analysis results for the diagnosis. Furthermore, a negative test for a suspected COVID-19 case is only considered genuine if no positive findings are recorded following the two weeks period of testing [8]. It might be stressful to patients and pricy for the healthcare owing to lack of these test kits in certain nations [9]. Early disease discovery increases the chances of effective treatment for afflicted individuals while also preventing the spreading of infectious viruses such as COVID-19 in the community. COVID-19 patients are identified using advanced wearable healthcare sensors and effective artificial neural networks associated with physiological and survey inputs [10]. Furthermore, several methods based on machine learning prediction were developed to foresee the infection rate, the plausibility of the pandemic's second, third, and fourth waves, and the danger of infection linked with travel. The chest X-ray examination and computed tomography exams are commonly used to detect lung-related disorders, including pneumonia and tuberculosis, and could also be used to detect COVID-19 [11–12]. One advantage of the chest X-ray is the simplicity with which it may be conducted using portable chest X-ray equipment, allowing quicker and much more reliable COVID-19 diagnostic system [13–15]. Chest X-ray has been found to detect COVID-19 employing artificial intelligence and to be less hazardous to the human body than computed tomography.

We list our objectives as follows:

- To use deep CNNs to categorize lung opacity, viral pneumonia, COVID-19, and healthy lung from a chest radiograph test and transfer learning to have more robust and efficient (computational cost) models.
- To implement an oversampling technique to resolve the imbalance problem with the dataset.

- To test MobileNet V3's, EfficientNet B3, Xception-Net, and Inception_ResNetV2 performance on the task of classifying multiple classes from one input.

This work is divided into six sections: Section 6.1 examines scholar's perspectives on the influence of the malignant COVID-19 between countries and peoples. Section 6.2 discusses the previous works and advances in the field of medical radiology imaging. Section 6.3 discusses the general architecture and dictates the implemented CNNs. Section 6.4 is dedicated to the data collection. Section 6.4 also discusses several matrices and methods. Section 6.5 discusses the evaluation of results during training and testing phases for utilized models. Section 6.6 concludes this study by discussing its potential scope.

6.2 RELATED WORKS

COVID-19, which itself is correlated to the symptoms of pneumonia, is detected using radiography examination. Therefore, the chest X-ray modality ought to be capable of distinguishing the novel COVID-19 symptoms from other pneumonia categories. The COVID-19 traces on a chest X-ray must be recognized from other designated forms of pneumonia. A variety of research activities reveal a distinguishing information about chest X-rays that best represents pneumonia from negative samples. In the assessment of pneumonia/COVID-19, classification from X-rays radiograph, machine learning methods, statistical approaches, deep learning architectures, transfer learning for pneumonia and lung opacity detection, sophisticated CNN models, and adversarial networks were utilized, as also big-data.

6.2.1 LUNG OPACITY AND PNEUMONIA DETECTION

Machine learning-based methods outline novel strategies, namely, the feature extraction strategies capable of successfully exploiting characteristics of interest from chest X-rays. These characteristics are often detected using a machine learning technique. In Ref. [18], the authors propose a novel process for automated pneumonia identification. The lungs' X-ray regions are extracted and then quantified using order one statistical parameters such the mean, kurtosis, and so on. To get classification labels, these feature encodings are discriminated against using logistic regressor classifier, multiple layer perceptron, and random forests classifier. Ambita [19] offered an approach for detecting pneumonia using adaptive regression descriptors and SVM. In Ref. [20], the authors suggested a technique for categorizing chest X-rays using neural networks that leverage texture-based statistical data from the GLCM to illustrate the randomized strategies variable as a feature for the classifier.

In Ref. [21], the authors examined the intensity distribution of infected and non-infected with pneumonia X-rays using the Earth mover's distance. To identify X-rays as having or not having pneumonia, thresholds are created from the fluctuation in EMD values.

CNN approaches rapidly learn the underlying latent vector representations, allowing them to differentiate between positive pneumonia data and normal data. In Ref.

[22], the authors demonstrate a customized CNN to classify pneumonia; the obtained performance of the trained model was examined under a range of conditions to validate the addition of dropouts and data augmentation process. Wu [23] provided convolutional neural network method to identify pneumonia by extracting deep features from denoised X-rays. Denoising is accomplished via adaptive median filtering, and RF classifier is trained on the resulting CNN features. Fathurahman [24] trained a one-dimensional convolutional network using the HOG and GCLM from a chest X-ray. In Ref. [25], a combination of blood examination and testicular screening to detect and diagnose this deadly virus is illustrated; in order to address dataset problems, they adopted the synthetic minority oversampling technique. Furthermore, the Shapley Additive Explanations method was also applied to determine the features' gravity. Stephen et al. [26] created a feedforward CNN model with an added Conv layer and also an FC layer. Li et al. [27] demonstrated a customized CNN that can detect pneumonia and was tested using a variety of convolutional layers.

Transfer learning is a method of reusing pretrained neural network weights to train the model on a new dataset by altering and retraining just the classification layer of the model, the modified CNN consume all of the architectural advantages of the basic CNN. In Ref. [27], the authors employed transfer learning with five neural architectures to build an ensemble model to detect pneumonia. In Ref. [28], the authors utilized Google's InceptionV3 model for deep transfer learning, integrating dropout, pooling, and FC layers at the network's end. Chen [29] addressed the use of trained model such as Inception ResNet, NASNet, and others. Table 6.1 resembles the described work. Yu-Xing [30] employed the RSNA pneumonia dataset to identify lung opacity cases. They picked a binary classifier (lung opacity or negative) and attained AUC and sensitivity values of 98% and 92.2%, respectively.

TABLE 6.1
Summary of the Presented Work to Detect Pneumonia

Reference	Dataset	Result
Wu [23]	COVID-19 image [34] RSNA [35] USNLM-NLM(MC) [36]	The models achieved 95% accuracy and 90% recall for NasNet Large for four classes
Chadaga [25]	5,644 patients for a blood test and other tests	Using feature extraction methodologies and traditional ML classifiers, the accuracy, specificity, and sensitivity attained were 95.95%, 95.13%, and 96%, respectively, for only the first dataset
Stephen [26]	The database provided by Jaime M et al. [36]	CNN achieves 94% training accuracy
Chouhan [27]	The data collection, a part of which comes from the data collective of Josef et al. [37]	The ensemble model obtained an accuracy of 96.4% with a recall of 99.62%
Huang Le [31]	Private CT data collection with a total of 126 patient	Computed tomography calculated opacification percentage (median [interquartile]: 3.6% [0.5%, 12.1%] vs. 8.7% [2.7%, 21.2%]; $P < .01$).

According to Huang [31], lung opacity percentage could be used to predict the prognosis of ILD and COVID-19. The deep learning technique used in this approach is a fully connected CNN architecture trained using COVID-19 annotated datasets. A deep learning technique was also utilized to provide quantitative feedback on lung opacity. This method is separated into three modules: lung segmentation, identifying opacity segmentation, and quantitative lung opacity analysis. Different novel architectures were used to detect multiple abnormalities. Souid. [32] provided a technique to identify 14 lung ailments, including pneumonia. The proposed method uses the MobileNet V2 [33] in combination with transfer learning and classifier block. This approach inspired us to improve his work by adding layers in the classifier block, and also by fine-tuning the model and adjusting the dataset to prevent data imbalance.

6.2.2 COVID-19 DETECTION

To describe the concept and performance of computer vision CT and chest X-ray-based disease detection, we present some recent novel studies that offer an overview of efficiency of these methods. It is worth emphasizing that they have been supplying many performance indicators and utilizing a broad range of visuals and data. Comparing them is challenging due to the design of these techniques. Some measures include accuracy metric, specificity, sensitivity, the area under the curve (AUC), and the F1 score. Table 6.2 depicts the comparable ideas in a more managed fashion.

TABLE 6.2
Summary of the Presented Work to Detect COVID-19

Reference	Dataset	Result
Li [43]	Private CT data collection of 4,356 CT scans from 3,322 subjects between 2016 and 2020	Private CT data collection of 4,356 CT scans from 3,322 patients between 2016 and 2020
Hemdan. [39]	Data collecting is provided in the research of Josef C.	Data collection comprises several small chest X-ray scans
P. Afshar [17]	The COVIDX dataset consists of 13,975 scans from 1,387 cases	This approach attains 95.7% accuracy, 95.9% sensitivity, and 0.97 AUC
Yu-Huan Wu [31]	The COVID-CS dataset comprises 144,167 scans from 750 subjects of whom 400 were COVID-19 positive	The COVID-CS dataset combines 144,167 images from 750 patients of which 400 are COVID-19 positive
Bhuyan [46]	Collection of COVID-19 CTs datasets	The model has 96.66% of F1 score with mass classification, and 98.75% COVID-19 detection
Bao N. [47]	Six sets of CTs of 512 × 512 dimensions	This method provides chest organ segmentation with Pareto optimization to help find optimal surgery paths
Dash S. [48]	Data collection from multiple resources	The model identifies five significant change points in the Florence curve of the COVID-19 confirmed cases with 85% MAPE

In Ref. [38], a CNN is suggested to extract visual characteristics from voxel CT applying transfer learning on a ReSNet50. As a preprocessing procedure, lung segmentation was accomplished using the U-Net model. Within the period of August 2016 until the month of February 2020, it studied 4,356 chest CT pictures from 3,322 patients at six hospitals. COVID-19 archives specificity and sensitivity of 90% and 95%, respectively, with a confidence interval of 95% and 96%, respectively. The model was open-sourced to the public as well.

Hemdan [39] introduced the COVIDX-Net design, which is constructed on five unique DCNN architectures: VGG19, DenseNet201 [40], InceptionResNetV2, Xception [41], and MobileNetV2 [33]. Joseph Cohen [37] provided COVID-19 cases for the development of these models. Also, in Ref. [11], the DeTraC architecture is proposed that includes a decomposer module followed by transfer module and composer for classifying COVID-19 data. For diagnosis, the scientists used CNN features from trained models on ImageNet. Biraj Ghoshal [42] proposed a drop-weight Bayesian Conv Net (BCNN) that integrates the transfer learning dataset provided in Ref. [37]. This approach achieves 95.57% accuracy. The Capsule Network Framework was developed in Ref. [17] to identify coronavirus instances from X-ray examination. Xen Li [43] propose a lightweight deep NN for smartphone software to process noisy X-ray pictures for point-of-care COVID-19 screening. The work of Farooq provides [44] a technique of refining a trained ResNet50 model to increase model performance. Chinmay [45] developed and boosted machine learning approach that embeds the hybrid grey wolf optimization to assess biomedical heart disorders from five gathered datasets. The outcome of the hybrid RFBT classifier reaches 99.26% of accuracy; this technique has 11.9% accuracy increase over the traditional model.

6.3   MATERIALS AND METHOD

Throughout this section, we will go over the intricacies of our process, in which we employed various strategies to attain our suggested outcome. We will start by talking about the basic model and then we approach toward model training using the method of altering data and fine-tuning the model.

6.3.1   MODEL GENERAL ARCHITECTURE

The goal of this study is to create a state-of-the-art deep learning model based on convolutional neural network, as illustrated in Figure 6.1. Our approach can correctly identify COVID-19 data with high efficiency. From the previously cited work, we did find that it is quite a challenge to find a useful dataset. Transfer learning approaches can improve the learning process in the new problem by transferring knowledge from a related problem that has been learnt and solved to overcome the issue of imbalanced data. The first block is the dataset block which is responsible for data cleaning, processing, and data augmentation. The second block is the training block which contains the transfer learning block, the additional layers, and the training methodology. Finally, once the model is trained, we perform an evaluation process to specify whether the model achieves the requested results.

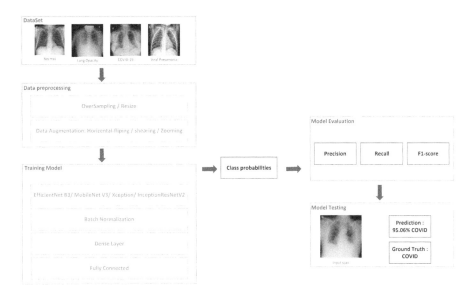

FIGURE 6.1 Block diagram of the model architecture.

TABLE 6.3
The Architecture of EfficientNet Basic Network: The B0 Net

Level Stage	Block Operator	Resolution	#Channels	Number of Layers
1	Conv (3,3)	(224,224)	32	1
2	Mobile Bottleneck Conv 1 (3,3)	(112,112)	16	1
3	Mobile Bottleneck Conv 6 (3,3)	(112,112)	24	2
4	Mobile Bottleneck Conv 1 (5,5)	(56,56)	40	2
5	Mobile Bottleneck Conv 6 (3,3)	(28,28)	80	3
6	Mobile Bottleneck Conv 1 (5,5)	(14,14)	112	3
7	Mobile Bottleneck Conv 1 (5,5)	(14,14)	192	4
8	Mobile Bottleneck Conv 1 (5,5)	(7,7)	320	1
9	Conv (1, 1) + Pooling	FC (7, 7)	1,280	1

6.3.2 The EfficientNet Architecture

The Conv Net family named EfficientNet composed from a set of approaches that rely on the network of the baseline [49] is given in Table 6.3. The key component has been the Mobile Inverted Bottleneck Conv (MB-Conv) block, which was introduced and illustrated in Figure 6.2 [33]. The EfficientNet family is built on the concept of beginning with a high-quality but compact baseline model and then uniformly scaling all its dimensions using a predetermined scaling factors set. The EfficientNet is an extremely resilient convolutional neural network that focuses on scaling, which is important since scaling aids in model efficiency. EfficientNet employs neural

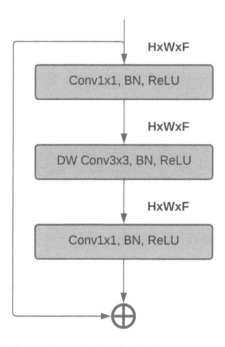

FIGURE 6.2   The DW-Conv refers to the Depthwise Conv.

architecture search to improve the accuracy as well as the FLOPS cost. For our study, we employed two Efficient Nets (B3) to scale the model in resolution.

6.3.3 MOBILENET V3

The deep convolutional neural network architectures have recently been introduced to handle a variety of challenges while enhancing speed of operation and size. Efficient convnets that utilize the depthwise-separable convolution structure, such as MobileNets [50] and EfficientNet [49], are recognized as a vital strategy in many computer vision applications that necessitate a rapid training phase. The depthwise conv block module is characterized with a learnable parameter that separates spatial information from each input channel of the training input. Furthermore, these blocks are shared across all input channels, enhancing model efficiency and cutting processing costs. However, the depthwise block size could be tough to learn, increasing the complexity of the depthwise convolutions training process. As illustrated in Figure 6.3, the MobileNet V3 block has a construction block termed the inverted residual block that comprises a depthwise separable conv block as well as a squeeze and excitation hinder [51]. The inverted residual module gets inspiration from the bottleneck blocks [52], which utilize the inverted residual connection to link input and output features on the same channels and increase feature representations while utilizing small memory amount. The depthwise separable conv module includes a depthwise conv block within channels, as well as an 11-pointwise conv kernel with batch normalization layer (BN) and ReLU or h-swish activation functions. The

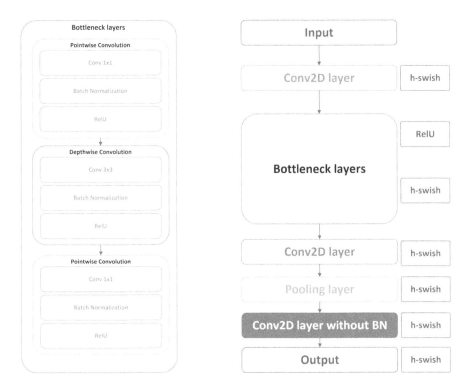

FIGURE 6.3 Block diagram of the MobileNet V3 architecture.

depthwise separable module is dedicated to enhancing model capacity by changing the classic convolutional. During training, the squeeze-and-excite (SE) block is utilized to concentrate on the major components of each channel.

6.3.4 XCEPTION-NET

The Xception Net architecture encompasses 36 conv layers that provide the feature extractor module of the network architecture; this architecture comprises a linear stack of extremely separable convolution operation and also has residual connections to make easy straightforward update and explain the infrastructure [41]. The model flow is shown in Figure 6.4, the data travels through the input flow. After it is done, the data gets injected through the middle flow and repeats the procedure eight times, finally going via the exit flow. All conv layers and separable conv layers are followed by batch norm layers; also depth expansion is not available in the separable conv module.

6.3.5 INCEPTION _ RESNETV2

The Inception-ResnetV2 [52] structure is generated by merging the Residual connection implemented within Inception-ResnetV2 structure. The Inception-Resnet

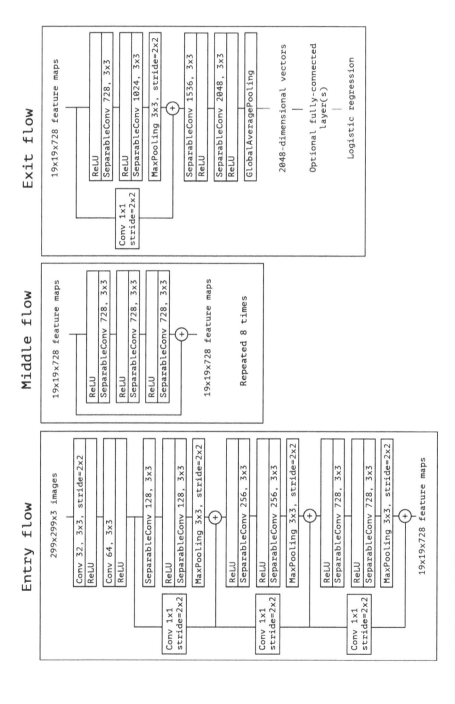

FIGURE 6.4 The Xception Net architecture.

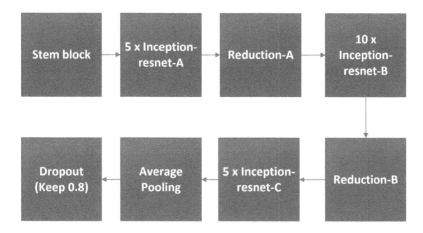

FIGURE 6.5   The fundamental architecture of the Inception-ResNetV2.

module distinguished with the different sized concatenated conv filters using residual connections. The incorporation of residual connections not only addresses the issue of gradient degradation caused by deep structures but also saves training time. Figure 6.5 illustrates the underlying network architecture of Inception-ResNetV2.

6.4   PROPOSED METHODOLOGY

Throughout this section, we provide the research and analysis of our model from the previous section. We split the section into two parts. The first part describes the data employed for the task, including data processing. The second part shows the suggested approach for training our proposed model.

6.4.1   DATASET

The following public coronavirus chest X-ray databases were used in this work as a collection from multiple resources, namely, the public COVID-19 chest X-ray datasets and the COVID-19 Radiography Database from chest X-rays [16, 53–56]. The COVID-19 Radiography Database comprises 219 COVID-19 positive scans, 1,341 negative scans, and 1,345 viral pneumonia scans. The COVID-19 chest X-ray dataset initiative comprises 55 positive COVID-19 photos. Figure 6.6 depicts the distribution of each class in further detail. This dataset was acquired by a team of researchers from several countries and partnering with medical practitioners. These datasets are open-sourced and also continually updated. The dataset consists of four categories: viral pneumonia, normal, COVID-19, and lung opacity. Figure 6.7 displays each class.

6.4.2   DATASET PREPARATION AND PREPROCESSING AND MODEL BUILDING

Toward training the model, dataset cleaning is an essential step, which is in our case was a time-consuming task since the images were not the same size. As

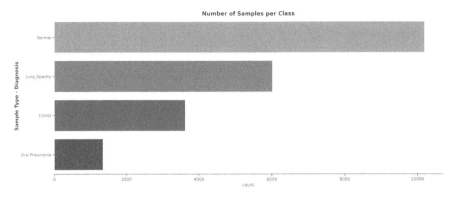

FIGURE 6.6   Class distribution in the dataset.

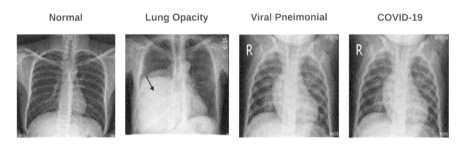

FIGURE 6.7   The dataset classes: COVID-19, normal, viral pneumonia, and lung opacity.

illustrated in Figure 6.6, the dataset was hugely imbanded by having the normal sample doubling the size of viral pneumonia, which can heavily infect the performance overall or even lead to overfitting the model. There are many methods addressing this problem; in our approach, we choose to oversample the model by 1,000 samples in each class. Such a method has its limitations, but it can help in creating the training random sequence. The dataset was also segregated into 70% training, 20% validating, and 10% to test the model. The medical images data are very sensitive data, both on a legal base and on a computer vision base. From the CV perspective, the data augmentation is a solid technique to agile the model; however, small changes in the CXR could change the meaning of the scans. Hence, we only used specific types of data augmentation, namely, horizontal flip, rotation with a range of 0.2, width shifting, height shifting with a 0.2 shifting parameter, and zooming range. The method illustrated in Figure 6.1 considers the transfer learning method to have an efficient and robust deep learning model. The transfer block consists of the following layers:

- **Base Model:** In our approach, the base model is one of the defined CNNs detailed in the previous section, namely, EfficientNetB3, MobileNetV3 [50], Xception [41], and Inception_ResNetV2 [52].

- **Batch Normalization Layer:** We included batch normalization layer to normalize the acquired weights, the parameters added to the Batch Norm layer are momentum equal to 0.99 and epsilon equal to 0.001.
- **Dense Layer 1:** We fix this dense layer with 256 kernels and a ReLU activation. We also applied L1 regularization to prevent overfitting.
- **Dropout Layer:** By adding dropout layer, we are more confident about the possibility of having overfitting in our model.
- **Fully Connected Layer:** We added the fully connected layer which has four kernels that represent the number of classes that we are trying to classify.

All the neural networks were compiled with the Adamax optimizer which is very much optimized to handle classification tasks. For the loss function, we used a categorical cross-entropy, and lastly each model experiment was trained for 50 epochs with an early stopping mechanism pointed to the validation loss.

6.4.3 EVALUATION METRICS

As for performance metrics, we utilized Equations (1)–(5) for accuracy (ACC), F1 score, and time consumption. The following are their definitions:

$$Accuracy = \frac{TP + TN}{TP + TN + FP + FN} \tag{6.1}$$

$$Precision = \frac{TP}{TP + FP} \tag{6.2}$$

$$Recall = \frac{TP}{TP + FN} \tag{6.3}$$

$$F_1 = \frac{TP}{TP + \frac{1}{2}(TP + FN)} \tag{6.4}$$

The true positive (TP) indicates the number of disease samples that are properly classified, whereas true negative (TN) refers to the number of misidentified disease samples. The number of disease samples that were falsely identified as disease-free in the sample is denoted by false positive (FP), whereas the number of disease-free samples that were not classified as disease samples is denoted by false negative (FN). The Xception model achieved 92% result.

6.5 RESULTS AND DISCUSSION

We examine the effectiveness of our proposed methodology using metrics obtained from the trials, and we investigate the fine-tuning technique of transfer learning by extracting features from pretrained CNNs. The experimental investigation was carried out using publicly accessible datasets, as stated in Section 6.4.1. The proposed system's efficacy is assessed using the performance measures outlined in Section

6.4; since our method uses a fine-tuning approach on top of the models, we used some settings for the four experiments.

6.5.1 EXPERIMENTAL RESULT

The first part contains the collective result after the training of the model. We first start with the accuracy metric, which was relevant for all the models. The EfficientNet B3 achieved a mean of accuracy of 95%, while Inception_ResNetV2 model achieved 95.64%, the Xception achieved 95.64%, and MobileNet V3 achieved 95.92%. The MobileNet V3 achieves the best accuracy overall.

The loss was less in all the models: the EfficientNet B3 achieved 0.301, the Inception_ResNetV2 model achieved 2.8301, the Xception achieved 0.3189, and the MobileNet V3 achieved 0.2958. The MobileNet V3 achieved the lowest loss.

Our models give great results from the recall metric, with 96% for both the Xception model and the MobileNet V3, the EfficientNet B3 achieved 96%, and the Inception_ResNet 93%. Summarized in Table 6.4, our models give great results with a precision metric of 96% for the Xception model, the MobileNet V3, and the EfficientNet B3. The Inception_ResNet achieved 93%. The F1 score did not show much difference in terms of value change.

- **Result MobileNet V3**

The obtained result is by far the highest of all the experiments. The MobileNet V3 model, as presented in the previous paragraph, achieved 95.91% accuracy, which is higher compared to the previously tested model. Also, as presented in Figure 6.8, this model finished 50 epochs with less noise in the accuracy curve. The best epoch was number 48. From this, we can presume that the model could get more improvement. Also, the model did not show an overfitting sign, as we can see clearly in the loss curve. The distance between the training and validation is fairly small. From this, we can interpret that the model shows similarity between training and validation.

There are some improvements compared to the EfficientNet model in the confusion matrix value presented in Figure 6.9 within the test set, with 200 detected COVID-19 samples and 7 samples that are misclassified, which explains the improvement in the precision metric and also the recall metric presented in Table 6.4.

TABLE 6.4
The Overall Results Obtained by the Proposed Models

Model	Accuracy	Loss	Precision	Recall	F1 Score
EfficientNet B3	0.9550	0.3010	0.96	0.96	0.96
MobileNet V3	0.9591	0.2958	0.96	0.96	0.96
Xception	0.9564	0.3189	0.96	0.96	0.96
Inception_ResNet	0.9292	2.8301	0.93	0.93	0.93

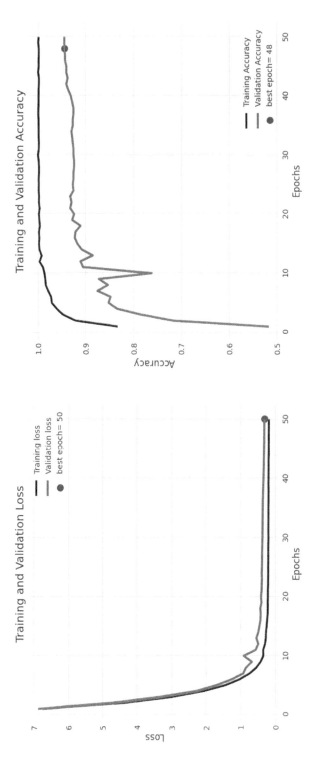

FIGURE 6.8 The acquired loss curve and accuracy curve during the training/validation process.

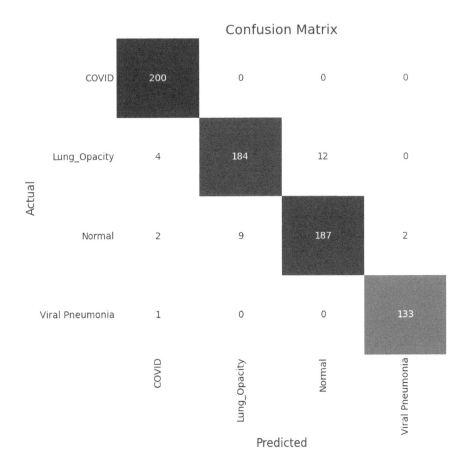

FIGURE 6.9 Confusing matrix for the MobileNet V3 prediction.

- **Result EfficientNet B3**

The EfficientNet B3 is considered one of the state-of-the-art neural networks achieving a solid result in the classification task, which is assessed by the embedded NAS models. However, the goal in medical diagnosis is to achieve a better recall value. This model provided a solid performance during training/validation, which includes accuracy and loss values. During training process, the gap between the training and validation gets bigger over time, which may lead to overfitting to manage the issues; also, an early stopping mechanism was implemented with the patients of ten adjustments on the learning rate. This model also had very consistent results in the other metrics that are included in Table 6.4. The confusion matrix shows some misclassification results. Overall, the model shows that the majority of the predictions were correct (197 COVID-19 samples were classified), which explains the good precision and recall values (both 96%).

- **Result Xception Net**

Based on the loss and accuracy presented in Table 6.4, the Xception Net model scored a result considered good. However, the models have some overfitting which could affect the overall performance. Also, we can see that this model results are similar to the values provided by the EfficientNet B3.

- **Result Inception_ResNetV2**

From the accuracy and loss values provided previously in Table 6.4, the Inception_ResNetV2 had the lowest result compared to the previous experiments.

The confusion matrix misclassified values are as follows: 21 misclassified COVID-19 samples out of 221, 19 misclassified lung opacity samples, and 21 misclassified normal samples. which can be congruent with the obtained results in Table 6.4. Although the model precision and recall scored 93% in both, he had several misclassified samples.

6.5.2 Experimental Result

The result of the four presented experiments is presented in Table 6.5, including a metrics comparison based on class. All the models achieved very good results. The MobileNet V3 shows the highest result without a sign of overfitting.

In this study, we investigated the performance of MobileNet V3, the EfficientNet B3, the Inception_ResNetV2, and the Xception architecture to design a solid predictive model. Our ensemble model shows very good results in recall and F1 score. Also, it is well-known that neural networks are computationally expensive to train. By applying transfer learning, we can leverage these large neural networks after applying oversampling and preprocessing as data augmentation to the dataset. The proposed approach to applying these NN with transfer learning to classify COVID-19,

---

TABLE 6.5

Details of the Four Experiments: Precision, Recall, and F1 Score for Each Pathology

| | Model Results | | | | | | | | | | | |
| | EffecientNet B3 | | | Mobilenet V3 | | | XceptionNet | | | Inception_ ResNetV2 | | |
Pathologies	P	R	F1	P	R	F1	P	R	F1	P	R	F1
COVID-19	0.98	0.98	0.98	0.97	1	0.98	0.98	0.98	0.98	0.95	0.95	0.95
Lung opacity	0.94	0.91	0.93	0.95	0.92	0.94	0.94	0.93	0.94	0.91	0.91	0.91
Normal	0.91	0.94	0.93	0.94	0.94	0.94	0.93	0.93	0.93	0.89	0.88	0.89
Viral pneumonia	0.99	1	1	0.99	0.99	0.99	0.99	1	0.99	0.99	1	1

Note: P: precision; R: recall; F1: F1 score.

in comparison to the state-of-the-art convolutional neural network, gets extremely respectable results.

6.6 CONCLUSION

The COVID-19 epidemic is spreading at a frightening rate. With nothing but an ever-growing number of instances, mass examination of patients quickly should be necessary. We used various CNN models that attempt to categorize coronavirus patients based on their chest X-ray exams. Furthermore, we decided that the MobileNet V3 net has the best performance and is best suited for use with these three models.

We effectively categorized COVID-19 images, demonstrating the potential use of such approaches in automating diagnostic chores. The great accuracy gained might be a reason for worry because it could be the consequence of overfitting. This may be validated by comparing it to fresh data that will be made available soon. In the future, we may use the enormous dataset of chest X-rays in order to examine our suggested model. It is also recommended that we need to speak with a medical facility before embarking on any real implementation of the proposed project.

Our proposed work purpose is not creating a flawless detection tool, but rather to investigate economically realistic approaches to battle this disease. Such approaches may be explored for additional study to demonstrate their real-world use.

While the study reveals that deep neural network training in the medical profession is a realistic option, deep learning deployment in clinical practice is still in the works until additional public databases become accessible.

REFERENCES

[1] C. I. Paules, H. D. Marston, and A. S. Fauci, "Coronavirus infections—more than just the common cold," *JAMA*, vol. 323, no. 8, p. 707, Feb. 2020, doi:10.1001/jama.2020.0757.

[2] Y. Chen, Q. Liu, and D. Guo, "Emerging coronaviruses: Genome structure, replication, and pathogenesis," *Journal of Medical Virology*, vol. 92, no. 4, pp. 418–423, Apr. 2020, doi:10.1002/jmv.25681.

[3] "Guidance-and-SOP-COVID-19-Testing-NHS-Laboratories.pdf." Accessed: Apr. 12, 2022 [Online]. Available: www.rcpath.org/uploads/assets/90111431-8aca-4614-b06633 d07e2a3dd9/Guidance-and-SOP-COVID-19-Testing-NHS-Laboratories.pdf

[4] "Snapshot." Accessed: Apr. 12, 2022 [Online]. Available: www.who.int/

[5] S. Boseley, editor, "WHO warns that few have developed antibodies to Covid-19," *The Guardian*, Apr. 20, 2020. Accessed: Jun. 3, 2022 [Online]. Available: www.theguardian.com/society/2020/apr/20/studies-suggest-very-few-have-had-covid-19-without-symptoms

[6] "Coronavirus disease (COVID-19)." Accessed: Jun. 03, 2022. Available: www.who.int/emergencies/diseases/novel-coronavirus-2019

[7] J.-L. He *et al.*, "Diagnostic performance between CT and initial real-time RT-PCR for clinically suspected 2019 coronavirus disease (COVID-19) patients outside Wuhan, China," *Respiratory Medicine*, vol. 168, p. 105980, Jul. 2020, doi:10.1016/j.rmed.2020.105980.

[8] H. Y. F. Wong *et al.*, "Frequency and distribution of chest radiographic findings in patients positive for COVID-19," *Radiology*, vol. 296, no. 2, pp. E72–E78, Aug. 2020, doi:10.1148/radiol.2020201160.

[9] S. Hassantabar *et al.*, "CovidDeep: SARS-CoV-2/COVID-19 test based on wearable medical sensors and efficient neural networks," *arXiv:2007.10497 [cs]*, Oct. 2020. Accessed: Apr. 12, 2022 [Online]. Available: http://arxiv.org/abs/2007.10497

[10] I. D. Apostolopoulos and T. A. Mpesiana, "Covid-19: automatic detection from X-ray images utilizing transfer learning with convolutional neural networks," *Physical and Engineering Sciences in Medicine*, vol. 43, no. 2, pp. 635–640, Jun. 2020, doi:10.1007/s13246-020-00865-4.

[11] A. Abbas, M. M. Abdelsamea, and M. M. Gaber, "Classification of COVID-19 in chest X-ray images using DeTraC deep convolutional neural network," *Applied Intelligence*, vol. 51, no. 2, pp. 854–864, Feb. 2021, doi:10.1007/s10489-020-01829-7.

[12] S. Minaee, R. Kafieh, M. Sonka, S. Yazdani, and G. Jamalipour Soufi, "Deep-COVID: predicting COVID-19 from chest X-ray images using deep transfer learning," *Medical Image Analysis*, vol. 65, p. 101794, Oct. 2020, doi:10.1016/j.media.2020.101794.

[13] J. Irvin *et al.*, "CheXpert: A large chest radiograph dataset with uncertainty labels and expert comparison," *AAAI*, vol. 33, pp. 590–597, Jul. 2019, doi:10.1609/aaai.v33i01.3301590.

[14] A. I. Khan, J. L. Shah, and M. M. Bhat, "CoroNet: A deep neural network for detection and diagnosis of COVID-19 from chest X-ray images," *Computer Methods and Programs in Biomedicine*, vol. 196, p. 105581, Nov. 2020, doi:10.1016/j.cmpb.2020.105581.

[15] E. Goldstein *et al.*, "COVID-19 classification of X-ray images using deep neural networks," *arXiv:2010.01362 [cs, eess]*, Oct. 2020. Accessed: Apr. 12, 2022 [Online]. Available: http://arxiv.org/abs/2010.01362

[16] N. K. Chowdhury, M. A. Kabir, M. M. Rahman, and N. Rezoana, "ECOVNet: An ensemble of deep convolutional neural networks based on EfficientNet to detect COVID-19 from chest X-rays," *PeerJ Computer Science*, vol. 7, p. e551, May 2021, doi:10.7717/peerj-cs.551.

[17] P. Afshar, S. Heidarian, F. Naderkhani, A. Oikonomou, K. N. Plataniotis, and A. Mohammadi, "COVID-CAPS: A capsule network-based framework for identification of COVID-19 cases from X-ray images," *Pattern Recognition Letters*, vol. 138, pp. 638–643, Oct. 2020, doi:10.1016/j.patrec.2020.09.010.

[18] R. Kundu, R. Das, Z. W. Geem, G.-T. Han, and R. Sarkar, "Pneumonia detection in chest X-ray images using an ensemble of deep learning models," *PLoS ONE*, vol. 16, no. 9, p. e0256630, Sep. 2021, doi:10.1371/journal.pone.0256630.

[19] A. A. E. Ambita, E. N. V. Boquio, and P. C. Naval, "Locally adaptive regression kernels and support vector machines for the detection of pneumonia in chest X-ray images," in *Intelligent Information and Database Systems*, vol. 12034, N. T. Nguyen, K. Jearanaitanakij, A. Selamat, B. Trawiński, and S. Chittayasothorn, Eds. Cham: Springer International Publishing, 2020, pp. 129–140, doi:10.1007/978-3-030-42058-1_11.

[20] S. Varela-Santos and P. Melin, "Classification of X-ray images for pneumonia detection using texture features and neural networks," in *Intuitionistic and Type-2 Fuzzy Logic Enhancements in Neural and Optimization Algorithms: Theory and Applications*, vol. 862, O. Castillo, P. Melin, and J. Kacprzyk, Eds. Cham: Springer International Publishing, 2020, pp. 237–253, doi:10.1007/978-3-030-35445-9_20.

[21] A. Khatri, R. Jain, H. Vashista, N. Mittal, P. Ranjan, and R. Janardhanan, "Pneumonia identification in chest X-ray images using EMD," in *Trends in Communication, Cloud, and Big Data*, vol. 99, H. K. D. Sarma, B. Bhuyan, S. Borah, and N. Dutta, Eds. Singapore: Springer Singapore, 2020, pp. 87–98, doi:10.1007/978-981-15-1624-5_9.

[22] H. Sharma, J. S. Jain, P. Bansal, and S. Gupta, "Feature extraction and classification of chest X-ray images using CNN to detect pneumonia," in *2020 10th International Conference on Cloud Computing, Data Science & Engineering (Confluence)*, Noida, India, Jan. 2020, pp. 227–231, doi:10.1109/Confluence47617.2020.9057809.

[23] H. Wu, P. Xie, H. Zhang, D. Li, and M. Cheng, "Predict pneumonia with chest X-ray images based on convolutional deep neural learning networks," *IFS*, vol. 39, no. 3, pp. 2893–2907, Oct. 2020, doi:10.3233/JIFS-191438.

[24] M. Fathurahman, S. C. Fauzi, S. C. Haryanti, U. A. Rahmawati, and E. Suherlan, "Implementation of 1D-convolution neural network for pneumonia classification based chest X-ray image," in *Recent Advances on Soft Computing and Data Mining*, vol. 978, R. Ghazali, N. M. Nawi, M. M. Deris, and J. H. Abawajy, Eds. Cham: Springer International Publishing, 2020, pp. 181–191, doi:10.1007/978-3-030-36056-6_18.

[25] K. Chadaga, C. Chakraborty, S. Prabhu, S. Umakanth, V. Bhat, and N. Sampathila, "Clinical and laboratory approach to diagnose COVID-19 using machine learning," *Interdisciplinary Sciences: Computational Life Sciences,* vol. 14, pp. 452–470, Feb. 2022, doi:10.1007/s12539-021-00499-4.

[26] O. Stephen, M. Sain, U. J. Maduh, and D.-U. Jeong, "An efficient deep learning approach to pneumonia classification in healthcare," *Journal of Healthcare Engineering*, vol. 2019, pp. 1–7, Mar. 2019, doi:10.1155/2019/4180949.

[27] V. Chouhan *et al.*, "A novel transfer learning based approach for pneumonia detection in chest X-ray images," *Applied Sciences*, vol. 10, no. 2, p. 559, Jan. 2020, doi:10.3390/app10020559.

[28] P. Chhikara, P. Singh, P. Gupta, and T. Bhatia, "Deep convolutional neural network with transfer learning for detecting pneumonia on chest X-rays," in *Advances in Bioinformatics, Multimedia, and Electronics Circuits and Signals*, vol. 1064, L. C. Jain, M. Virvou, V. Piuri, and V. E. Balas, Eds. Singapore: Springer Singapore, 2020, pp. 155–168, doi:10.1007/978-981-15-0339-9_13.

[29] X. Chen *et al.*, "PIN92 pediatric bacterial pneumonia classification through chest X-rays using transfer learning," *Value in Health*, vol. 22, pp. S209–S210, May 2019, doi:10.1016/j.jval.2019.04.962.

[30] Y.-X. Tang *et al.*, "Automated abnormality classification of chest radiographs using deep convolutional neural networks," *NPJ Digital Medicine*, vol. 3, no. 1, p. 70, Dec. 2020, doi:10.1038/s41746-020-0273-z.

[31] L. Huang *et al.*, "Serial quantitative chest CT assessment of COVID-19: A deep learning approach," *Radiology: Cardiothoracic Imaging*, vol. 2, no. 2, p. e200075, Apr. 2020, doi:10.1148/ryct.2020200075.

[32] A. Souid, N. Sakli, and H. Sakli, "Classification and predictions of lung diseases from chest X-rays using MobileNet V2," *Applied Sciences*, vol. 11, no. 6, Art. no. 6, Jan. 2021, doi:10.3390/app11062751.

[33] M. Sandler, A. Howard, M. Zhu, A. Zhmoginov, and L.-C. Chen, "MobileNetV2: inverted residuals and linear bottlenecks," *arXiv:1801.04381 [cs]*, Mar. 2019. Accessed: Mar. 29, 2022 [Online]. Available: http://arxiv.org/abs/1801.04381.

[34] "RSNA pneumonia detection challenge." Accessed: Apr. 12, 2022. Available: https://kaggle.com/competitions/rsna-pneumonia-detection-challenge.

[35] "Two public chest X-ray datasets for computer-aided screening of pulmonary diseases—PMC." Accessed: Apr. 12, 2022. Available: www.ncbi.nlm.nih.gov/pmc/articles/PMC4256233/.

[36] J. Melendez *et al.*, "A novel multiple-instance learning-based approach to computer-aided detection of tuberculosis on chest X-rays," *IEEE Transactions on Medical Imaging*, vol. 34, no. 1, pp. 179–192, Jan. 2015, doi:10.1109/TMI.2014.2350539.

[37] J. P. Cohen, P. Morrison, and L. Dao, "COVID-19 image data collection," *arXiv: 2003.11597 [cs, eess, q-bio]*, Mar. 2020. Accessed: Apr. 12, 2022 [Online]. Available: http://arxiv.org/abs/2003.11597.

[38] L. Li *et al.*, "Using artificial intelligence to detect COVID-19 and community-acquired pneumonia based on pulmonary CT: Evaluation of the diagnostic accuracy," *Radiology*, vol. 296, no. 2, pp. E65–E71, Aug. 2020, doi:10.1148/radiol.2020200905.

[39] E. E.-D. Hemdan, M. A. Shouman, and M. E. Karar, "COVIDX-Net: A framework of deep learning classifiers to diagnose COVID-19 in X-ray images," *arXiv:2003.11055 [cs, eess]*, Mar. 2020. Accessed: Apr. 12, 2022 [Online]. Available: http://arxiv.org/abs/2003.11055.

[40] G. Huang, Z. Liu, L. van der Maaten, and K. Q. Weinberger, "Densely connected convolutional networks," *arXiv:1608.06993 [cs]*, Jan. 2018. Accessed: Mar. 29, 2022 [Online]. Available: http://arxiv.org/abs/1608.06993.

[41] F. Chollet, "Xception: Deep learning with depthwise separable convolutions," *arXiv:1610.02357 [cs]*, Apr. 2017. Accessed: Mar. 29, 2022 [Online]. Available: http://arxiv.org/abs/1610.02357.

[42] B. Ghoshal and A. Tucker, "Estimating uncertainty and interpretability in deep learning for coronavirus (COVID-19) detection," *arXiv:2003.10769 [cs, eess, stat]*, Mar. 2020. Accessed: Apr. 12, 2022 [Online]. Available: http://arxiv.org/abs/2003.10769.

[43] X. Li, C. Li, and D. Zhu, "COVID-MobileXpert: On-device COVID-19 patient triage and follow-up using chest X-rays," *arXiv:2004.03042 [cs, eess]*, Sep. 2020. Accessed: Apr. 12, 2022 [Online]. Available: http://arxiv.org/abs/2004.03042.

[44] M. Farooq and A. Hafeez, "COVID-ResNet: A deep learning framework for screening of COVID19 from radiographs," *arXiv:2003.14395 [cs, eess]*, Mar. 2020. Accessed: Apr. 12, 2022 [Online]. Available: http://arxiv.org/abs/2003.14395.

[45] C. Chakraborty, A. Kishor, and J. J. P. C. Rodrigues, "Novel Enhanced-grey Wolf Optimization hybrid machine learning technique for biomedical data computation," *Computers and Electrical Engineering*, vol. 99, p. 107778, Apr. 2022, doi:10.1016/j.compeleceng.2022.107778.

[46] H. K. Bhuyan, C. Chakraborty, Y. Shelke, and S. K. Pani, "COVID-19 diagnosis system by deep learning approaches," *Expert Systems*, vol. 39, no. 3, p. e12776, 2022, doi:10.1111/exsy.12776.

[47] N. Bao, Y. Chen, Y. Liu, and C. Chakraborty, "Multi-objective path planning for lung biopsy surgery," *Multimedia Tools and Applications*, vol. 81, pp. 36153–36170, Jan. 2022, doi:10.1007/s11042-021-11476-w.

[48] S. Dash, C. Chakraborty, S. K. Giri, and S. K. Pani, "Intelligent computing on time-series data analysis and prediction of COVID-19 pandemics," *Pattern Recognition Letters*, vol. 151, pp. 69–75, Nov. 2021, doi:10.1016/j.patrec.2021.07.027.

[49] M. Tan and Q. V. Le, "EfficientNet: Rethinking model scaling for convolutional neural networks," *arXiv*, vol. 97, pp. 6105–6114, May 2019, doi:10.48550/arXiv.1905.11946.

[50] A. Howard *et al.*, "Searching for MobileNetV3," *arXiv:1905.02244 [cs]*, Nov. 2019. Accessed: Apr. 12, 2022 [Online]. Available: http://arxiv.org/abs/1905.02244.

[51] M. Tan *et al.*, "MnasNet: Platform-aware neural architecture search for mobile," *arXiv:1807.11626 [cs]*, May 2019. Accessed: Apr. 12, 2022 [Online]. Available: http://arxiv.org/abs/1807.11626

[52] C. Szegedy, S. Ioffe, V. Vanhoucke, and A. Alemi, "Inception-v4, Inception-ResNet and the impact of residual connections on learning," *arXiv:1602.07261 [cs]*, Aug. 2016. Accessed: Apr. 12, 2022 [Online]. Available: http://arxiv.org/abs/1602.07261.

[53] A. M. Tahir *et al.*, "COVID-19 infection localization and severity grading from chest X-ray images," *Computers in Biology and Medicine*, vol. 139, p. 105002, Dec. 2021, doi:10.1016/j.compbiomed.2021.105002.

[54] Anas M. Tahir *et al.*, "COVID-QU." *Kaggle.* doi:10.34740/KAGGLE/DSV/3122898.

[55] T. Rahman *et al.*, "Exploring the effect of image enhancement techniques on COVID-19 detection using chest X-ray images," *Computers in Biology and Medicine*, vol. 132, p. 104319, May 2021, doi:10.1016/j.compbiomed.2021.104319.

[56] A. Degerli *et al.*, "COVID-19 infection map generation and detection from chest X-ray images," *Health Information Science and Systems*, vol. 9, no. 1, p. 15, Dec. 2021, doi:10.1007/s13755-021-00146-8.

7 Trends in Malware Detection in IoHT Using Deep Learning
A Review

Merve Varol Arisoy

CONTENTS

DOI: 10.1201/9781003315476-7

7.1   INTRODUCTION

The Internet of Things (IoT) is a type of network that integrates various types of sensors and communication protocols, allowing many devices such as smartphones, home appliances, and medical devices to be included in a network structure and output these devices to the Internet. Due to the wide benefits it offers, this technology has found the opportunity to be used in many areas today. Smart homes, energy, health, agricultural applications, automation, and industrial systems are among the areas where IoT technology is used [1]. The advances in the infrastructure of IoT have been noticed on the basis of studies carried out, where the adaptation of this technology to the health field brings great convenience in terms of both early diagnosis and treatment of diseases and easing the burden on the health sector, especially during the pandemic period [2–4]. Thereupon, IoHT (Internet of Healthcare Things), a subbranch of IoT, was born due to the confidentiality of the data transferred from various sensors and the necessity of considering its security first.

IoHT is a network structure in which many devices such as smart pacemakers, smart glucose meters, smart heart rate monitors are connected and interact to transfer medical data to healthcare professionals [5, 6]. Figure 7.1 shows the IoHT architecture. The medical devices and sensors in this architecture form the detection layer of the IoHT network. Through this layer, medical data is collected from patients and transferred to gateways. Meanwhile, standards such as BLE (Bluetooth Low Energy), NFC (Near-Field Communication), and RFID (Radio-Frequency Identification) are used for communication [7].

In the IoHT network, patient information is stored in the cloud service and transmitted to end users via a separate gateway. Thanks to the use of IoHT technology, wearable sensors, and the introduction of many devices such as surgical robots, we come across many subbranches of health such as remote monitoring of patients' blood values and surgical interventions [8].

The increase in the usage area of IoHT day by day has led to the emergence of large amounts of data whose privacy is essential. The insufficient level of protection of the IoHT network may cause the system to become vulnerable to various cyberattacks. As a result, patient data can be disclosed, and even by remote access to sensors, results leading to the death of the patient can be achieved [8]. Therefore, the first point to be taken care of during the establishment of the IoHT network is the security of the system. To secure the IoT network, many studies have previously been carried out, including technologies such as fuzzy logic and fog information services [9–11]. But later, IoT security measures, which are carried out using machine learning and its subbranch, deep learning methods, have become an area that is more researched and applied on due to its effectiveness.

Intrusion detection systems (IDS) are among the methods frequently used in order to eliminate the attacks that threaten the IoT network. In Ref. [12], a framework design for improving edge computing is mentioned [13]. In Ref. [14], an IDS system was developed to detect DoS, Botnet, and web attacks. In the study using the CICIDS dataset, they detected botnet attacks with 97.93% accuracy. In Ref. [15], the authors mentioned an IoHT frame structure working on NSL-KDD dataset by combining FFDNN and FBFSA to detect anomaly attack in wireless networks. In Ref.

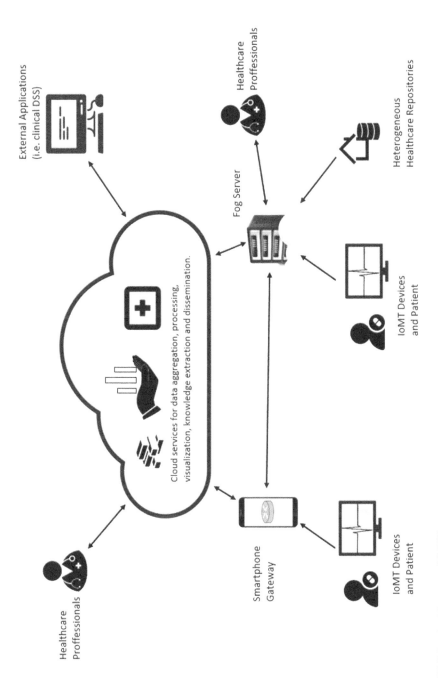

FIGURE 7.1 Architecture of IoHT.

[16], an IDS system based on mobile agents was applied to the healthcare field. In their systems, they used machine learning and regression methods to catch anomalies in wearable sensors and attacks at the network level. In Ref. [17], an IDS system using the two-stage deep learning method was developed. They used the probability model to classify the network traffic and then performed the classification of the data. In Ref. [18], an IDS system was developed based on the detection of WBAN jamming attacks. In Ref. [19], penetration detection was performed based on the combination of a variational autoencoder and DNN. In another study [20], in which network leak detection was performed, they mentioned the deep adversary learning (DAL) method using statistical learning and data augmentation. In its work, the SVM classifier rejected the intrusion requests, and at the same time, data augmentation was done to create datasets developed with unauthorized access. In Ref. [21], a cybersecurity IDS for smart cities was created using deep-pass supervised learning. In Ref. [22], the authors mentioned the RBM model to detect DDoS attacks in smart city applications. They used RF (random forest) and SVM for classification. They used the RBM model to process the K-means approach while learning the properties of the datasets. In Ref. [23], GDM and GDM/AG are integrated with DLNN architecture to detect intrusions in the automotive industry. In Ref. [24], the authors mentioned a hybrid model that detects violations using MLP, IBK, and SVM classifiers on NSL-KDD, Kyoto 2006+, and ISCX 2012 datasets. In Ref. [25], CNN and Softmax were used to detect anomalous cyberattack threats.

In Ref. [26], a model was developed using deep learning algorithms for the detection of cyberattacks in the IoT network, and the detection success obtained was compared with the rate obtained from machine learning methods. In Ref. [27], the authors proposed a hybrid approach for detecting suspected attacks in cyberphysical systems (CPS) and industrial IoT. Their approach includes controlling and reconfiguring the cyberattacks that occur in the input data of CPS systems in shared networks by intelligent systems. In Ref. [28], the authors proposed a real-time automatic attack detection approach using machine learning algorithms to detect attacks that may occur in the SDN (software-defined networking) application layer. In Ref. [29], a framework structure on securing a virtual machine in cloud computing is mentioned. In Ref. [30], an authentication method is proposed for the security of cloud servers in the IoT network. It is stated in Ref. [31] that the use of artificial intelligence-assisted IDS in IoT and IoHT networks provides a great improvement in providing security. In this context, in Ref. [32], reinforcement learning is used to detect cyberattacks. In Ref. [33], the authors used semi-supervised learning in fog computing-based intrusion detection systems, and they also suggested an extreme learning machine (ELM)-based semisupervised fuzzy method to attain a high performance in serial detection. In Ref. [34], the authors used a feedforward deep neural network for wireless IDSs. The summary of other existing DL-based attack detection solutions is given in Tables 7.1 and 7.2.

7.1.1 Motivation of Survey

The better understanding of the benefits brought by the use of IoT systems in the health field has led to the desire to adapt this technology to many subcategories of health. In order to meet the demand, nonstandard devices with heterogeneous

TABLE 7.1

Performances and Limitations of Existing DL-Based Studies

Reference	Method	Obtained Results	Limitations
[87]	CNN	Accuracy: 92.0 F1:94	It has problems with accuracy
[88]	LCNN	Accuracy: 94.0	Other metrics such as MCC, F1, and precision should also be considered
[91]	AE (autoencoder) IDS	Accuracy: 80.0 F1: 79.08	Low accuracy High training time
[19]	VAE + DNN IDS	Accuracy: 89.08 F1: 90.61 FPR: 19.01	Low detection accuracy High training time
[92]	CCN + VAE + LSTM anomaly-based network IDS	Accuracy: 99	Resource-consuming High computational complexity

TABLE 7.2

DL-Based Different Attack Detection Solutions in IoT/IoHT Environments

Reference	Methods	Attack Detection Type	Strength	Weakness
[44]	Deep learning	False alarm detection based on anomaly	High accuracy	High computation Burden and excessive FPR
[89]	Neural network-based Mlp	False alarm detection based on anomaly	Real-time energy-efficient high accuracy	High memory requirement
[43]	Deep learning classification	Attack prediction	Reduction in training time	Accuracy information is missing
[90]	Cryptography, convolutional neural network (CNN)	Authentication and access control	Strong against multiple attacks Real time	Communication and high training overhead
[46]	Deep-Q-Network (LDQN)	Based on signature Malware detection	High determination rate Low-energy consumption	FPR Training overhead
[14]	Deep belief network (DBN)	Anomaly-based Network IDS	High accuracy, precision and F1	High training overhead
[91]	AE (autoencoder)	Network IDS	Lightweight	Low determination accuracy Long training time
[19]	VAE (variational autoencoder) + DNN	Network IDS	Lightweight Low resource excise	Low determination accuracy Long training time
[92]	CCN + VAE + LSTM	Anomaly-based network IDS	Lightweight high-determination accuracy	Resource consuming high computational complexity

connection protocols and multiple data transmission standards have started to be produced. The fact that each of the devices has separate vulnerabilities and is not sufficiently protected has led to the launch of different types of attacks in IoMT [7].

Another reason for security problems in the IoMT network is the growth in the number of devices connected to the network or the number of networks connected to each other. This increase causes compatibility problems. In addition, expansion in the network raises additional concerns about whether privacy, integrity, and usability factors can be fully met. Due to the privateness of the health data streamed in IoHT systems, the necessity of protecting its confidentiality requires having a large amount of data processing capacity to prevent authorization violations. These factors, which make the IoHT network vulnerable to attacks, have led to the understanding that the system should be protected and controlled by an intelligent model, and, as a result, many machine and deep learning-based researches have been carried out [8].

7.1.2 CONTRIBUTIONS OF SURVEY

This chapter aims to review the latest research on deep learning–based IoT security systems used in healthcare. The point that distinguishes the research conducted here is that it includes analysis and evaluation of research that covers especially deep learning, IoHT, and a combination of both technologies.

The following are the main topics discussed in this chapter:

- Various uses of deep learning–based IoT in medical services
- The architectures of IoHT environment
- The importance of various security requirements of IoT communication environment
- The latest malware attacks and their impact
- Deep learning–based IoT applications in health sector
- Malware detection applications based on IoT and deep learning in health sector
- Recent DL methods used in detecting malware of the IoT environment
- The performance of current DL-based detection methods
- Future research challenges and inclinations toward IoHT

The remainder of the chapter is organized as follows. Section 7.2 describes studies conducted on deep learning applications for IoHT. Section 7.3 offers a review about deep learning–based studies on malware detection in IoT/IoHT environment. In Section 7.4, architectures of IoT/IoHT communication environment are given. In Section 7.5, Internet of Healthcare Things (IoHT)–enabling technologies are provided. In Section 7.6, usage areas of IoT systems in the health sector are specified. In Section 7.7, security requirements of IoT/IoHT systems are highlighted. In Section 7.8, malware types in IoT/IoHT environment are discussed. In Section 7.9, results and future challenges of malware detection in IoT/IoHT are provided. Finally, the chapter is concluded in Section 7.10.

7.2 DEEP LEARNING–BASED RELATED STUDIES IN IoHT

In this section, literature studies on IDS, health monitoring, activity monitoring, disease diagnosis, patient identity verification, which are carried out using deep learning methods in IoHT networks, are mentioned. In Ref. [35], a deep learning–based health monitoring system approach was proposed. This work was created using four different deep learning architectures: autoencoder, restricted Boltzmann machines, CNN, and RNN. The dataset scale they used had a limiting effect on the performance of the model they created. In Ref. [36], human activities were monitored through wearable sensors and these features were processed with deep learning methods: restricted Boltzmann machines, autoencoder, deep mixture models approaches. In the discriminatory models part, CNN, RNN, and deep neural models were used. It has been stated that feature learning can be improved, thanks to hybrid models in which generative and discriminatory deep learning methods are combined. In Ref. [37], which includes approaches for collecting and combining vital signs data in hospitals, the authors presented a strategy on vital signs processing using smart algorithms. The positive side of IoHT approaches, which includes data collection, storage, processing, and delivery stages, is that service downtime can be reduced and limited resources can be allocated efficiently. In Ref. [38], a research is presented that evaluates the new edge computing frameworks, effective technologies in the field of smart healthcare, and the challenges of different scenarios concerned to applications. In addition, an evaluation was made on the monitoring of vital signals and classification of health data using deep learning technology in an IoHT network to which many end devices are connected. In Ref. [39], the authors developed an IoHT system that can identify six different activity types with a three-layer CNN network followed by a deep neural network (DNN) architecture with an LSTM network. In Ref. [40], the authors developed a convolutional neural networks (CNN)–based model for real-time detection of heart diseases. They compared the responsiveness of their systems to a traditional cloud-based IoT system and noted that their proposed framework can improve usability, especially when connectivity is poor. In Ref. [41], a two-stage framework structure for patient authentication was mentioned. Accordingly, in the first stage, combined RFID and finger vein (FV) features were created to raise security levels. In the second phase, a unified technique consisting of AES encryption, blockchain, and PSO steganography was used for the secure conduction of data. Thanks to their systems, an improvement of 55.56% has been achieved in secure biometric data transfer.

7.3 DEEP LEARNING–BASED STUDIES ON MALWARE DETECTION IN IoT/IoHT ENVIRONMENT

In this section, literature studies in which various attacks are detected by using deep learning methods in IoHT networks are included. In Ref. [42], which includes the detection of attacks in the IoHT network, attacks from each node were considered as input features to be given to the model, and then these data were given to the deep belief network (DBN) model, which is a part of the deep learning algorithm. In order to increase the detection success, a hybrid algorithm was created by combining the grasshopper optimization algorithm (GOA) and spider monkey optimization (SMO) algorithms. In Ref. [43], a deep learning methodology is presented to predict different types of attacks in deep brain stimulants (DBSs). In their proposed study, they used the LSTM network to estimate palpitation rate, a type of trait observed to assess the intensity of neurological diseases. Its predictions are intended to diagnose false alerts versus real alerts. With the study tested on patients with Parkinson's disease, different types of attacks could be detected and the patient was warned about a possible attack. In another study dealing with the safety of signals from deep brain stimuli [44], they classified the attacks using Raspberry Pi3 and used deep learning to distinguish false alarms. They concluded that deep learning achieves a high accuracy rate in learning and diagnosing false signals. In Ref. [45], the authors developed an approach to classify and predict unpredictable cyberattacks in the healthcare field. Here, a hybrid PCA–GWO algorithm is applied for feature selection, and DNN classifier is used to classify network attacks. The method they propose is suitable for use with IoHT devices with a unique IP. They stated that while the hybrid feature selection algorithm increases the detection accuracy, it also shortens the time spent on training and classification. In Ref. [46], a suggestion was made on providing a secure data transmission in IoHT using the Deep-Q-Network (DQN) method. Their systems were first analyzed by the deep neural network to verify and eliminate malware attacks, and then the traffic characteristics of each request were recorded in the database. After evaluating the output behavior of the demand using the state feature and the associated behavior, classification was performed using a deep neural network. In Ref. [8], RNN and SML (supervised machine learning models: random forest, decision tree, KNN, and ridge classifier) were used to detect attacks such as DoS, research attacks, and u2R in the NSLKDD dataset, which includes attacks against the IoHT environment–based detection system. They used PSO (particle swarm optimization) algorithm for feature reduction and extraction of effective features in the sampled data. Finally, they divided the data into classes using the ML- and DL-based algorithms mentioned earlier. In Ref. [47], the performance of RNN models in detecting IoT malware was examined: an accuracy rate of 98.18% was achieved in detecting new malware samples. The success of the models with different machine learning methods was also compared.

In Ref. [48], a unified deep learning approach for detecting malware and infected files in the IoT network is presented. TensorFlow-based deep neural network has been used to define pirated software using source code plagiarism. In Ref. [49], the authors compared the success of the model they built with self-normalizing neural network (SNN), another version of feedforward neural networks (FNN), with FNN to classify intrusion attacks in an IoT network. As a result of their experiments on the BoT-IoT dataset, they observed that FNN gave more successful results than SNN in infiltration detection. When evaluated on the basis of resistance to attacks, they found that SNN showed better resilience against hostile attack patterns in the IoT dataset.

In Ref. [50], the authors proposed an adaptive deep forest–based method to detect complicated SQL injection attacks in IoHT networks. They first combined the input of each layer in the deep forest structure with the raw feature vector and the average of the previous outputs and then created the deep forest–based

AdaBoost model, which uses the error proportion to update the weights of the features in each layer. In Ref. [14], the authors suggested the use of deep belief network (DBN) for the detection of attacks in IoHT environments. They suggested that their model, which they applied on the CICIDS dataset, could be extended to detect various forms of attacks against IoT devices and different databases. In Ref. [51], the authors proposed a new network-based anomaly detection method for IoT called N-BaIoT that takes snapshots of network behavior and uses deep autoencoders to detect anomalous network traffic from IoT devices. They tested their method by infecting the IoT device with two broadly known IoT-based botnets, Mirai and BASHLITE. As a result of the assessment, they affirmed the ability to exactly and instantly detect attacks launched from the IoT device running as part of the botnet. In Ref. [52], the authors proposed a CNN-based deep learning model, CNN-DMA, to detect malware attacks in the IoHT network. As a result of their experiments on the Malimg dataset, they detected the "Alueron.gen!J" malware and achieved an accuracy rate of 99% with the CNN-DMA model. In Ref. [53], a research on the anonymizing algorithm of sensitive information about the health dataset operating in the IoHT environment was presented. Its algorithms (Deep Q-Network) identify unrecoverable records, protecting the privacy of users interacting online during the data session. In addition, its algorithms include an encryption process that ensures the anonymity of health data. Their results indicated that the anonymization algorithm guarantees security features for the IoHT system. In Ref. [54], the authors proposed an intrusion detection system for an IoT network and arranged the IoT environment to detect attacks such as spoofing and sinkholes. In Ref. [55], a model was developed using two different deep learning algorithms—CNN (Convolutional Neural Networks) and DNN (Deep Neural Networks)—to process data from smartphones and wearable devices. Symmetric encryption protocols in Ref. [56] and lightweight encryption protocols in Ref. [57] provide solutions for access control and protection against spoofing in healthcare. In the compilation study in Ref. [58], the authors proposed a deep belief network (DBN)–based intelligent intrusion detection request to inspect suspicious network traffic. Here, they have integrated the virtual network with a deep learning algorithm. They stated that their proposed solution is most suitable for black hole attacks, DDoS attacks, sinkhole, and wormhole attacks.

In the study in Ref. [59], which was carried out to follow a series of applications running on Android and IoT devices, the authors developed a deep learning–based feature detector that can be used with different classifiers for malware detection. To test the correctness and validity of the feature detector, the extracted features are first fed into a fully connected network (FCN) with Softmax activation, and then is determined whether the application is harmful using attention-based RNN. In Table 7.3, a comparison based on recent existing DL methods in detecting malware of the IoT environment is given.

7.4 ARCHITECTURES OF IOT/IOHT COMMUNICATION ENVIRONMENT

In this section, IoT/IoHT communication network architectures are discussed.

TABLE 7.3

Comparison Based on Recent Existing DL Methods in Detecting Malware of the IoT Environment

DL Method	Advantage	Limitation	Sample Application Area
CNN	• Robust supervised DL method • High competitive performance • Training time complexity is improved	• High computational burden	[96]
AE (autoencoder)	• Effective feature extraction • Feature size reduction	• High computational time	[97, 98]
DRL (deep reinforcement learning)	• Sequential actions with limited knowledge so it is adaptable for adversarial environments	• It needs a set of assumptions	[99]

7.4.1 GENERIC IoT/IoHT ARCHITECTURE

The generic architecture of the IoT communication network is given in Figure 7.1. This architecture can be applied in many areas, from smart health systems to smart traffic applications and industrial applications, with the same configuration [60]. In each of the different application areas, devices such as smart sensors and AC controllers are used. Smart devices in the IoT/IoHT communication network have their own unique IP address and send the data they collect to servers over gateway for processing.

7.4.2 FOG-BASED IoT/IoHT ARCHITECTURE

There are various fog servers and cloud servers in this architecture type. Fog-based IoT architecture is given in Figure 7.2.

There are cloud servers in the "cloud layer," which is the top layer of this architecture. Fog servers are distributed in the "Fog Layer." At the bottom layer, it includes end user devices (such as smart pacemakers, smart machines, and devices). The widespread use of the IoT communication network causes an increase in the amount of data collected and processed by smart devices in these networks. Therefore, the data must be processed simultaneously and their security must be ensured. In order to meet this need, the method of processing the data obtained from IoT devices with cloud computing technology was applied, but when the security of the data could not be met sufficiently, "Fog Computing" technology was created [61]. The existence of this technology has facilitated the operation of cloud servers. Fog informatics processes the data collected from IoT devices like a proxy. It also serves to increase performance by reducing end-to-end latency. The working logic of Fog informatics is simple calculation processes by fog servers; it is based on the principle that the more complex ones are resolved by cloud servers [62].

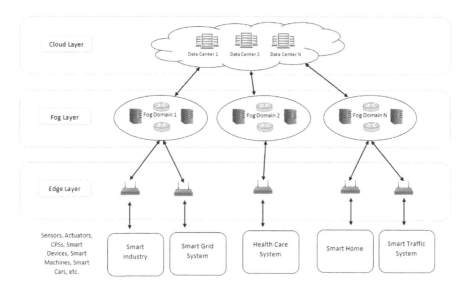

FIGURE 7.2   Fog-Based IoT/IoHT architecture.

7.5   INTERNET OF HEALTHCARE THINGS (IoHT)– ENABLING TECHNOLOGIES

In this section, the technologies used in IoHT systems are mentioned [7, 63–66].

7.5.1   Cloud/edge Computing

Due to resource limitations during the processing and storage of data from various sensors in IoHT infrastructure, these systems need cloud support during their operation. Although cloud computing is a solution to resource limitation problems, it adds a particular amount of delay in the transfer of data to the cloud environment and from the cloud environment to the end users. However, this is seen as a disadvantage since IoHT systems require real-time processing because the data they work with is health related. To meet this challenge, edge computing technology has been developed. In this way, data collection, evaluation, and analysis were carried out at the edge of IoHT systems. In edge computing technology, there is a coordinated work with the central cloud.

7.5.2   Software-Defined Networking (SDN)

SDN is a technology that separates the network control and routing planes. In this way, dynamic management of network traffic and flexible control of resources can be achieved. The SDN structure has three separate planes. These are the control plane, the data plane, and the application plane. While the majority of computations are performed on the control plane, there are routing devices in the data plane that are only responsible for transmitting traffic. At the top, the application plane contains applications developed to apply network policies, security solutions, and custom traffic routing. When IoHT systems are created with traditional network structures, confusion arises as the number of devices added to the network increases. In such cases, SDN technology provides a centralized network view that provides control over the network by removing the management complexities.

7.5.3 Federated Learning

In the unified learning method, it is a matter of training a shared model using deployed data without sharing the data itself. Thus, the confidentiality of the data is preserved. There are two main parts in FL operation: cloud/server and edge devices. First, the cloud model deploys to all edge devices. Then, each end device trains this model with its local data, and the learned network parameters are shared with the cloud server again without sharing the real data. After the cloud server creates the weight pool of the parameter updates it receives, it shares these parameters with all end devices again. This operation continues until performance improvement is achieved.

7.6 USAGE AREAS OF IoT SYSTEMS IN THE HEALTH SECTOR

In this section, some application areas of IoHT systems are provided [7, 67–72].

7.6.1 Patient's Medicine Management

In particular, IoHT systems are very useful in tracking the drugs that should be taken by middle-aged and older people. Thus, the extent to which the patient follows the treatment steps given by the doctor can be determined by monitoring the patient's activities. Body sensors that capture the patient's movement, body temperature, heart rate, and pulse data transfer the collected data to the end node. Then, the home gateway analyzes this data coming to it from the end nodes and looks for anomalies between the normal runtime and the current data.

7.6.2 Remote Patient Monitoring

Real-time monitoring of critical patients can be done through IoHT devices and sensors. With remote patient monitoring, individuals' lives are facilitated by providing general health services such as online checkups, diagnoses, and prescriptions.

7.7 SECURITY REQUIREMENTS OF IOT/IOHT SYSTEMS

In this section, some security requirements that must be present in the IoT/IoHT communication network are included [9, 11, 73–74].

7.7.1 Authentication

Authentication is a very important step in ensuring that data is transmitted securely and to the right person. Many devices such as smart device, fog-cloud server, and gateways in the IoT/IoHT network require authentication in order for the communication to proceed securely.

7.7.2 INTEGRITY

Integrity means that the data transmitted in the IoT/IoHT communication environment contains complete and accurate information, and is free from unauthorized deletion and modification.

7.7.3 CONFIDENTIALITY

It is to prevent the data transmitted in the IoT/IoHT communication environment from being disclosed to unauthorized persons.

7.7.4 NONREPUDIATION

It is a situation where the validity of a message cannot be denied. The nonrepudiation feature is a proof of the integrity of the message data and that the message was sent by the right person.

7.7.5 AUTHORIZATION

This feature is used to determine the permission status of devices and people to use system resources.

Figure 7.3 presents the attack types for each of the earlier listed security requirements of IoHT/IoT networks.

7.8 MALWARE CHARACTERISTICS

Malware are pieces of malicious code, usually transmitted over the network, that allow performing operations such as deleting, modifying, or running a desired program. By providing remote access to the system to be damaged, malware is sent to other target systems via this system. With this attack, personal information such as identity number and credit card information can be obtained. It is possible to see strange icons and programs on the home screen of system devices that have been subjected to a malware attack. In addition, there are situations such as running unauthorized programs on devices, changing the working order of an existing program, and automatic mail sending. Considering that malware attacks are carried out on an IoHT system (for example, the undesirable release of insulin from a blood glucose monitoring system, changing the settings of the pacemaker), it is possible that this could have life-threatening consequences [9, 72, 75–79]. Malware types and their attacks are summarized in Table 7.4. Also, DL/ML-based solutions developed against some types of malware are given in Table 7.5.

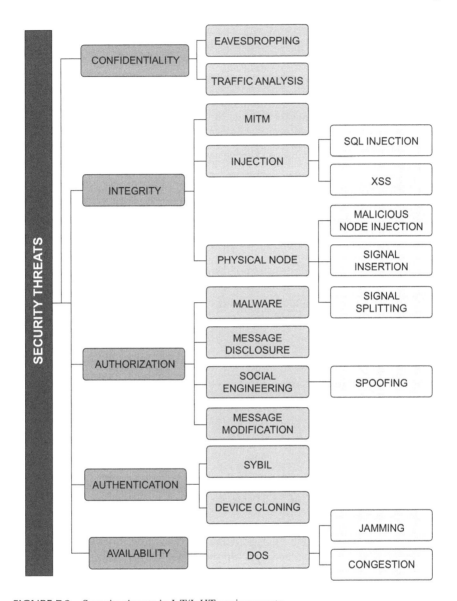

FIGURE 7.3   Security threats in IoT/IoHT environments.

7.8.1   Malware Types in IoT/IoHT Environment

The following are the types of malware targeting IoT/IoHT networks [9, 72, 80–84]:

- **Spyware:** In this attack type, the users' own activities are monitored without their knowledge. Applications such as tracking which keys are pressed on the keyboard, monitoring activity, stealing identity-credit card information can be evaluated under this type. This type of attack can transfer itself to the system by taking advantage of the vulnerabilities in the software or by adding it to some regular programs.

- **Keylogger:** It is a fragment of code developed specifically for users to listen to keyboard strokes. When the link in the e-mail from an unknown person is clicked, it infects the system.
- **Trojan Horse:** It hides itself inside a normal program and when users install this program, they automatically install the malicious software hidden in the program. In this way, it is possible for the hacker to monitor the target system in an authorized manner and to install the desired programs.
- **Virus:** This software spreads by copying itself to another program. It can be used to thieve personal information, damage the system, and create botnets.
- **Worm:** It spreads over the network by finding the gap of the operating system. Bandwidth expenditure and overloading of web servers are among its damages. While a human intervention is required for the spread of viruses (such as installing virus software.), worms can spread independently.
- **Adware:** It is a type of software that automatically displays or downloads undesirable advertising materials that the user encounters while browsing the web pages. In this software, which aims to generate revenue, every click of the user on the relevant advertisement makes money for the adware developer. In addition, by capturing users' browsing information, ads compatible with this data are opened.
- **Ransomware:** It is a type of software that locks the infected system and demands a ransom to solve it. It restricts the users' access to the files on the hard disk by putting encryption from the moment they enter the system. In order to remove this restriction, money is requested and after the payment is made, the encryption is removed and the user is granted access again.
- **Rootkit:** Hackers use rootkits for remote access to the system (IOHT device) in this attack type. After the rootkit is installed, confidential data can be stolen and even the settings of the system and security software can be changed. The rootkit's ability to hide itself prevents it from being detected by security software.
- **Botnets:** These are also known to carry out malware attacks on IoT/IoHT communication networks [9, 85].
- **Mirai Botnet:** Here, the control of the network device with the Linux operating system is left to the remote bots. The Mirai botnet specifically aims to take control of devices such as IP cameras and smart home appliances. By using the IoT devices they have seized, they can also carry out other attacks with a wider scope.
- **Reaper (IoTroop) Botnet:** This botnet can crash the entire system infrastructure much faster than the Mirai botnet. Reaper specifically targets the vulnerability in devices from different manufacturers such as DLink, Netgear, and Linksys. After the system is taken over, the botnet code

can be changed by the attacker, increasing the destructive effect of the software.

- **Echobot Botnet:** Using 26 scripts for its propagation, this botnet aims to damage the entire system by exploiting vulnerabilities in unpatched smart IoT devices.
- **Emotet Botnet:** This botnet aims to hijack the target's email account.
- **Gamut Botnet:** It aims to capture the target device with spam emails.
- **Necurs Botnet:** It was developed to launch digital extortion attacks such as ransomware attack.

Table 7.4 gives information about the types of malware and the damages they can cause; Table 7.5 presents a list of deep and machine learning–based solution references developed against these attacks.

TABLE 7.4
Malware Types and Their Damages

Malware Type	Damages of the Attacks
Spyware	Confidentiality, integrity, and authenticity of available resources
Keylogger	Confidentiality, integrity, and authenticity of various resources
Trojan horse	Confidentiality and availability of system resources
Virus	Integrity and availability of system resources
Worm	Availability of the data or other network resources
Ransomware	Availability of system resources
Rootkit	Confidentiality, integrity, authenticity, usability of the data or system resources

TABLE 7.5
Malware Attacks and DL/ML-Based Solutions

Attack Type	Property	Solution Reference
Emotet	This botnet aims to hijack the target's email account	[93, 51]
Echobot	This botnet aims to damage the entire system by exploiting vulnerabilities in unpatched smart IoT devices	[93, 51]
Reaper	This botnet can crash the entire system infrastructure much faster than the Mirai botnet	[94, 95]
	Reaper specifically targets the vulnerability in devices from different manufacturers such as DLink, Netgear, and Linksys	
	After the system is taken over, the botnet code can be changed by the attacker, increasing the destructive effect of the software	
Mirai	The control of the network device with the Linux operating system is left to the remote bots	[93, 51]
	The Mirai botnet specifically aims to take control of devices such as IP cameras and smart home device	
Gamut	It aims to capture the target device with spam emails	[93, 51]
Necurs	It launches digital extortion attacks such as ransomware attack	[93, 51]

7.9   RESULTS AND FUTURE DIFFICULTIES OF MALWARE DETECTION IN IOT/IOHT

It is known that intrusion detection studies in the literature do not provide adequate detection toward various types of malware. Therefore, it is necessary to develop a detection system that can be effective against all malware attacks. In addition, the low computing and storage capacities of the devices in the IoT/IoHT environment make it impossible to run algorithms that require intensive processing power on these devices. Detection should be provided by using algorithms with low processing volume. The IoT/IoHT environment has a heterogeneous structure that brings together many devices with different communication protocols. The malware detection system to be developed should be capable of evaluating the data coming from all these devices and providing security to all devices at the same time. The heterogeneity of the IoT network structure creates difficulties in developing an effective malware detection mechanism. Therefore, there is a need for the developed detection system to provide a compatible and fluent communication environment between different IoT platforms.

Recently developed blockchain technology is promising in terms of security for IoT/IoHT environments [86]. The decentralization of the blockchain structure makes it more secure at the point of data communication and storage. It is predicted that by keeping data about malware in blockchains, it will enable all devices in the IoHT environment to have prior knowledge of these software and to design themselves to detect these attacks.

As a result of this work, based on the reviewed studies, power governance, confidence and confidentiality, fog computing, and source administration are the problems that need to be resolved first for IoHT environments. Innovative solutions that can solve the security problems of IoHT environments are considered to be technologies such as big data analytics, SDN, nano-Internet of Things, and blockchain. Further challenges that require further study are interoperability, real testbed enforcement, scalability, and motility [100–102].

7.10   CONCLUSION

The fact that the IoHT communication network offers innovative solutions to the healthcare field is the foremost factor that encourages the use of this technology. But besides the benefits offered by the IoHT environment, this system must also ensure the confidentiality of patient data. In order to eliminate the devastating effects of malware attacks of different types and characteristics, which are developed day by day, it is expected that systems that will resist these software can be developed at the same speed, and while doing this, the computational load will be minimized and be able to resist all attacks. In this study, the types of malware that pose a threat to IoHT environments and the damage they can cause were examined, and a research was carried out on the solution methods that can be brought to this problem with deep learning methods. At the same time, IoHT architecture and technologies used in this field are discussed. Future research challenges in the IoHT environment and solutions that will bring a new approach to malware detection are also highlighted.

REFERENCES

1. Singh, S., Sheng, Q. Z., Benkhelifa, E., & Lloret, J. (2020). Guest editorial: Energy management, protocols, and security for the next-generation networks and Internet of Things. *IEEE Transactions on Industrial Informatics*, 16(5), 3515–3520.
2. Yadav, P., Kumar, P., Kishan, P., & Raj, P. (2021, August). Development of pervasive IoT based healthcare monitoring system for Alzheimer patients. In *Journal of Physics: Conference Series* (Vol. 2007, No. 1, p. 012035). IOP Publishing.
3. Sula, A., Spaho, E., Matsuo, K., Barolli, L., Miho, R., & Xhafa, F. (2013, October). An IoT-based system for supporting children with autism spectrum disorder. In *2013 Eighth International Conference on Broadband and Wireless Computing, Communication and Applications* (pp. 282–289). IEEE.
4. Sumathy, B., Kavimullai, S., Shushmithaa, S., & Anusha, S. S. (2021). Wearable non-invasive health monitoring device for elderly using IOT. In *IOP Conference Series: Materials Science and Engineering* (Vol. 1012, No. 1, p. 012011). IOP Publishing.
5. Lokshina, I., & Lanting, C. (2019). A qualitative evaluation of IoT-driven eHealth: knowledge management, business models and opportunities, deployment and evolution. In *Data-Centric Business and Applications* (pp. 23–52). Springer, Cham.
6. Sikarndar, M., Anwar, W., Almogren, A., Din, I. U., & Guizani, N. (2020). IoMT-based association rule mining for the prediction of human protein complexes. *IEEE Access*, 8, 6226–6237.
7. Rasool, R. U., Ahmad, H. F., Rafique, W., Qayyum, A., & Qadir, J. (2022). Security and privacy of internet of medical things: A contemporary review in the age of surveillance, botnets, and adversarial ML. *Journal of Network and Computer Applications*, 103332.
8. Othman, S. Ben, Bahattab, A. A., Trad, A., & Youssef, H. (2016, November). Lightweight and confidential data aggregation in healthcare wireless sensor networks. *Transactions on Emerging Telecommunications Technologies, Wiley*, 26(11).
9. Saheed, Y. K., & Arowolo, M. O. (2021). Efficient cyber attack detection on the Internet of Medical things-smart environment based on deep recurrent neural network and machine learning algorithms. *IEEE Access*, 9, 161546–161554.
10. Wazid, M., Das, A. K., Rodrigues, J. J., Shetty, S., & Park, Y. (2019). IoMT malware detection approaches: Analysis and research challenges. *IEEE Access*, 7, 182459–182476. doi:10.1109/ACCESS.2019.2960412.
11. Liaqat, S., Akhunzada, A., Shaikh, F. S., Giannetsos, A., & Jan, M. A. (2020). SDN orchestration to combat evolving cyber threats in Internet of Medical Things (IoMT). *Computer Communications*, 160, 697–705.
12. Papaioannou, M., Karageorgou, M., Mantas, G., Sucasas, V., Essop, I., Rodriguez, J., & Lymberopoulos, D. (2020). A survey on security threats and countermeasures in internet of medical things (IoMT). *Transactions on Emerging Telecommunications Technologies*, e4049.
13. Kurte, R., Salcic, Z., Kevin, I., & Wang, K. (2019). A distributed service framework for the internet of things. *IEEE Transactions on Industrial Informatics*, 16(6), 4166–4176.
14. Abdullahi, M., Baashar, Y., Alhussian, H., Alwadain, A., Aziz, N., Capretz, L. F., & Abdulkadir, S. J. (2022). Detecting cybersecurity attacks in Internet of Things using artificial intelligence methods: A systematic literature review. *Electronics*, 11(2), 198.
15. Manimurugan, S., Al-Mutairi, S., Aborokbah, M. M., Chilamkurti, N., Ganesan, S., & Patan, R. (2020). Effective attack detection in internet of medical things smart environment using a deep belief neural network. *IEEE Access*, 8, 77396–77404.
16. Usman, M., Jan, M. A., He, X., & Chen, J. (2019). P2DCA: A privacy-preserving-based data collection and analysis framework for IoMT applications. *IEEE Journal on Selected Areas in Communications*, 37(6), 1222–1230.

17. Thamilarasu, G., Odesile, A., & Hoang, A. (2020). An intrusion detection system for internet of medical things. *IEEE Access*, 8, 181560–181576.
18. Khan, F. A., Gumaei, A., Derhab, A., & Hussain, A. (2019). A novel two-stage deep learning model for efficient network intrusion detection. *IEEE Access*, 7, 30373–30385.
19. Bengag, A., Moussaoui, O., & Moussaoui, M. (2019, October). A new IDS for detecting jamming attacks in WBAN. In *2019 Third International Conference on Intelligent Computing in Data Sciences (ICDS)* (pp. 1–5). IEEE.
20. Yang, Y., Zheng, K., Wu, C., & Yang, Y. (2019). Improving the classification effectiveness of intrusion detection by using improved conditional variational autoencoder and deep neural network. *Sensors*, 19(11), 2528.
21. Zhang, H., Yu, X., Ren, P., Luo, C., & Min, G. (2019). Deep adversarial learning in intrusion detection: A data augmentation enhanced framework. *arXiv preprint arXiv:1901.07949*.
22. Li, D., Deng, L., Lee, M., & Wang, H. (2019). IoT data feature extraction and intrusion detection system for smart cities based on deep migration learning. *International Journal of Information Management*, 49, 533–545.
23. Ren, J., Guo, J., Qian, W., Yuan, H., Hao, X., & Jingjing, H. (2019). Building an effective intrusion detection system by using hybrid data optimization based on machine learning algorithms. *Security and Communication Networks*, 2019.
24. Zhang, J., Li, F., Zhang, H., Li, R., & Li, Y. (2019). Intrusion detection system using deep learning for in-vehicle security. *Ad Hoc Networks*, 95, 101974.
25. Salo, F., Nassif, A. B., & Essex, A. (2019, January). Dimensionality reduction with IG-PCA and ensemble classifier for network intrusion detection. *Computer Networks*, 148, 164–175, doi:10.1016/j.comnet.2018.11.010.
26. Khan, R. U., Zhang, X., Alazab, M., & Kumar, R. (2019, May). An improved convolutional neural network model for intrusion detection in networks. In *2019 Cybersecurity and Cyberforensics Conference (CCC)* (pp. 74–77). IEEE, doi:10.1109/CCC.2019.000-6.
27. Diro, A. A., & Chilamkurti, N. (2018). Distributed attack detection scheme using deep learning approach for Internet of Things. *Future Generation Computer Systems*, 82, 761–768.
28. Farivar, F., Haghighi, M. S., Jolfaei, A., & Alazab, M. (2019). Artificial intelligence for detection, estimation, and compensation of malicious attacks in nonlinear cyber-physical systems and industrial IoT. *IEEE Transactions on Industrial Informatics*, 16(4), 2716–2725.
29. Sarica, A. K., & Angin, P. (2020). Explainable security in SDN-based IoT networks. *Sensors*, 20(24), 7326.
30. Patil, R., Dudeja, H., & Modi, C. (2020). Designing in-VM-assisted lightweight agent-based malware detection framework for securing virtual machines in cloud computing. *International Journal of Information Security*, 19(2), 147–162.
31. Dang, T. K., Pham, C. D., & Nguyen, T. L. (2020). A pragmatic elliptic curve cryptography-based extension for energy-efficient device-to-device communications in smart cities. *Sustainable Cities and Society*, 56, 102097.
32. Bland, J. A., Petty, M. D., Whitaker, T. S., Maxwell, K. P., & Cantrell, W. A. (2020). Machine learning cyberattack and defense strategies. *Computers & Security*, 92, 101738.
33. Rathore, S., & Park, J. H. (2018). Semi-supervised learning based distributed attack detection framework for IoT. *Applied Soft Computing*, 72, 79–89.
34. Kasongo, S. M., & Sun, Y. (2020). A deep learning method with wrapper based feature extraction for wireless intrusion detection system. *Computers & Security*, 92, 101752.
35. Zhao, R., Yan, R., Chen, Z., Mao, K., Wang, P., & Gao, R. X. (2019). Deep learning and its applications to machine health monitoring. *Mechanical Systems and Signal Processing*, 115, 213–237.

36. Nweke, H. F., Teh, Y. W., Al-Garadi, M. A., & Alo, U. R. (2018). Deep learning algorithms for human activity recognition using mobile and wearable sensor networks: State of the art and research challenges. *Expert Systems with Applications*, 105, 233–261.

37. Da Costa, C. A., Pasluosta, C. F., Eskofier, B., Da Silva, D. B., & da Rosa Righi, R. (2018). Internet of health things: Toward intelligent vital signs monitoring in hospital wards. *Artificial Intelligence in Medicine*, 89, 61–69.

38. Amin, S. U., & Hossain, M. S. (2020). Edge intelligence and Internet of Things in healthcare: A survey. *IEEE Access*, 9, 45–59.

39. Fridriksdottir, E., & Bonomi, A. G. (2020). Accelerometer-based human activity recognition for patient monitoring using a deep neural network. *Sensors*, 20(22), 6424.

40. Azimi, I., Takalo-Mattila, J., Anzanpour, A., Rahmani, A. M., Soininen, J. P., & Liljeberg, P. (2018, September). Empowering healthcare IoT systems with hierarchical edge-based deep learning. In *CHASE '18: Proceedings of the 2018 IEEE/ ACM International Conference on Connected Health: Applications, Systems and Engineering Technologies* (pp. 63–68). https://doi.org/10.1145/3278576.3278597

41. Mohsin, A. H., Zaidan, A. A., Zaidan, B. B., Albahri, O. S., Albahri, A. S., Alsalem, M. A., & Mohammed, K. I. (2019). Based blockchain-PSO-AES techniques in finger vein biometrics: A novel verification secure framework for patient authentication. *Computer Standards & Interfaces*, 66, 103343.

42. Santhi, J. A., & Saradhi, T. V. (2021, October). Attack detection in medical Internet of things using optimized deep learning: Enhanced security in healthcare sector. *Data Technologies and Applications*, 55, 33–52.

43. Rathore, H., Al-Ali, A. K., Mohamed, A., Du, X., & Guizani, M. (2019). A novel deep learning strategy for classifying different attack patterns for deep brain implants. *IEEE Access*, 7, 24154–24164.

44. Abdaoui, A., Al-Ali, A., Riahi, A., Mohamed, A., Du, X., & Guizani, M. (2020). Secure medical treatment with deep learning on embedded board. In *Energy Efficiency of Medical Devices and Healthcare Applications* (pp. 131–151). Elsevier, Amsterdam.

45. Swarna Priya, R. M., Maddikunta, P. K. R., Parimala, M., Koppu, S., Reddy, T., Chowdhary, C. L., & Alazab, M. (2020). An effective feature engineering for DNN using hybrid PCA-GWO for intrusion detection in IoMT architecture. *Computer Communications*, 160, 139–149.

46. Mohamed Shakeel, P., Baskar, S., Sarma Dhulipala, V. R., Mishra, S., & Jaber, M. M. (2018). Maintaining security and privacy in health care system using learning based deep-Q-networks. *Journal of Medical Systems*, 42(10), 1–10.

47. HaddadPajouh, H., Dehghantanha, A., Khayami, R., & Choo, K. K. R. (2018). A deep recurrent neural network based approach for internet of things malware threat hunting. *Future Generation Computer Systems*, 85, 88–96.

48. Ullah, F., Naeem, H., Jabbar, S., Khalid, S., Latif, M. A., Al-Turjman, F., & Mostarda, L. (2019). Cyber security threats detection in internet of things using deep learning approach. *IEEE Access*, 7, 124379–124389.

49. Ibitoye, O., Shafiq, O., & Matrawy, A. (2019, December). Analyzing adversarial attacks against deep learning for intrusion detection in IoT networks. In *2019 IEEE Global Communications Conference (GLOBECOM)* (pp. 1–6). IEEE.

50. Li, Q., Li, W., Wang, J., & Cheng, M. (2019). A SQL injection detection method based on adaptive deep forest. *IEEE Access*, 7, 145385–145394.

51. Meidan, Y., Bohadana, M., Mathov, Y., Mirsky, Y., Shabtai, A., Breitenbacher, D., & Elovici, Y. (2018). N-BaIoT—network-based detection of iot botnet attacks using deep autoencoders. *IEEE Pervasive Computing*, 17(3), 12–22.

52. Anand, A., Rani, S., Anand, D., Aljahdali, H. M., & Kerr, D. (2021). An efficient CNN-based deep learning model to detect malware attacks (CNN-DMA) in 5G-IoT health-care applications. *Sensors*, 21(19), 6346.
53. Yin, X. C., Liu, Z. G., Ndibanje, B., Nkenyereye, L., & Riazul Islam, S. M. (2019). An IoT-based anonymous function for security and privacy in healthcare sensor networks. *Sensors*, 19(14), 3146.
54. Iqridar Newaz, A. K. M., Sikder, A. K., Ashiqur Rahman, M., & Selcuk Uluagac, A. (2020). A survey on security and privacy issues in modern healthcare systems: Attacks and defenses. *arXiv e-prints, arXiv-2005.*
55. Lane, N. D., Bhattacharya, S., Georgiev, P., Forlivesi, C., & Kawsar, F. (2015, November). An early resource characterization of deep learning on wearables, smartphones and internet-of-things devices. In *IoT-App '15: Proceedings of the 2015 International Workshop on Internet of Things Towards Applications* (pp. 7–12). https://doi.org/10.1145/2820975.2820980
56. Malasri, K., & Wang, L. (2009). Design and implementation of a secure wireless mote-based medical sensor network. *Sensors*, 9(8), 6273–6297.
57. Rahman, M. A., Hossain, M. S., Islam, M. S., Alrajeh, N. A., & Muhammad, G. (2020). Secure and provenance enhanced internet of health things framework: A blockchain managed federated learning approach. *IEEE Access*, 8, 205071–205087.
58. Thamilarasu, G., & Chawla, S. (2019). Towards deep-learning-driven intrusion detection for the internet of things. *Sensors*, 19(9), 1977.
59. Amin, M., Shehwar, D., Ullah, A., Guarda, T., Tanveer, T. A., & Anwar, S. (2020). A deep learning system for health care IoT and smartphone malware detection. *Neural Computing and Applications*, 1–12.
60. Aman, A. H. M., Hassan, W. H., Sameen, S., Attarbashi, Z. S., Alizadeh, M., & Latiff, L. A. (2021). IoMT amid COVID-19 pandemic: Application, architecture, technology, and security. *Journal of Network and Computer Applications*, 174, 102886.
61. Razdan, S., & Sharma, S. (2021). Internet of Medical Things (IoMT): Overview, emerging technologies, and case studies. *IETE Technical Review*, 1–14.
62. Dilibal, Ç. (2020, October). Development of edge-IoMT computing architecture for smart healthcare monitoring platform. In *2020 4th International Symposium on Multidisciplinary Studies and Innovative Technologies (ISMSIT)* (pp. 1–4). IEEE.
63. Bhuiyan, M. N., Rahman, M. M., Billah, M. M., & Saha, D. (2021, July). Internet of Things (IoT): A review of its enabling technologies in healthcare applications, standards protocols, security and market opportunities. *IEEE Internet of Things Journal*, 8(13), 10474–10498. doi: 10.1109/JIOT.2021.3062630
64. Islam, S. M., Lloret, J., & Zikria, Y. B. (2021). Internet of Things (IoT)-based wireless health: Enabling technologies and applications. *Electronics*, 10(2), 148.
65. Čolaković, A., & Hadžialić, M. (2018). Internet of Things (IoT): A review of enabling technologies, challenges, and open research issues. *Computer Networks*, 144, 17–39.
66. Mahmoud, M. M., Rodrigues, J. J., Ahmed, S. H., Shah, S. C., Al-Muhtadi, J. F., Korotaev, V. V., & De Albuquerque, V. H. C. (2018). Enabling technologies on cloud of things for smart healthcare. *IEEE Access*, 6, 31950–31967.
67. Scarpato, N., Pieroni, A., Di Nunzio, L., & Fallucchi, F. (2017). E-health-IoT universe: A review. *Management*, 21(44), 46.
68. Wu, F., Wu, T., & Yuce, M. R. (2018). An Internet-of-Things (IoT) network system for connected safety and health monitoring applications. *Sensors*, 19(1), 21.
69. Milovanovic, D., & Bojkovic, Z. (2017). Cloud-based IoT healthcare applications: Requirements and recommendations. *International Journal of Internet of Things and Web Services*, 2, 60–65.

70. Kashani, M. H., Madanipour, M., Nikravan, M., Asghari, P., & Mahdipour, E. (2021). A systematic review of IoT in healthcare: Applications, techniques, and trends. *Journal of Network and Computer Applications*, 192, 103164.

71. Mohammed, C. M., & Askar, S. (2021). Machine learning for IoT healthcare applications: A review. *International Journal of Science and Business*, 5(3), 42–51.

72. Joyia, G. J., Liaqat, R. M., Farooq, A., & Rehman, S. (2017). Internet of medical things (IoMT): Applications, benefits and future challenges in healthcare domain. *Journal of Communication*, 12(4), 240–247.

73. Koutras, D., Stergiopoulos, G., Dasaklis, T., Kotzanikolaou, P., Glynos, D., & Douligeris, C. (2020). Security in IoMT communications: A survey. *Sensors*, 20(17), 4828.

74. Ghubaish, A., Salman, T., Zolanvari, M., Unal, D., Al-Ali, A., & Jain, R. (2020). Recent advances in the internet-of-medical-things (IoMT) systems security. *IEEE Internet of Things Journal*, 8(11), 8707–8718.

75. Ngo, Q. D., Nguyen, H. T., Le, V. H., & Nguyen, D. H. (2020). A survey of IoT malware and detection methods based on static features. *ICT Express*, 6(4), 280–286.

76. Vinayakumar, R., Alazab, M., Soman, K. P., Poornachandran, P., & Venkatraman, S. (2019). Robust intelligent malware detection using deep learning. *IEEE Access*, 7, 46717–46738.

77. Kim, T., Kang, B., Rho, M., Sezer, S., & Im, E. G. (2018). A multimodal deep learning method for android malware detection using various features. *IEEE Transactions on Information Forensics and Security*, 14(3), 773–788.

78. Zhou, W., & Yu, B. (2018). A cloud-assisted malware detection and suppression framework for wireless multimedia system in IoT based on dynamic differential game. *China Communications*, 15(2), 209–223.

79. Wu, B., Lu, T., Zheng, K., Zhang, D., & Lin, X. (2014). Smartphone malware detection model based on artificial immune system. *China Communications*, 11(13), 86–92.

80. Yan, P., & Yan, Z. (2018). A survey on dynamic mobile malware detection. *Software Quality Journal*, 26(3), 891–919.

81. Takase, H., Kobayashi, R., Kato, M., & Ohmura, R. (2020). A prototype implementation and evaluation of the malware detection mechanism for IoT devices using the processor information. *International Journal of Information Security*, 19(1), 71–81.

82. Azmoodeh, A., Dehghantanha, A., & Choo, K. K. R. (2018). Robust malware detection for internet of (battlefield) things devices using deep eigenspace learning. *IEEE Transactions on Sustainable Computing*, 4(1), 88–95.

83. Rudd, E. M., Rozsa, A., Günther, M., & Boult, T. E. (2016). A survey of stealth malware attacks, mitigation measures, and steps toward autonomous open world solutions. *IEEE Communications Surveys & Tutorials*, 19(2), 1145–1172.

84. Aboosh, O. S. A., & Aldabbagh, O. A. I. (2021, September). Android adware detection model based on machine learning techniques. In *2021 International Conference on Computing and Communications Applications and Technologies (I3CAT)* (pp. 98–104). IEEE.

85. Othman, Soufiene Ben, Almalki, Faris A., Chakraborty, Chinmay, & Sakli, Hedi (2022). Privacy-preserving aware data aggregation for IoT-based healthcare with green computing technologies. *Computers and Electrical Engineering*, 101, 108025. https://doi.org/10.1016/j.compeleceng.2022.108025.

86. Othman, Soufiene Ben, Bahattab, Abdullah Ali, Trad, Abdelbasset, & Youssef, Habib (2020). PEERP: A priority-based energy-efficient routing protocol for reliable data transmission in healthcare using the IoT. *The 15th International Conference on Future Networks and Communications (FNC) August 9–12*, 2020, Leuven, Belgium, 2020.

87. Othman, Soufiene Ben, Bahattab, Abdullah Ali, Trad, Abdelbasset, & Youssef, Habib (2020). LSDA: Lightweight secure data aggregation scheme in healthcare using IoT. *ACM — 10th International Conference on Information Systems and Technologies*, Lecce, Italy. June 2020.

88. Othman, Soufiene Ben, Bahattab, Abdullah Ali, Trad, Abdelbasset, & Youssef, Habib (2019). RESDA: Robust and efficient secure data aggregation scheme in healthcare using the IoT. *The International Conference on Internet of Things, Embedded Systems and Communications (IINTEC 2019)*, HAMMAMET, Tunisia from 20–22 December 2019.

89. Vignau, B., Khoury, R., Hallé, S., & Hamou-Lhadj, A. (2021). The evolution of IoT Malwares, from 2008 to 2019: Survey, taxonomy, process simulator and perspectives. *Journal of Systems Architecture*, 116, 102143.

90. Gürfidan, R., & Ersoy, M. (2022). A new approach with blockchain based for safe communication in IoT ecosystem. *Journal of Data, Information and Management*, 1–8.

91. Nguyen, H. T., Ngo, Q. D., & Le, V. H. (2018, September). IoT botnet detection approach based on PSI graph and DGCNN classifier. In *2018 IEEE International Conference on Information Communication and Signal Processing (ICICSP)* (pp. 118–122). IEEE.

92. Su, J., Vasconcellos, D. V., Prasad, S., Sgandurra, D., Feng, Y., & Sakurai, K. (2018, July). Lightweight classification of IoT malware based on image recognition. In *2018 IEEE 42nd annual computer software and applications conference (COMPSAC)* (Vol. 2, pp. 664–669). IEEE.

93. Rathore, H., Wenzel, L., Al-Ali, A. K., Mohamed, A., Du, X., & Guizani, M. (2018). Multi-layer perceptron model on chip for secure diabetic treatment. *IEEE Access*, 6, 44718–44730.

94. Mohsen, N. R., Ying, B., & Nayak, A. (2019, July). Authentication protocol for real-time wearable medical sensor networks using biometrics and continuous monitoring. In *2019 International Conference on Internet of Things (iThings) and IEEE Green Computing and Communications (GreenCom) and IEEE Cyber, Physical and Social Computing (CPSCom) and IEEE Smart Data (SmartData)* (pp. 1199–1206). IEEE.

95. Lopez-Martin, M., Carro, B., Sanchez-Esguevillas, A., & Lloret, J. (2017). Conditional variational autoencoder for prediction and feature recovery applied to intrusion detection in iot. *Sensors*, 17(9), 1967.

96. Malaiya, R. K., Kwon, D., Kim, J., Suh, S. C., Kim, H., & Kim, I. (2018, March). An empirical evaluation of deep learning for network anomaly detection. In *2018 International Conference on Computing, Networking and Communications (ICNC)* (pp. 893–898). IEEE.

97. Sinanović, H., & Mrdovic, S. (2017, September). Analysis of Mirai malicious software. In *2017 25th International Conference on Software, Telecommunications and Computer Networks (SoftCOM)* (pp. 1–5). IEEE.

98. Kumar, A., & Lim, T. J. (2019, April). EDIMA: Early detection of IoT malware network activity using machine learning techniques. In *2019 IEEE 5th World Forum on Internet of Things (WF-IoT)* (pp. 289–294). IEEE.

99. Kelley, T., & Furey, E. (2018, June). Getting prepared for the next botnet attack: Detecting algorithmically generated domains in botnet command and control. In *2018 29th Irish Signals and Systems Conference (ISSC)* (pp. 1–6). IEEE.

100. McLaughlin, N., Martinez del Rincon, J., Kang, B., Yerima, S., Miller, P., Sezer, S., . . . & Joon Ahn, G. (2017, March). Deep android malware detection. In *CODASPY '17: Proceedings of the Seventh ACM on Conference on Data and Application Security and Privacy* (pp. 301–308). https://doi.org/10.1145/3029806.3029823

101. Yousefi-Azar, M., Varadharajan, V., Hamey, L., & Tupakula, U. (2017, May). Autoencoder-based feature learning for cyber security applications. In *2017 International joint conference on neural networks (IJCNN)* (pp. 3854–3861). IEEE.
102. Li, Y., Ma, R., & Jiao, R. (2015). A hybrid malicious code detection method based on deep learning. *International Journal of Security and Its Applications*, 9(5), 205–216.

8 IoT-Based Wrist Attitude Sensor Data for Parkinson's Disease Assessment for Healthcare System

*Amarendranath Choudhury,
Sathish E., Dhilleshwara Rao Vana,
and L. Ganesh Babu*

CONTENTS

DOI: 10.1201/9781003315476-8

8.1 INTRODUCTION

The Internet of Things is based on the existing telecommunications and Internet infrastructures. It enables the autonomous treatment of all common physical items, creating a web of related objects [1]. The Internet of Things is built on globally standardized standards and technology, which enables worldwide coverage and large-scale applications. The Internet of Things, which is closely linked to new technologies like cloud computing and big data, solves a number of problems, such as fragmentation in technology, network, application, and industry. Using IoT-related technologies like sensors, short-range communication, the Internet, and so on with medical and health technologies is called medical and health IoT. This allows doctors, residents, patients, and medical care to be connected in a whole way. To provide intelligent medical and health services, equipment, drugs, the environment, and other service factors must be able to automatically identify, track, collect, manage, and share medical data, advance the medical and health industry's comprehensive informatization, improve service efficiency, and keep the patient at the center of everything. The Internet of Things process for medical and healthcare has been incorporated into total-person, total-process, and total-process management. As a summary of its core notions, the following three points apply:

(a) The term "objects" refers to medical entities such as patients, physicians, nurses, medical devices, and medical information. (b) "Link" refers to the process interaction engine, which includes, but is not limited to, the medical information integration platform, Internet of Things middleware, data collecting sensors, automated workflow engines, management and monitoring platforms, and data processing platforms. (c) The term "Net" refers to standardized medical processes such as nursing procedures, inspection procedures, diagnosis procedures, traceability procedures, and quality control and management procedures, to name but a few.

In our country, Parkinson's disease affects about 1.7% of people who are over 65 years old [2]. Parkinson's disease can cause a variety of movement disorders [3], cognitive impairment, and mental problems such as depression and anxiety [4], and the quality of life gradually declines. Currently, drugs are mainly used to control various symptoms of Parkinson's disease, but drugs will appear an "on-off" phenomenon over time [5]; that is, after the patient takes the drug, the symptoms of various movement disorders around the body will gradually reduce, At this time, it is medically defined as the patient in the "on period"; after that, the patient's symptoms gradually worsen, which is defined as the "off period." Timely and accurate detection of the on-off period can help doctors more scientifically arrange the dosage and frequency. Currently, the unified Parkinson disease's rating scale (UPDRS) is mainly used clinically to assess Parkinson's motor symptoms to determine the on-off state of patients, but the scale is not a continuous quantitative assessment of patient's status and symptom severity. A mainstream objective detection method of Parkinson's disease on-off period is to use wearable devices to capture the patient's muscle stiffness, frozen gait, and tremor and other motion features. These methods usually look at the raw data in terms of time and frequency of accelerometer, gyroscope, and magnetometer (magnetic, angular rate, and gravity—MARG) motion IoT-based sensors to characterize the motor symptoms of Parkinson's disease. In current research, multiple IoT-based sensors are usually used. Although the number of IoT-based sensors is more, the information obtained will be richer, but it will bring more inconvenience to the patient. In the process of UPDRS assessment of hand movement, doctors mainly rely on the posture of the patient's wrist. By assessing the severity of symptoms, by requiring patients to complete specific actions, the wrist posture of patients with different symptoms will show significant differences. This chapter proposes a single-handed-based on-off detection method for Parkinson's disease in a hospital environment, focusing on patient's movement. When the wrist posture changes, the MARG motion IoT-based sensor data is used for posture calculation, and the Parkinson's disease on-off state detection is realized based on the posture information. Through the verification results in the actual use of nine Parkinson's disease clinical patients, the proposed detection method based on single dominant hand is practical and effective.

8.2 EVALUATION OF PARKINSON'S DISEASE MOTOR SYMPTOMS AND ON-OFF PERIOD

It has become the most common way to measure clinical Parkinson's disease symptoms and has been used for more than 30 years. The MDS-UPDRS revised in 2019 is the latest version of the UPDRS scale, including four parts of daily non-motor symptoms, daily motor symptoms, motor function, and motor complications. Section 8.3 corresponds to the Parkinson's disease severity assessment of motor symptoms. Clinical on-off state judgment has 18 items, covering motor symptoms in speech, expression, rigidity, limb flexibility, gait, tremor, etc. Each item is scored from 0 to 4. The scores are all integers. Finally, the current exercise state of the patient is assessed according to the total score of all items [6]. One UPDRS evaluation was performed before as the baseline score, and after completion, the patient took an appropriate amount of levodopa preparation; the total score of each UPDRS evaluation after that would be compared with the baseline total score, and when the evaluation score decreased by more than 30%, it would be judged as entry on-stage, and when the difference from the baseline is small, it will be judged to be in off-stage. Scale-based assessment has a large time cost; even if an experienced medical staff completes a UPDRS score, it takes at least 15 minutes; for ordinary or medical staff, this process may take 20 minutes or even longer. If the evaluation is performed once an hour, each doctor can only be responsible for four patients, which not only causes a great waste of medical staff time, but also brings heavy burden to patients. However, it is far from meeting the daily testing needs of patients. The description of symptoms on the UPDRS scale for 0–4 points is not completely objective and quantifiable, such as "slightly slowed movement" and "moderately slowed movement." Such ambiguous descriptions make medical staff only rely on their own experience to give corresponding scores, resulting in differences in scores between different medical staff, which eventually leads to a weakening of the reference of scores and affects the diagnosis and treatment of patients. Find a simple, efficient, real-time approach. It is particularly important to have an objective and accurate detection method of Parkinson's disease on-off period.

In view of the situation that the on-off period of Parkinson's disease is mainly based on the severity of motor symptoms, the medical community has continued to conduct a large number of studies and proposed a variety of assessments for Parkinson's disease and equipment and methods for motor symptoms such as tremor and stiffness [7], but these methods are insufficient in convenience, practicability, and accuracy. For example, the Parkinson's disease tremor detection equipment designed in Ref. [7] is based on electromagnetic fields. The effect requires the subject's entire arm to be placed in a device with multiple IoT-based sensors and a wired connection to a computer to work.

In Ref. [8], a laser-based Parkinson's disease tremor detection device is designed. The patient needs to fix a reflective sheet on the index finger and place the index finger. In Refs [9], the data were used when the patient turned the turntable to detect Parkinson's disease stiffness and bradykinesia. The straps secure the patient's arm to the device, and the patient grips the turntable and turns it hard, turning it in the process. The movement angle and horizontal axis movement speed reflect the severity of symptoms of stiffness and bradykinesia, respectively, but this detection method has obvious shortcomings in accuracy. Devices designed by the traditional medical community exist in both accuracy and ease of use. It is obviously insufficient to meet the needs of Parkinson's disease patients for convenient and real-time detection of motor symptoms and on-off periods. With the vigorous development of wearable technology in recent years, wearable devices have gradually become miniaturized and practical, and have been successfully applied to the evaluation of Parkinson's disease symptoms and the detection of on-off states, attracting extensive attention from many researchers at home and abroad. Movement worn by the patient IoT-based sensors collect motion features and input them into machine learning models to get diagnosis. The on-off state of the user is currently a common method for on-off detection based on wearable devices. Wearing the IoT-based sensor on different body parts can obtain different motion characteristics, so choose the wearing position reasonably and design corresponding on-off period detection model. These are the two most concerned issues in the current research work.

8.2.1 WEARING POSITION OF MOTION IoT-BASED SENSOR

Parkinson's disease on-off state is directly reflected by motor symptoms, so how to design a combination of wearable IoT-based sensors to obtain more motion characteristics of patients is an important work of most studies. In Ref. [10], six acceleration motion IoT-based sensors were worn on the patient's chest, bilateral upper arms, bilateral thighs, and the wrist with the most severe symptoms to detect the patient's symptoms of tremor and bradykinesia, so as to judge the patient's on-off state. In Ref. [11], six wearable motion IoT-based sensors were used, but the wearing positions were located on the bilateral wrists and ankles, as well as on the chest and waist, while the six-axis acceleration gyroscope IoT-based sensors were used on the chest and waist of the upper limbs to record the rotation of the limb's information. Too many IoT-based sensors cause some inconvenience to patients, so they choose to wear two more IoT-based sensors in subsequent work [12]: wearing motion IoT-based sensors on the ankles of patients [13–14] and wearing motion IoT-based sensors on both wrists of the patient; in Ref. [15], patients chose to wear one IoT-based sensor on each of the unilateral wrist and ankle. Existing medical studies [9] have shown that repetitive motion at the wrist is related to the motor symptoms of Parkinson's disease. There is a strong correlation with the severity, and at the same time, the movement is affected by dopamine drugs, and the characteristics such as the amplitude, frequency, and completion of the movement after taking the medicine are significantly different from those before taking the medicine, which is indicative of the on-off period. The results of the study show that there is great correlation and redundancy between the multi-IoT-based sensor data on the limbs and the trunk, and only the motion IoT-based sensor worn on the unilateral wrist can be used to classify the upper extremity motor symptoms of Parkinson's disease. In conclusion, in this chapter, the patient is only required to wear the motion IoT-based sensor in the unilateral dominant hand, which improves the wearing convenience of the patient by reducing redundant data and realizes the convenient detection of the on-off state.

8.2.2 ALGORITHMIC MODEL OF ON-OFF PERIOD DETECTION BASED ON STATISTICAL MACHINE LEARNING

Xi's model method has shown excellent performance in motion IoT-based sensor applications such as behavior recognition, fall detection, and movement disorder assessment. At present, most of the research work on Parkinson's disease on-off state detection uses machine learning technology. In Refs [12, 16], the support vector machine (SVM) model is used to build an on-off period classification algorithm and achieve an accuracy of more than 80%. In Refs [10, 11], a multilayer perception (multilayer perception—MLP) is built, and it achieved similar accuracy. Compared with traditional machine learning, deep learning has received extensive attention due to its stronger representation learning ability and generalization ability and has been applied to the on-off period detection task. In Ref. [13], restricted Boltzmann machines are used to achieve continuous detection of on-off periods in an unrestricted environment; in Ref. [14] the performance of deep learning CNN models and traditional machine learning algorithms SVM, AdaBoost, etc., are compared on the symptoms of bradykinesia, and the results showed that CNN-based methods are able to achieve on average more than 5% higher accuracy than traditional machine learning methods. To sum up, we choose to build an on-off state classification model based on CNN network, mine the hidden layer features of motion IoT-based sensors, and achieve high accuracy detection of on-off state. Based on the aforementioned research results, the hospital interior on-off detection method for Parkinson's disease is based on a single dominant hand in the environment. Using the IoT-based sensor worn by the patient's dominant hand as the data source, a deep neural network is constructed to realize the convenient and efficient detection of the on-off state.

8.3 ON-OFF PERIOD DETECTION METHOD BASED ON WRIST POSTURE

The designed on-off period detection method based on a single dominant wrist posture is introduced according to the process. During hospitalization, the MARG

IoT-based sensor is worn on the patient's dominant hand every morning to collect the patient's wrist motion data and posture information. The resident doctor will evaluate the patient's UPDRS score on time and judge the current on-off state. Preprocessing operations such as cleaning, aligning, and windowing are performed on the posture information of the whole process of patient collection, and the processed data is used as input. The on-off period state of α is used as a label to train the on-off period detection model. Using the trained on-off period detection model for on-off period prediction, the proposed method based on a single conventional wrist posture is evaluated through a variety of metrics performance of the on-off period detection method.

8.3.1 DATA COLLECTION AND PREPROCESSING

All data collected were from hospitalized patients. Patients were used to wear the MARG motion IoT-based sensor on the hand and conduct UPDRS evaluation under the guidance of the doctor. During this process, the raw data generated by the IoT-based sensor will be transmitted to the storage gateway in real time through Wi-Fi; after the evaluation is completed, the doctor will use the mobile phone to enter the scoring information and the corresponding on-off state of the data is uploaded to the storage gateway together as the calibration data for the subsequent algorithm. The MARG IoT-based sensor used for data acquisition integrates a three-axis accelerometer with a range of $8g$, a three-axis gyroscope with a range of $\pm2,000/s$, and a three-axis magnetometer with a range of $\pm4,800\ \mu T$, which can fully cover the range of human motion state; IoT-based sensor size is 34 mm × 34 mm × 25 mm and has a mass of 21 g, which can capture the tremor and stiffness of Parkinson's patients and other motor symptoms details. The IoT-based sensor module can directly filter and solve the attitude into quaternions, and output nine-axis raw measurement data and quaternion attitude information at the same time. The output frequency of IoT-based sensor measurement is 100–120 Hz. In order to transmit data quickly, the communication between the IoT-based sensor and the gateway is through the UDP protocol, which causes the actual received data frequency to be 81–108 Hz. In order to maintain the consistency of the data, the data recording files were preprocessed after the experiment, and all IoT-based sensor data were down sampled to 80 Hz. All data were windowed with 5 s as the window size and 50% overlap, that is, each window contains 400 data, each data consists of nine-axis IoT-based sensor raw data and four-dimensional quaternion data, the window size is (400, 13). The data in each window is filtered by a four-order Butterworth filter; among them, a 0.5-Hz high-pass filter is applied to the three-axis acceleration data to remove the influence of gravity [11], and a 3–8 Hz band-pass filter is applied to the three-axis acceleration and three-axis gyroscope data to extract the Parkinson's disease characteristics of motor symptoms [11, 13].

8.3.2 ATTITUDE AND QUATERNION DESCRIPTION

The attitude of a rigid body refers to the angular position relationship between the rigid body's own coordinate system and the reference coordinate system, which is described in mathematics by the process of three-dimensional space rotation. The rotation in three-dimensional space can be represented by a 3 × 3 rotation matrix, but in computer applications, in order to reduce the computational complexity, Euler angles and quaternions [6] are usually used for two representations. The rotation is regarded as the rotation along the three orthogonal coordinate axes of the rigid body itself, and the three coordinates. The rotation angle of the axis constitutes a set of Euler angles for three-dimensional rotation. Select a vector in the three-dimensional space as the axis, and regard the rotation as a rotation around this axis, which is the parameterization method of the axis angle. In order to facilitate the calculation, the quaternion is usually used to represent the axis coordinates and the rotation angle (see Figure 8.1).

For the Euler angle representation, once the rotation angle encountered by the second coordinate axis causes the third coordinate axis to coincide with the first coordinate axis, the third rotation becomes a rotation angle on the first coordinate axis, so that the overall rotation process loses 1 degree of freedom. This phenomenon is called gimbal lock [7]. Due to the existence of gimbal lock, Euler angles are rarely used in high-speed motion systems, and the MARG motion IoT-based sensor is used. It has a frequency close to 100 Hz, so the Euler angle is not suitable for this chapter. Different from the Euler angle, the axis angle is represented by the basic coordinate system, which does not change with the rotation of the rigid body, so there is no problem of Vientiane lock, which is suitable for the application scenario of this chapter (Figure 8.2). The axis angle has four parameters, which are the coordinates of the reference axis and the rotation angle around the reference axis. The definition of a quaternion is very similar to that of a complex number. One imaginary part of

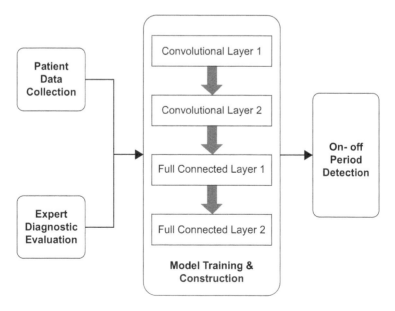

FIGURE 8.1 The overall flow of the on-off period detection method.

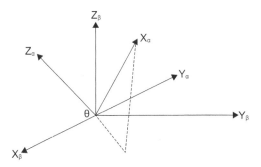

FIGURE 8.2 Schematic diagram of the rotation from the coordinate system to the coordinate system.

a complex number is expanded to 3, and the following quaternion representation is obtained:

$$Q = q_0 + q_1 i + q_2 j + q_3 k \qquad (8.1)$$

$$i^2 = j^2 = k^2 = ijk = -1 \qquad (8.2)$$

Rigid bodies have two coordinate systems: one for their own bodies, one for the world around them. If this is true, then the rigid body's attitude with respect to this world is like this: the coordinate system rotates this angle around this vector to the coordinate system.

8.3.3 On-Off Period Detection Algorithm Model

In the process of on-off period detection, it is necessary to deal with the challenges brought by the large difference between the action categories and the large individual symptoms of the patients in the UPDRS score and choose to use the end-to-end neural network model to solve. There are many kinds of movements, and the symptoms of patients are quite different. It is a huge task to manually design feature groups for different movements and symptoms to construct multiple classifier combinations [12, 16]; in an unrestricted daily life environment, the patient will inevitably make unexpected actions, which eventually leads to the failure of the model to produce accurate on-off period classification for unknown scenarios. The end-to-end deep neural network is used as the on-off period detection model. The original pose information or simply filtered MARG IoT-based sensor data is used as the input of the neural network, and the hidden layer feature extraction task is completed through a large number of convolution kernels, and finally calculated through the fully connected layer. On-off period classification results; when training the model, the model optimizer directly targets the on-off period classification results, so both the convolution kernel for feature extraction and the fully connected layer for final classification in the process can be used in large amounts of data. It is fully iteratively optimized to obtain better generalization ability, so as to achieve the effect of adapting the model to different patients and different symptoms. In order to facilitate the deployment of the model on devices with limited computing resources in edge computing and mobile computing environments, to realize the real-time detection of the patient's on-off period by doctors, the designed on-off period detection model will minimize the number of hidden layers of the neural network to reduce the computational amount. Based on the above analysis of model requirements and motion characteristics, a lightweight convolutional neural network with four trainable layers (denoted as CNN-4) is constructed to discriminate Parkinson's disease on-off state architecture. The network consists of two convolutional layers, each convolutional layer is connected to a maximum pooling layer, the last two layers of the network are fully connected layers, and Dropout is used to prevent overfitting; the output layer uses softmax. As an activation function, the final classification result is output. The input of the network uses a window of data, each dimension of data is used as a channel, and the size of each channel is 1×400 for the input layer. Flat features are used in the convolutional neural network. The size of the convolution kernel is 132, and the size of the pooling layer is set to 14 and 16. Adam optimization is used in the network training process, the learning rate is 0.001; the network training period is set to 200. Although the designed convolutional neural network with only four trainable layers is well controlled in the model structure and parameter quantity, deeper neural networks can often get more hidden layer features to obtain better classification results. In order to maximize the hidden features of IoT-based sensor data, five deeper convolutional neural networks are constructed for comparison: AlexNet, ResNet20, ResNet56, ResNet101, and ResNet155. AlexNet [11] is a neural network with five layers of convolutional layers plus the last three layers of fully connected layers, a total of eight trainable network layers (see Figure 8.3).

The network adopts the ResNet network structure, the single channel size of the network input layer is 1×400, the number of layers of the network is 20, 56, 101, and 155 layers, and the corresponding residual modules are 2, 6, 11, and 17, respectively. By calculating the number of trainable parameters of the target network, CNN-4 and each comparison network can be obtained. It can be seen that the number of parameters of the proposed CNN-4 network is increased by more than an order of magnitude for the deeper comparison network. Among them, AlexNet is mainly

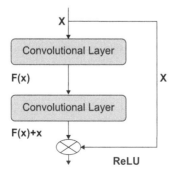

FIGURE 8.3　Residual learning module for ResNet.

composed of traditional convolutional layers, resulting in a higher number of model trainable parameters than ResNet20, which has more network layers; this indicates that it is more and more difficult to train a network that deepens layers by stacking convolutional layers alone. ResNet's residual structure advantages gradually appear. The ResNet155 network with the largest number of layers has about 80 times the parameters of the CNN-4 network. Higher parameters will bring better representation learning effect, which requires a lot of training and prediction time.

8.3.4 EVALUATION INDICATORS

For the classification performance of the model, the accuracy rate A is the most commonly used indicator, and the commonly used evaluation indicators in medicine are the sensitivity Sen and the specificity Sp. The calculation methods are as follows:

$$A = \frac{TP + TN}{TP + FP + TN + FN}$$

$$Sen = \frac{TP / TP}{FN}$$

$$Sp = \frac{TN}{TN + FP}$$

In the formula, TP and FP are the true and false positive rates, respectively; TN and FN are respectively true and false negative rates.

In most classification problems, using accuracy as a performance metric can comprehensively evaluate the quality of the model. In Parkinson's disease on-off phase detection, when the drug starts to work into the on-phase and when it declines into the off-phase, the model's two main tasks, the performance of the model on their respective tasks cannot be reflected only from the accuracy rate. So in this case, only using the accuracy rate cannot reflect the true value of the classification model. Using the sensitivity, that is, the true positive rate, can effectively evaluate the accuracy of the classification model's judgment on the open period; using the specificity, that is, the true negative rate, can truly evaluate the accuracy of the classification model accuracy of closing time judgment. Decreasing the positive class judgment threshold can increase the positive class judgment ratio, thereby improving the sensitivity of the model; lowering the negative class judgment threshold can improve the specificity of the model, so there is an obvious conflict between sensitivity and specificity. This way, we can get a full picture of how things are going. Often in medicine, the performance of the model in two different types of tasks in the on-off period is drawn. The receiver operating characteristic curve (ROC) is often drawn, and the area under the receiver operating characteristic (AUROC) is used as a comprehensive evaluation. This is how you would explain it. False positive rates and true positive rates can be changed by changing the threshold for making a judgment. This means that the false positive rate can go from 0 to 1. It is easy to figure out how to fit these points to the coordinate system so that the true positive rate is on the vertical axis and the false positive rate is on the horizontal axis. Obtain the ROC curve; integrate the ROC curve to obtain the area, which is the AUROC of the test model. AUROC is 0–1.0; the larger the AUROC, the smaller the sensitivity that needs to be reduced to improve the specificity, which means that the model can maintain high sensitivity and high sensitivity at the same time. In the Parkinson's on-off detection problem, comparing AUROC can comprehensively evaluate the detection effect of the model on the on-phase and off-phase. Compared with the individual sensitivity or specificity, AUROC has more important significance for the performance evaluation of the on-off phase detection model.

8.4   EXPERIMENTAL VERIFICATION

8.4.1   Experimental Data

A total of nine patients with Parkinson's disease participated in the experimental study. All the patients are over 55 years old; the data are the mean ± standard deviation. Since the history of Parkinson's disease in each patient ranges from two to eight years, the disease stage is different, resulting in a big difference in the UPDRS score; some patients' on-stage UPDRS score is higher than the off-stage score of patients with mild symptoms, and the symptoms are that the tremor symptoms are relieved after taking the drug, but it is more severe than other patients; this situation is classified as a classification. Algorithms bring greater challenges. Common features such as exercise intensity and frequency can no longer be used to correctly classify the on-off state. All Parkinson's disease patients participating in the study are inpatients, and their daily life is fully taken care of by medical staff, except that you must leave the ward when completing medical items such as CT or blood tests, all activities are limited to the ward on this floor. Patients will wear a posture IoT-based sensor in their dominant hand after getting up in the morning and complete many tasks under the guidance of medical staff. UPDRS assessments occur until the end of the drug effect and then enter the off-period, the patient can perform any activities during this time, such as eating, going to the toilet, indoor activities, using electronic devices such as mobile phones, and sleeping. MARG exercise for nine participants. The IoT-based sensor data was preprocessed, and a total of 9,452 windows of data were obtained. The UPDRS evaluation results of the medical staff showed that the patients were generally in the open phase for 1–3 hours after taking the drug, and the drug effect disappeared after 3 hours, and recovered to off-state. The patients were in the off-phase state during at least four evaluations (baseline and 0.5 hour, 1 hour, and 4 hours after taking the drug), so 61.3% of the obtained data window was in the off-period, and there was a certain imbalance in the data. The experimental code is built with TensorFlow 2.1.0 and runs on Ubuntu 18.04.4 system. The main configuration of the system is Xeon Gold 6145@2.0 GHz, the memory is 192 GB, and the training process is accelerated by 4 RTX 2080 Ti. In the experiment, a tenfold crossover is used. Verify that the All-index values are taken as the mean value of cross-validation to better reflect the generalization ability in the statistical sense.

8.4.2 THE INFLUENCE OF FEATURE INFORMATION ON THE PREDICTION OF THE ON-OFF PERIOD

In order to verify the validity of the posture information for the prediction of the on-off period of Parkinson's disease, the posture information (posture quaternion) was used as the input of the CNN model for training and testing. It was compared with the original MARG motion IoT-based sensor data without attitude information calculation. The attitude compared with the benchmark results using accelerometer data, the accuracy and specificity of the state information are more than 20% higher, and the AUROC of 0.948 is about 23% higher than the benchmark results (Table 8.1). The results show that the on-off period detection model is based on attitude information. It can maintain a good detection rate and a low false alarm rate, indicating the possibility of wearing a posture IoT-based sensor on the wrist to detect the on-off state of Parkinson's disease patients and comprehensive use of accelerometers, gyroscopes, and magnetic. The strong meter extracts attitude information, which has a greater performance improvement than the existing methods that only use the accelerometer, indicates the angular velocity of the wrist joint movement.

The geomagnetic direction of the wrist can be used as supplementary data for motion acceleration in Parkinson's on-off period detection, and multi-IoT-based sensor fusion is carried out to improve the detection accuracy. When using all the raw data of the MARG motion IoT-based sensor as the input of the CNN network, the classification accuracy is only 55.5%. Analyzing the specific test results, it is found that the classifier obtained by training will judge all the data as on or off, losing the ability to classify (see Figure 8.4). This can explain the use of acceleration data in the introduced work, while discarding the collected angular velocity and geomagnetic intensity data. Attitude information is sensed by Kalman filter to MARG motion (see Tables 8.2 and 8.3).

A feasible explanation is that although the original data contains more information, the shallow CNN network cannot directly learn the implicit features required for classification; the pose solution results are used as a more intuitive representation. In this way, it is convenient for the classifier to learn the features, so as to obtain a higher detection accuracy (Figure 8.5).

TABLE 8.1
Patient Demographics

Attributes	Statistics
Gender (male:female)	(5:4)
Age (years)	62.9
Dominant hand (left:right)	(1:8)
Parkinson's disease duration (years)	3.8
Duration of levodopa preparations (years)	1.5
Open UPDRS score	38.2
The UPDRS score in the off-period	20.3

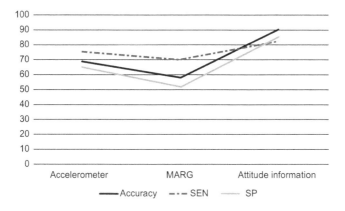

FIGURE 8.4 Graphs for different parameters.

TABLE 8.2
Data for Different Parameters

Parameter	Accelerometer	MARG	Attitude Information
Accuracy	69	58	90
Sensitivity	75	70	82
Specificity	65	52	85

TABLE 8.3
Data for AUROC

Methods	AUROC
Accelerometer	78
MARG	61
Attitude Information	91

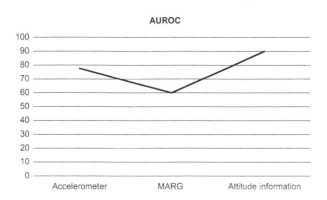

FIGURE 8.5 Graphs for ROC curve.

8.4.3   THE EFFECT OF THE NUMBER OF NETWORK LAYERS ON THE PREDICTION OF THE ON-OFF PERIOD

In order to deal with the problem of the convergence of the deep neural network training, the neural network with 20 layers and above uses the ResNet structure (see Table 8.4). After increasing the number of network layers, about 88% detection accuracy can be obtained using the MARG motion IoT-based sensor, which is similar to the accuracy of the pose information; this indicates that increasing number of network layers can extract more hidden layer features of the MARG motion IoT-based sensor. Even if the deepest ResNet155 only improves the accuracy by 0.5% and the AUROC of 0.003 compared to ResNet20, it can be considered that the 20-layer ResNet network can provide more stable Parkinson's disease on-off detection capabilities (see Figure 8.6 and Table 8.5).

The attitude information in the accuracy of the deeper network has always been greater than 88%, which is close to the IoT-based sensor data. This is because the

TABLE 8.4
Data for Validation Set of Accuracy

Methods	MARG	Attitude Information
CNN	0.55	0.9
AlexNet	0.75	0.8
ResNet20	0.85	0.87
ResNet56	0.86	0.86
ResNet101	0.85	0.87
ResNet155	0.86	0.84

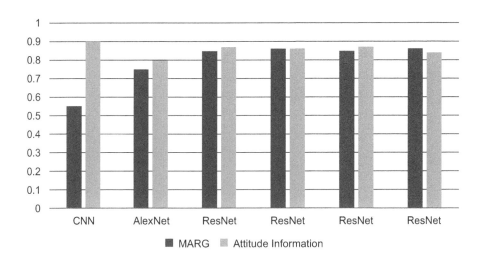

FIGURE 8.6   Validation set of accuracy.

TABLE 8.5

Raw Data and Attitude Information in Training Performance Analysis

CNN-4 + MARG	ResNet20 + MARG	CNN-4 + Attitude Information	ResNet20 + Attitude Information
0.32	0.6	0.7	0.72
0.2	0.75	0.75	0.78
0.3	0.8	0.82	0.82
0.4	0.87	0.84	0.87
0.34	0.84	0.85	0.84
0.4	0.82	0.87	0.85
0.5	0.83	0.84	0.83

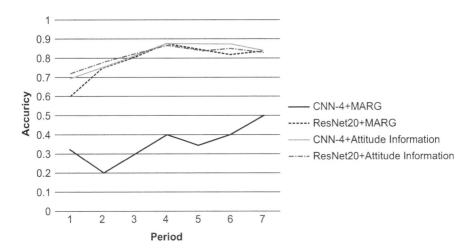

FIGURE 8.7 Performance analysis of IoT-based sensor raw data and attitude information in training.

attitude calculation does not bring additional information supplements, and the results of the shallow CNN network basically reach the maximum accuracy (see Figure 8.7). The state information can make the network reach a more stable accuracy earlier. From the accuracy of the validation set during the training process, it can be seen that whether it is the CNN network or the ResNet network, when using the pose information, it can be achieved after 25 training cycles. To achieve an accuracy rate of greater than 85%, using MARG motion IoT-based sensor data on the ResNet network, requires more than 50 training cycles to achieve a similar accuracy rate. Statistics on the running time can show that the training time of the CNN model is less than the training time of the ResNet model: 1/120, the prediction time is 32.5% of the ResNet model. The process of attitude calculation from the raw data of the nine-axis IoT-based sensor through filtering can be completed in real time on the embedded system-on-a-chip STM32. In conclusion, the CNN model using attitude data can greatly reduce the amount of calculation and training prediction time, it maintains good classification performance of Parkinson's disease on-off state, and posture information is used in Parkinson's disease and other movement disorders. It has potential application value in the diagnosis and detection of diseases.

8.4.4 The Detection Results of the Patient's Free Motion On-Off Period

In the process of training and verification, the data generated when the patients completed the UPDRS assessment were used. The proposed CNN network based on pose information on unrestricted free movements, nine patients were used within 4 hours after taking the medicine. The complete data of the test is tested, and the prediction results of the on-off period are output every minute to simulate the real-time detection of the on-off period when the patient performs free movements in the daily ward environment. The prediction accuracy of the overall on-period was 0.915 ± 0.110, and the prediction accuracy of the overall off-period was 0.944 ± 0.048. The on-off period state by using the patient's daily actions is the detection data. Corresponding to the results in the UPDRS test ratio, the improvement of the accuracy of free motion detection is mainly due to the reduction of the output frequency, which is determined by the majority of the 24 data windows per minute, clustering points, improving the overall accuracy. For example, the prediction results within 4 hours are plotted. In Figure 8.7, P is the predicted switching period probability, the scatter points represent the predicted value given by the model every minute, 0 means the closing period, and 1 means the opening period. Scattered points for the fitted curve present an obvious low-increase–high-decrease trend, indicating that the patient's motor symptoms gradually improved from the off-period to after taking the drug, entered the open period, and returned to the back-off period after the efficacy of the drug declined. The light-colored represents the off-period as indicated by the doctor, the dark part represents the on-period, and the gray in the middle indicates that the doctor believes that the patient is in the process of improving/deteriorating but has not yet reached the on-period/off-period. There are some fluctuations in the prediction results at the intermediate stage, which is consistent with the patient's UPDRS assessment during this period. The results of the on-off period are similar, and the judgment of the on-off period cannot be drawn. In the final stage of the test, the prediction confidence of the off-period is lower than that at the beginning of the test. By analyzing the UPDRS score of the patient at this time, it can be determined that the patient is in this period. Some improvement in motor symptoms is relative to the start of the test. This results in that the model infers the off-period state, but the confidence is not as high as at the beginning. The prediction results of the entire testing process show that the proposed on-off period detection method for Parkinson's disease can effectively predict the patient's pre- and post-medication conditions. It can continuously and stably give the correct on-off period prediction results, especially in the obvious on-period and off-period states.

8.5 CONCLUSION

This chapter proposes a detection method for Parkinson's disease on-off state based on wrist posture information. Using the MARG motion IoT-based sensor worn on the wrist, the posture calculation is carried out, and the wrist posture information is obtained. The motion IoT-based sensor worn on the wrist can be used for Parkinson's disease on-off state detection, and the pose information can achieve good on-off phase detection performance with lower complex model design. In the future, we will further excavate and explore from the following perspectives:

(a) The experiment will be extended to the daily environment and all-day time, including in-hospital wards, outpatient clinics, and home environments.
(b) Consider introducing transfer learning to build a personalized model or adopt an adaptive method to reduce the impact of individual patient differences on the model.
(c) The data group composed of nine patients is small, and more data are needed to improve the experiment to further confirm the effectiveness of posture information for detection.

REFERENCES

[1] A. Mohawish, R. Rathi, V. Abhishek, T. Lauritzen and R. Padman, "Predicting Coronary Heart Disease Risk Using Health Risk Assessment Data," *2015 17th International Conference on E-health Networking, Application & Services (HealthCom)*, 2015, pp. 91–96, doi:10.1109/HealthCom.2015.7454479.

[2] L. Cunningham, S. Mason, C. Nugent, G. Moore, D. Finlay and D. Craig, "Home-Based Monitoring and Assessment of Parkinson's Disease," in *IEEE Transactions on Information Technology in Biomedicine*, vol. 15, no. 1, pp. 47–53, Jan. 2011, doi:10.1109/TITB.2010.2091142.

[3] T. Wang, Y. Tian and R. G. Qiu, "Long Short-Term Memory Recurrent Neural Networks for Multiple Diseases Risk Prediction by Leveraging Longitudinal Medical Records," *IEEE Journal of Biomedical and Health Informatics*, vol. 24, no. 8, pp. 2337–2346, Aug. 2020, doi:10.1109/JBHI.2019.2962366.

[4] C. Wang, L. Peng, Z. -G. Hou, Y. Li, Y. Tan and H. Hao, "A Hierarchical Architecture for Multi-symptom Assessment of Early Parkinson's Disease via Wearable Sensors," *IEEE Transactions on Cognitive and Developmental Systems*, vol. 13, pp. 444–452, 2021, doi:10.1109/TCDS.2021.3123157.

[5] M. van Gils, J. Koikkalainen, J. Mattila, S. Herukka, J. Lötjönen and H. Soininen, "Discovery and Use of Efficient Biomarkers for Objective Disease State Assessment in Alzheimer's Disease," *2010 Annual International Conference of the IEEE Engineering in Medicine and Biology*, 2010, pp. 2886–2889, doi:10.1109/IEMBS.2010.5626311. https://ieeexplore.ieee.org/document/5626311

[6] Shi, W. Zuo, W. Chen, L. Yue, Y. Hao and S. Liang, "DMMAM: Deep Multi-source Multi-task Attention Model for Intensive Care Unit Diagnosis," *Proceedings of International Conference on Database Systems for Advanced Applications. LNCS*, vol. 11447, pp. 53–69, 2019,

[7] R. Patankar, "A Survey on Computer-aided Breast Cancer Detection Using Mammograms," *Journal of Applied and Natural Science*, vol. 2, no. 1, pp. 1–6, 2019.

[8] Soufiene Ben Othman, Faris A. Almalki, Chinmay Chakraborty, Hedi Sakli, "Privacy-Preserving Aware Data Aggregation for IoT-Based Healthcare with Green Computing Technologies," *Computers and Electrical Engineering*, vol. 101, p. 108025, 2022, doi:10.1016/j.compeleceng.2022.108025.

[9] Soufiene Ben Othman, Abdullah Ali Bahattab, Abdelbasset Trad and Habib Youssef, "PEERP: A Priority-Based Energy-Efficient Routing Protocol for Reliable Data Transmission in Healthcare using the IoT," *The 15th International Conference on Future Networks and Communications (FNC) August 9–12, 2020*, Leuven, Belgium, 2020.

[10] A. V. Demidov, E. V. Udaltsova and S. M. Gerashchenko, "Development of the System for Assessment of Periodontal Tissue State," *2021 Ural Symposium on Biomedical Engineering, Radioelectronics and Information Technology (USBEREIT)*, 2021, pp. 0027–0029, doi:10.1109/USBEREIT51232.2021.9455109. https://ieeexplore.ieee.org/document/9455109

[11] Z. Shi, W. Zuo, S. Liang, X. Zuo, L. Yue and X. Li, "IDDSAM: An Integrated Disease Diagnosis and Severity Assessment Model for Intensive Care Units," *IEEE Access*, vol. 8, pp. 15423–15435, 2020, doi:10.1109/ACCESS.2020.2967417.

[12] M. Pavel et al., "Continuous Assessment of Gait Velocity in Parkinson's Disease from Unobtrusive Measurements," *2007 3rd International IEEE/EMBS Conference on Neural Engineering*, 2007, pp. 700–703, doi:10.1109/CNE.2007.369769. https://ieeexplore.ieee.org/document/4227374

[13] T. Kurata et al., "The Usefulness of a Simple Computerized Touch Panel-type Screening Test for Alzheimer's Disease Patients," *2012 ICME International Conference on Complex Medical Engineering (CME)*, 2012, pp. 215–217, doi:10.1109/ICCME.2012.6275655. https://ieeexplore.ieee.org/abstract/document/6275655

[14] H. Similä and M. Immonen, "Disease State Fingerprint for Fall Risk Assessment," in *2014 36th Annual International Conference of the IEEE Engineering in Medicine and Biology Society*, 2014, pp. 3176–3179, doi:10.1109/EMBC.2014.6944297. https://ieeexplore.ieee.org/document/6944297

[15] A. Nawar, F. Rahman, N. Krishnamurthi, A. Som and P. Turaga, "Topological Descriptors for Parkinson's Disease Classification and Regression Analysis," *2020 42nd Annual International Conference of the IEEE Engineering in Medicine & Biology Society (EMBC)*, 2020, pp. 793–797, doi:10.1109/EMBC44109.2020.9176285. https://ieeexplore.ieee.org/document/9176285

[16] Z. Li, H. Suk, D. Shen and L. Li, "Sparse Multi-Response Tensor Regression for Alzheimer's Disease Study With Multivariate Clinical Assessments," *IEEE Transactions on Medical Imaging*, vol. 35, no. 8, pp. 1927–1936, Aug. 2016, doi:10.1109/TMI.2016.2538289.

9 Robotics and the Internet of Health Things to Improve Healthcare
Especially during the COVID-19 Pandemic

Leila Ennaceur, Ben Othman Soufiene, Chinmay Chakraborty, and Sakli Hedi

CONTENTS

9.1 INTRODUCTION

Healthcare organizations around the world face the challenge of improving the quality and access to care while controlling costs in a context of growth and population aging, increased life expectancy, and tightening public spending on health. Improving care remains a major challenge, from the point of view of both patients and stakeholders. Of course, there is healthcare personnel, but above all, it is the patient in the first place. It is to him that they are addressed with care. These and other considerations motivate companies operating in the extended and complex health ecosystem to accelerate their digitization and digital transformation while making them see the opportunities that such transformation is likely to engender. Digitization certainly contributes to promoting patient involvement in their health.

DOI: 10.1201/9781003315476-9

With digital innovation, patients have the tools to become more actively involved throughout the care pathway. In other words, it empowers the patient. Care centers must have the right infrastructure that helps doctors and other stakeholders optimize processes for medical and administrative staff, leaving them more time to focus on patient follow-up. In addition, intelligent infrastructures allow patients to better control their environment to live their situation with less stress, and thus potentially improve their state of health [1].

Among the technologies that accompany this transition, we can mention the Internet of Things (IoT), with all types of machine-to-machine (M2M) interactions and communications between devices, smart sensors, etc., cloud computing, analytics, virtual reality, nanotechnology, and robotics. The development of digital in health will be a major lever to reduce overall health expenditure and help caregivers to provide quality care [2].

Nowadays, individuals are increasingly bound to live indoors, investing less energy outdoors. They rely even more on new technologies to bring a more comfortable life. Various technologies have proven to be of considerable progress in recent years. The advancement of the Internet of Things (IoT) and robotics, for example, will greatly encourage analytical and monitoring procedures in various fields. That health is proving to be a cheap field for this said technology [3]. The patients are well-controllable and treated, thanks to the advanced technologies that are characterized day after day by an excellent evolution. In the IoT, wireless IP sensors are attached to patients. Depending on the case of the patient, the doctor specifies the clinical parameters to be measured, for example, blood pressure and coronary heart rate. The IoT marks the most significant developments of this century. The IoT is a network of physical objects attached to send and receive data to other devices and systems on the Internet using sensors, software, and other technologies. The number of connected objects reaches approximately 10 billion devices, and this number will increase to 25.4 billion by 2030 [4]. This requires a more efficient protocol and method to correctly transmit a large amount of information [5].

On the other part, the impressive advances in robotics and computer science influence all activities human. Applied to medicine and surgery, such a technology bubble has made it possible to conceptualize a revolutionary paradigm known as precision medicine. In this concept of precision, the entire patient health journey is digital and controlled by automated approaches, from screening and diagnosis to treatment and follow-up. The level of precision required to optimize healthcare exceeds the limits of evidence-based medicine and the capacity of the best healthcare professionals. Robots in healthcare play an important role in doing procedures and other tasks, which previously were made by humans [6]. Robots assist patients and help the medical profession in various ways to improve people's health and well-being. They have greatly simplified many complex surgical procedures.

Technological progress is moving so fast, and the growth of medicine has progressed. However, the emergence of COVID-19 has created a huge need for even faster change, and new needs are emerging. This pandemic has turned the world upside down. In addition, increasingly, populations are growing in need of more reliable and robust health services [7]. The increase in demand for expanding healthcare capacities coincides with the progressive needs, and the new technologies are very well consumable since they have proven efficiency and the desired security.

This chapter aims to understand the use of IoT and examine the role of a robot in healthcare management. We detail how IoT and wireless systems work to achieve reliable healthcare applications at lower cost. Therefore, we begin this chapter with the challenges faced by health centers in the treatment of patients with contagious diseases and highlight the physical and mental influence of the COVID-19 pandemic on caregivers. Faced with these challenges, governments around the world have felt the need for new technologies. In the next section, we discuss the role of new technologies in care and the benefit that can be presented. The following section describes IoT technology in healthcare with main applications and uses cases as well as the components of an intelligent IoT-aided system. In the last section, the role of robotic technology and how robots improve healthcare outcomes are discussed.

9.2   A PARTICULARLY EXCEPTIONAL PANDEMIC DUE TO ITS IMPACT ON CAREGIVERS

The disease spread rapidly across the planet from January 2020, filling hospitals overwhelmed by massive arrivals of patients with severe forms of the disease and resulting in a dramatic increase in death in the world, even within the care services. The indirect health issues of such a pandemic are at least twofold: the potential physical impact of hard work on a huge flow of seriously affected patients and the psychological impact on caregivers. Health services are strained by the pandemic, caregivers are on the front lines. They sounded the alert, and some died of the disease.

Frontline caregivers face many challenges: contact with patients with a high viral load, and therefore a high risk of contamination, physical fatigue, layout of workspaces, adaptation to rigid working conditions, lack of equipment, enormous number of deaths among the patients, colleagues, or relatives; ethical issues related to decision-making in an unstable health system [8]. The health system should provide a healthy working environment for caregivers.

As part of the response to COVID-19, health workers may be exposed to various occupational risks of illness, injury, and in some cases even death. These occupational hazards vary by work setting and may be contamination with the COVID-19 virus, skin conditions, stress, discomfort from prolonged use of personal protective equipment (PPE), exposure to toxins due to the misuse of disinfectants, psychological distress, chronic fatigue, as well as the risk of being the victim of physical and psychological violence and harassment.

According to the interim guidelines of the World Health Organization [9], to mitigate these dangers and ensure the safety and well-being of health workers, it is mandatory to put in place correct and well-functioning measures: coordinate for the control of hygiene and the follow-up of the disinfection of the premises, to make the good management of the health personnel, and to ensure the mental health and psychosocial support.

Healthcare workers are subject to an increased risk of occupational diseases in the absence of adequate safety measures, which consequently causes a high rate of absenteeism and a decline in productivity and quality of care.

9.3 SMART HEALTHCARE AND NEW TECHNOLOGIES

As one of the main drivers of developed economies, healthcare is undergoing a major revolution propelled by the increasingly personalized needs of patients. Knowledge has become the engine of change and technology for health will play a key role in this development. New advances in the field of medical imaging, for example, would enable various industrial and research players to play a central role. They would be the main beneficiaries of the new trends [10]. e-Health will play an increasingly important role in the way we receive medical care [11].

The use of new information and communication technologies (ICT) will make it possible to evolve toward a new model offering a smarter and much more patient-centered approach to health services [12].

Here are some examples of new information and communication technologies that have the potential to radically transform healthcare, as we know it today.

- **Artificial Intelligence:** Integrated into healthcare management, artificial intelligence will play an important role in the evolution of diagnostic and therapeutic processes [13]. Allowing the analysis of huge amounts of information, records, imaging results, etc. will significantly speed up searches. Robots will also play a leading role in the use of new technologies applicable to medicine. They already make it possible to improve the communication skills of autistic children and to carry out remote operations.
- **Mobile Apps:** The use of mobile devices to complement medical care can improve the relationship between healthcare professionals and, of course, the relationship between doctor and patient. Other applications, which will allow patients to store their information and monitor their health from mobile devices, are in development.
- **Telehealth:** It consists of using computer technologies to access health services remotely. The word telehealth refers to the entire health system that encompasses all kinds of activities such as education, awareness, and prevention programs, as well as diagnosis, self-care, and treatment. Providing access to these various services is particularly useful for people with reduced mobility, isolated, or living in rural areas. Examples of telehealth services include portals for making doctor appointments or viewing test results as well as videoconferencing systems between doctors and specialists or between doctor and patient.
- **Telemedicine:** It is one of the main branches of telehealth. In particular, it makes it possible to exchange medical information using electronic communication systems. Telemedicine makes it possible to provide health services when distance is a problem.
- **Wearable Devices:** These are biosensors allowing the surveillance and monitoring of different aspects of patient health. It is thus possible to detect diseases and control them in a much less intrusive way, which is one of the foundations of this new concept of technology for health.

The development of digital and its uses has led to the digitization of the health sector. Thanks to this, a change is taking place. The objective goes beyond treating the patient, but also to prevent the diseases that will take place. The patient is also placed at the heart of the care process. The development of the Internet and connected devices have changed the behavior of patients who now go online for information.

It is therefore important to be able to prevent diseases and to be able to educate people about their health. Scientific progress will thus make it possible to discuss new care methodologies based on prevention to improve services and the success rate of medical interventions. Prevention can also be achieved with artificial intelligence integrated with robots and the IoT (Internet of Things).

9.4 IOT INTEGRATED IN HEALTHCARE: USE CASES AND APPLICATIONS

The Internet of Things (IoT) can be applied everywhere, and it influences the quality of life. Broadband Internet is available in most homes and is becoming a necessary tool in our daily lives. Wi-Fi connections and sensors have been integrated into many ranges of home appliances. All these factors have paved the way for the IoT to become even more integrated into people's daily lives, as well as in many fields such as economics, especially health.

Today, everyday objects can be monitored remotely via an Internet connection. Machine learning algorithms can detect anomalies in monitored objects, send alerts, and trigger programmable solutions.

IoT technology has already begun to transform the health sector, various needs and applications are emerging, based on the great potential that this technology promises; its integration is taking place at a considerable pace. This technological portal has enabled patients to become more involved in digital health. They become able to access their medical records, choose appointments, and communicate with their doctors. Patients who suffer from long-term assignments are more comfortable because their health is monitored in real time from their homes. This is advantageous for the care services since it ensures permanent monitoring of the condition of the patients.

IoT integrates with electronic devices that harvest information and transmits it to the appropriate destination. These devices will then be able to automatically trigger certain events. These devices can be a thermometer, blood pressure monitors, glucometers, and even smart beds, mobile X-ray machines, and ultrasound units [14].

In general, medical devices are grouped into three major kinds [15]:

- **Fixed Medical Devices:** Here we are talking about devices used in various clinical applications in surgery, imaging, laboratory, monitoring, etc.
- **Portable External Devices:** These are biosensors devices that control physiological data. These devices measure temperature, blood pressure, glucose, oxygen level, electrocardiogram (ECG) [16], etc.
- **Integrated Medical Devices:** These devices are integrated into the human body that replaces, follow, or correct a biological structure, for example, an integrated infusion pump.

9.4.1 IoT-Healthcare Use Cases

IoT in healthcare is growing rapidly. In particular, the ability of connected devices to monitor health constants, route data, provide alerts, administer medications, and automate critical processes are the reasons for this rapid integration. In the medical industry, the Internet of Things technology is included in all care applications, whether it is medical clothing, patient monitoring or access to care, temperature monitoring of pharmaceutical products to improve precision, to give more efficiency with less expensive costs, to meet even more standards that results in more safety.

The term "Health IoT" or HIoT or IoMT for the Internet of Medical Things has been coined to describe this rich and buoyant market for healthcare applications that are attracting the attention of the medical industry and consequently that of governments throughout the world [17]. This vision is still well-supported by the appearance of rapidly transmissible diseases between individuals. The prime example here is the COVID-19 pandemic, which has in one way or another required a solicitous use of new technologies to deal with its spread. Technological innovations here, such as IoT, are called to play a crucial role in different fields.

IoT is embedded in various healthcare applications, whether for clinical care or remote monitoring [15].

- **Remote Clinical Control:** Hospitalized patients, especially those in critical conditions, must be under constant and close supervision. Thus, the medical profession can react as quickly as possible in the event of an emergency, and therefore contributes to increasing the chances of saving a patient's life. Necessary patient health information is collected through medical sensors based on Internet Protocol IP. For further examination and analysis, caregivers using the Internet connection can read clinical parameters collected from the patient.
- **Remote Monitoring:** The elderly and people with chronic diseases, cases of cardiovascular disease, for example, must be monitored all the time. Thus, people with disabilities lead increasingly independent and simple lives. The remote-control solution avoids the movement of patients to the care center and provides security because their health is monitored by specialists [18].
- Indeed, it happens that certain variations in the patient's clinical parameters go unnoticed and may cause a subsequent emergency point. Thanks to sensors and control platforms, the history of clinical parameter values shared on dedicated backup servers can be used for a diagnosis that specifies the exact condition of the patient, and therefore leads to the right treatment. Alerts can be submitted from monitoring platforms indicating severity.
- **Hygiene Control in Health Centers**. Many sanitary applications require hygiene control, and this has become fundamental during the COVID-19 pandemic that has taken over the world. Internet of Things technology is proving to have good capabilities for contactless applications and remote connectivity. The IoT is included in medical health applications without or with low contact: monitoring of air quality, temperature, control of hand hygiene, sterilization of work instruments, control of vital parameters of patients, pathogen detection, etc.

An example of this is the Clean Hands Safe Hands product in sanitary stations, which is based on Bluetooth technology. The stations are activated by sensors and trigger hygiene reminders to staff. The system records hand hygiene activities throughout the healthcare system and based on sensors can uniquely identify each employee. This system allows a specific time for hand disinfection before the sensor registers the event for any person entering a room.

9.4.2 IoT-Healthcare Applications

Today, healthcare is not just about treatment. The goal here is to promote healthy habits to improve worker health and safety. Health monitoring solutions that promote injury reduction are now being designed. These solutions in day-to-day practice save companies' huge amounts of money each year in lost productivity and workers' compensation due to injuries and workplace accidents in general.

- **Contact Detection:** Wearable devices mark a huge growth velocity for IoT in healthcare, thanks to advancements in wireless technologies such as Bluetooth. The KINETIC company has designed an intelligent work garment REFLEX to improve worker safety through self-feedback [19]. It is an ultra-compact device with a very small size. During the movement of the worker, the device triggers a low vibration if the worker performs an improper lifting or movement that could cause damage. This device is specially designed for companies whose employees perform physical movements with more muscular effort. At the end of the work session, the employee and the supervisor can view the saved report, which presents the data recorded during the work period of the day. This technology, once adopted, marks a dramatic reduction in dangerous movements. It is based on communication technologies that offer high performance and low power consumption for increased efficiency and reliability. This portable solution can be applied to care centers, nurses, and technicians mainly when caring for patients.
- **Autonomous Drug Distribution Solution**: Nowadays, the use of IoT in the field of health meets a very vast need. For example, the permanent control and management of the correct intake of medication in clinics, hospitals, and care establishments are now possible. We cite the example of the Medication on Demand (MOD) product, which is the first Patient Managed Analgesic Device (PCA) developed by Avancen. It is a healthcare IoT solution that reliably dispenses painkillers using a PRN (abbreviation of the Latin word "pro re nata," which means as needed) dispensing mode. Patients can then self-administer their oral analgesics [20]. This product is well secured. It is obviously subject to clinical examinations to avoid problems related to safety or overdoses. The patient swipes an RFID wristband close to the locked device configured to administer the necessary treatment dose as part of the medical prescription written by the doctor.
- **3D Imaging Technology:** IoT technology in the field of medical imaging has evolved rapidly. Faster processors process and deliver medical images

at higher resolutions. An innovative use case is the need to accurately measure wounds, whether new wounds or wounds in the process of healing. British medical imaging company Eykona has designed a system called Wound Measurement System. This system monitors the evolution of injuries over time. It is in fact equipped with cameras and promotes 3D images to photograph the progression of the injury. Clinicians observe the changes in the shape of the tissues and therefore judge the effectiveness of the treatment [21].

- **Pharmaceutical Temperature Monitoring and Compliance:** During the COVID-19 pandemic, the world has experienced a new and emerging need to maintain strict temperatures for medicines, vaccines, and pharmaceuticals in general. Smart Sense is part of Digi International that provides IoT-based monitoring solutions for supply chain monitoring in specific medical applications [22]. Their solution, Digi's Smart Sense for Healthcare, enables temperature monitoring and thus fills a critical need. With the COVID-19 pandemic, the development of vaccines to combat the spread of the COVID-19 virus has faced new manufacturing challenges that required certain specific conditions. Smart Sense said its pharmaceutical monitoring solution meets Centers for Disease Control and Prevention (CDC) requirements for handling COVID-19 vaccines throughout the vaccine cycle, right from the cold chain, from manufacturers to end suppliers.

- **For Emergency Response:** First responders play a fundamental role in the cycle of care and the effectiveness of interventions. They take care of the injured and guide the ambulances along the route to get patients to hospital services as soon as possible. This requires a fast and reliable GPS connection. The purpose of the FirstNet wireless networking site is to provide emergency personnel with the ability to make priority and preventative mobile calls during large-scale public emergencies when networks are congested. This FirstNet solution has been integrated by IoT solution providers like Digi International into cellular devices and certifies them for use on networks [23]. These devices are further deployed for critical communications in emergency vehicles such as ambulances and civil protection and again in intelligent traffic management systems.

- **IoT for Remote Surgery**: With the innovation of faster processors, fast data transfer speeds, and reduced latency, thanks to the fifth generation of standards for mobile telephony, 5G networks, the speed of innovation in medical technologies, and more security, the use of IoT in the health sector promotes a radical change in this sector [24].

Today, the medical industry and technological innovations are focused on the development of next-generation medical devices that increase the precision of care, improve remote healthcare and telemedicine cases, and promote robotic and further assisted surgeries by video. Thanks to this automation of medical acts, health professionals will have advanced diagnostic possibilities, thanks to IoT technology and other innovative technologies such as robotics, artificial intelligence, and machine learning.

9.4.3 Components of Intelligent Healthcare IoT-Aided System

In the general context of healthcare, IoT devices work together to improve the habitual activity in question. The IoT devices, which have just replaced the control carried out by the human being, must give various information on the patients' state, their activities, their environment, and a clear idea of the patient's condition and thus specify the nature of the medical intervention that must be carried out. IoT technology in healthcare is represented through a model, which brings into play the various components integrated from the sensors placed on the patient side, whether admitted to a care center or at home. This model [25] is organized into four layers: starting with the sensor layer which dialogues directly with the network layer. This is made up of equipment equipped with wireless technologies to collect data and transfer it to equipment in the cloud layer. At this level, the data is saved on dedicated servers to transmit it to the health applications developed adapted to computers or installed on smartphones or tablets. At this stage, the information is used by the medical staff who can finally monitor the patients concerned in real time. Again, the history of clinical parameters can be viewed as needed. It is a vast database for further scientific research.

9.5 ROBOTS IMPROVE HEALTHCARE OUTCOMES

Medical surgery has had radical changes with the appearance of robots in the health sector, which allow delivery, disinfection, and thus promote more time for caregivers to be even more close to the sick. The Intel Company is working on technologies that ensure the development of robotics in the medical field [21]. Robotic arm technologies in surgery appeared for more than 40 years and represent the first robots in the medical field. Subsequently, several innovative technologies have brought new advancements to healthcare robotics. The use of medical robotics, a growing field in the health industry, presents added value in certain surgical procedures and greater efficiency in health centers. Nowadays, robots are used in the operating room as well as in clinical settings to improve the care services offered to patients. In the period of pandemic caused by the coronavirus, many health centers are resorting to use robots in broad use cases to reduce exposure to pathogens. The robots are endowed with an operational efficiency that allows the reduction of risks. Again, robots can prepare and clean patient rooms autonomously, thereby reducing interpersonal contact in some cases of easily transmitted diseases. Robots equipped with AI-based drug identification software save time in identifying, matching, and dispensing drugs to admitted patients [22]. Advancement in technology has allowed robots to operate more autonomously and in some use cases, they perform certain tasks completely autonomously. As a result, hospitalized patients will be surrounded with greater empathy. In this way, the benefits of robotics in the field of health are varied. Robotics provides healthcare with improved quality, effective clinical interventions, and a healthy work environment for caregivers.

- **Patient Care:** Medical robots allow personalized and permanent monitoring of patients with chronic diseases, and social monitoring of the elderly. In this way, robots reduce workloads, and caregivers can pay more attention to patients and more human interaction.

- **Efficiency at Work:** These robots can follow the inventory to make the necessary orders, and thus ensure that supplies, equipment, and medicines are available according to the work schedule. For disinfecting and preparing hospital rooms for new admissions, robots runs faster and more reliably.
- **A Safe Working Environment:** Service robots transport supplies and linens to hospitals where exposure to pathogens is a risk. For cleaning and disinfection robots, the exposure to pathogens becomes reduced which helps to reduce nosocomial infections. While social robots also help lift heavy loads of bed fittings or patients, thereby reducing the physical burden on healthcare workers. In the field of health, robotics thus provides high-quality healthcare for patients, and a safer work environment for patients and caregivers. Robotics is now integrated into various medical procedures.
- **Surgical Robots:** They help surgeons perform more procedures that are specific. Robots equipped with AI can reach specific areas of the human body. Surgeons have the ability in some cases to monitor surgical operations from a console and entrust robots with the ability to perform tasks autonomously with almost no human intervention. This regenerated video stream can be broadcast allowing surgeons to benefit from communication with professionals in their field. In this way, patients benefit from being followed in the operation by experts.
- AI is even more involved in robotics, which brings more evolution. On the other hand, computer tracking allows robots to distinguish tissue types and thus avoid nerves and muscles that appear in the field of view during surgery. It is a computerized "high-definition 3D vision" that provides specific information and increased performance during medical interventions. Robotics also plays a major role in the training of surgeons. For example, during the simulation, artificial intelligence makes it possible to train new surgeons in surgical robotics. They are then able to perform surgical procedures and improve their skills.
- **Modular Robots**: They are therapeutic robots and are configured to perform several functions. Therapy robots can be used, for example, after a stroke. These robots, equipped with AI and surveillance cameras can control and measure movements in various positions and monitor progress. They can also communicate with patients to offer moral support, guidance, and encouragement.
- **Service Robots:** They lighten the heavy daily workload of healthcare workers. Most of these robots work autonomously and send a report when they complete a task. These robots prepare patient rooms, track supply delivery, and classify purchase orders, restock cabinets with medical supplies, and transport laundry. Having service robots perform a few routine tasks allows healthcare staff to focus on the urgent needs of patients.
- **Social Robots:** They communicate directly with humans. They are used in care facilities to provide social and moral monitoring. They can encourage patients to fit into their treatment regimens, keeping patients alert and optimistic. They can also be used in care centers to guide visitors and

patients. Overall, tireless social robots reduce the workload of caregivers and improve the emotional health of patients.

- **Mobile Robots**: These robots move along a programmed path in hospitals and clinics. They are used for a wide variety of purposes: disinfecting rooms, accompanying patients, or moving heavy machinery. These robots use ultraviolet (UV) light to help disinfect high-use areas.
- **Autonomous Robots**. Autonomous robots with a robust set of cameras move toward patients in exam rooms or patient rooms, allowing clinicians to interact with them remotely. Robots controlled by a remote third party can also be next to doctors during their visits. These robots monitor their levels of electrical charges and move to charging stations as needed. These robots are used in infectious disease departments, operating theaters, analytical laboratories, and hospital waiting rooms. The start-up Akara has developed an autonomous robot prototype used to disinfect contaminated surfaces using UV light, thus contributing to the fight against COVID-19. Industrial robot has quickly become commonplace in factories around the world. With the integration of the robotic aspect in the IoT, it continues to gain popularity. The robot and the Internet of Things become two related technologies. Until now, the robotics and IoT communities have been driven by varied, but very related goals. The IoT is all about supporting services for ubiquitous sensing, monitoring, and tracking. The robotic community focuses on production action, interaction, and autonomous behavior. Broader situational awareness is given to the robot through IoT sensor technologies. This leads to better task performance. By creating a robotic Internet of Things, a high added value would be increased.

9.6 ROBOTIC AND IOT TO DEAL WITH COVID-19 CASES

The Internet of Things improves robot-to-robot or robot-to-human learning in which robots interact and adapt their behaviors through shared programs and data collected from IoT sensors. The latter is used in robotics to help and manage their movements, such as detecting an obstacle or manipulating the objects for which they are responsible. Many tasks requiring contact with a dangerous environment are entrusted to robots.

Today, IoT sensors are connected to robots in an innovative way, say IoRT Robotic Internet of Things. The latter brings together huge piles of sensor data assembled from different objects to increase the detection capabilities of robots. The robots will be able to process huge data using reliable and inexpensive advanced computing that allows them to make appropriate decisions in real time. The coupling of robotics and IoT in the healthcare industry proves to have several advantages [23].

- **Safe Working Environment:** In recent years, the demand for the use of robots has been increasing in medicine. In the workplace, the use of robots brings benefit, whether in terms of efficiency, precision, or even additional safety. IoT-enabled robots can identify and diagnose problems and react with more performance. The integration of IoT with robotics makes it possible to track various objects and collect remotely controllable parameters.

- **Quality Care Service:** Medical robots can help medical staff provide scheduled and permanent monitoring of patients with chronic diseases, contagious diseases, and social monitoring for the elderly. As a result, robots minimize workload, and caregivers can give patients more attention and moral support.
- **Operational Efficiency:** These tireless robots automate daily tasks, minimizing the physical demands of workers while guaranteeing a reliable quality of service. These robots can deliver supplies, equipment, and medicines to patients, for example, in health services. Easily disinfectable robots quickly clean and disinfect hospital rooms.

As technology evolves, areas of IoT robotics integration will further advance, aiming for new perspectives for healthcare services, especially in response to the coronavirus disease. Noncontact technology can ensure people's safety and quickly determine product contamination and sick people. The IoRT analyzes and improves disinfection procedures using a range of installed sensors. The robots carry out contactless disinfection of areas and objects in a robust and reliable manner. The IoT-assisted robotic system is a wireless solution that provides advanced robotic services by interconnecting multiple robots with the intelligent environment. This is an example treated in Ref. [24], which highlights an intelligent system based on robotics and IoT, applicable in the field of health. The solution is very useful for treating patients with COVID-19 in an extended care center, as is the case when treating a huge flow of infected patients every day. Let's now talk about subsystems consisting of a single robot that communicates directly with the COVID-19 patient. The permanent monitoring and control of the condition of COVID-19 patients exposes medical personnel to the risk of contamination. The robot become a relay between the doctor and the patient. Mixing IoT and robotic technology gives birth to an "Internet of Robotic Things" (IoRT) system; these different technologies are developing in parallel. This intelligent system to fight the propagation of the coronavirus diseases ensures body distancing in hospitals and quarantine houses. We seek through this solution to benefit from [26]:

- A permanent control of patients infected with the virus of COVID-19 and monitoring the progress of processing from a dashboard.
- Ensure physical distancing that minimizes the risk of contamination.
- Intervention at the right time when needed.

The system is modeled through a three-layer architecture.

Patients infected with the COVID-19 virus are placed together separated by 3 m. Each patient is equipped with portable sensors (PPA for Patient Personal Agregater) that detect the biomedical parameters and communicate them to a Collector (Rc for Room Collector) placed in each patient room. On the second level, the robot moves through the corridor of the sick rooms. Going back and forth, it receives information from the Rc of each room. The robot acts as a relay between the subsystem installed in the hospital represented by the biomedical sensors and the cloud servers, which record the database of each patient. Robots combined with IoT technology form an intelligent system that safeguards the health of caregivers. Being a relay between caregivers and patients, this solution guarantees a healthy working environment in the COVID-19 departments of hospitals. The robot (Ro) moves along a well-defined path programmed to be able to communicate with the RCs. The RO moves in the service corridor near the sick rooms and ensures that these values are sent to the appropriate cloud servers. The doctor from the monitoring room and with a permanent Internet connection (HS) can follow the situation of the patients in real time. Through this system, when some values are achieved, alerts can be generated indicating the seriousness of a patient's situation.

9.7   CONCLUSION

This raises the question of the future use of robotics and IoT in the field of health. These healthcare technologies are evolving alongside advances in deep learning, computer vision, big data, and other technologies. These various innovations provide robots with new functionalities to perform tasks more autonomously and reliably. The medical industry collaborates with technology providers and research labs to profile the next generation of robotic solutions. By providing technical and research support, these companies help uncover innovative implications for AI and IoT technologies in medical robotics.

These contributions are the foundation of progressive innovations that increase automation, improve efficiency, and find solution for some of the biggest challenges in healthcare.

REFERENCES

1. Banu Çalış Uslu, Ertuğ Okay, Erkan Dursun, "Analysis of factors affecting IoT-based smart hospital design", *Journal of Cloud Computing*, vol. 9, pp. 1–23, November 2020, https://doi.org/10.1186/s13677-020-00215-5.
2. Alessandro Monaco, Katie Palmer, Nicolaj Holm Ravn Faber, Irene Ohler, Mitchell Ilva, Anita Vatland, Joop van Griensven, Mariano Votta, Donna Walsh, Vincent Clay, Mehmet Cuneyt Yazicioglu, Danute Ducinskiene, "Digital Health Tools for Managing Noncommunicable Diseases During and After the COVID-19 Pandemic: Perspectives of Patients and Caregivers", JMIR Publications, January 2021.
3. Mostafa Haghi, Andre Geissler, Heidi Fleischer, Norbert Stoll, Kerstin Thurow, "Ubiqsense: A Personal Wearable in Ambient Parameters Monitoring Based on IoT Platform", IEEE, 2019.
4. Lionel Sujay Vailshery, "Number of Internet of Things (IoT) Connected Devices Worldwide from 2019 to 2030", available at: www.statista.com/statistics/1183457/iot-connected-devices-worldwide/, March 17, 2022.
5. H.H. Attar, A.A.A. Solyman, A. Alrosan, C. Chinmay, R.K. Mohammad, "Deterministic Cooperative Hybrid Ring-mesh Network Coding for Big Data Transmission Over Lossy Channels in 5G Networks", *EURASIP Journal on Wireless Communications and Networking*, vol. 1–18, p. 159, 2021, https://doi.org/10.1186/s13638-021-02032-z
6. Meshal Alotaibi, Mohammad Yamin, "Role of Robots in Healthcare Management", IEEE, 2019.

7. Sera Whitelaw, Mamas A. Mamas, Eric Topol, Harriette G. C. Van Spall, "Applications of Digital Technology in COVID-19 Pandemic Planning and Response", Elsevier, March 2021.

8. Maria Cohut, "Heightened Challenges: How the Pandemic Impacts Caregivers", available at: www.medicalnewstoday.com/articles/heightened-challenges-how-the-pandemic-impacts-caregivers, May 29, 2020.

9. "COVID-19: Occupational Health and Safety for Health Workers", *Interim Guidance*, February 2, 2021.

10. S. Yogesh, C. Chinmay, "Augmented Reality and Virtual Reality Transforming Spinal Imaging Landscape: A Feasibility Study", *IEEE Computer Graphics and Applications*, vol. 41, issue 3, pp. 124–138, 2021, doi:10.1109/MCG.2020.3000359

11. Raazia Saher, Madiha Anjum, "Role of Technology in COVID-19 Pandemic", Elsevier, April 2021.

12. G.S. Fischer, R.D.R. Righi, V.F. Rodrigues, C.A. da Costa, "Use of Internet of Things with Data Prediction on Healthcare Environments: A Survey", *International Journal of E-Health and Medical Communications (IJEHMC)*, vol 11, issue 2, pp. 1–9, April 2020.

13. Rushabh Shah, Alina Chircu, "IOT and AI in Healthcare: A Systematic Literature Review", *Issues in Information Systems*, vol 19, issue 3, pp. 33–41, 2018.

14. Vinay Chamola, Vikas Hassija, Vatsal Gupta, Mohsen Guizani, "A Comprehensive Review of the COVID-19 Pandemic and the Role of IoT, Drones, AI, Blockchain, and 5G in Managing Its Impact", *IEEE Access*, vol. 8, pp. 90225–90265, May 2020, http://doi.org/10.1109/ACCESS.2020.2992341.

15. Twana Mustafa, Asaf Varol, "Review of the Internet of Things for Healthcare Monitoring", *2020 8th International Symposium on Digital Forensics and Security (ISDFS)*, 1–6, June 2020, http://doi.org/10.1109/ISDFS49300.2020.9116305.

16. K.R. Sravanth, P. Anudeep, S. Sudha, C. Chinmay, "Comparison of Attention and Meditation based Mobile Applications by Using EEG Signals", *IEEE: Global Wireless Summit (GWS-SS)*, 260–265, 25–28 November 2018, http://doi.org/10.1109/GWS.2018.8686634

17. Jorge Calvillo-Arbizu, Isabel Román-Martínez, Javier Reina-Tosina, "Internet of Things in Health: Requirements, Issues, and Gaps", Elsevier, 2021.

18. C. Chinmay, B. Gupta, S.K. Ghosh, "Tele-wound Monitoring through Smartphone", IEEE: International Conference on Medical Imaging, m-Health and Emerging Communication Systems (MedCom), 197–201, November 2014.

19. "Kinetic Creates an Innovative Wearable That Reduces Workplace Injuries and Increases Safety Using Digi IoT Solutions", available at: www.digi.com/customer-stories/kinetic-wearable-reduces-workplace-injuries.

20. "Avancen Transforms Delivery of Oral Pain Medications with Digi System on Module", available at: www.digi.com/customer-stories/avancen-transforms-delivery-oral-pain-medication.

21. Soufiene Ben Othman, Abdullah Ali Bahattab, Abdelbasset Trad, Habib Youssef, "PEERP: A Priority-Based Energy-Efficient Routing Protocol for Reliable Data Transmission in Healthcare using the IoT", *The 15th International Conference on Future Networks and Communications (FNC) August 9–12, 2020*, Leuven, Belgium, 2020.

22. "Dispositifs médicaux & progrès en robotique, les innovations technologiques médicales", Snitem - Décembre 2017 N° 12 - Page 1–28. https://www.snitem.fr/

23. R. Kevunie, "Robot est Internet des Objets: La technologie en évolution rapide", available at: www.objetconnecte.com/robot-iot-evolution-rapide/, September 2020.

24. Soufiene Ben Othman, Faris A. Almalki, Chinmay Chakraborty, Hedi Sakli, "Privacy-Preserving Aware Data Aggregation for IoT-Based Healthcare with Green Computing Technologies", *Computers and Electrical Engineering*, vol 101, p. 108025, 2022, https://doi.org/10.1016/j.compeleceng.2022.108025.

25. Ali Behmanesh, Nasrin Sayfouri, Farahnaz Sadoughi, "Technological Features of Internet of Things in Medicine: A Systematic Mapping Study", *Wireless Communications and Mobile Computing,* vol. 2020, Article ID 9238614, 27 pages, July 2020, https://doi.org/10.1155/2020/9238614.

26. Ennaceur Leila, Soufiene Ben Othman, Hedi Sakli, "An Internet of Robotic Things System for Combating Coronavirus Disease Pandemic (COVID-19)", *International Conference on Sciences and Techniques of Automatic Control and Computer Engineering (STA)*, IEEE, March 2022.

10 Artificial Intelligence at the Service of the Detection of COVID-19

Rabiaa Tbibe, Ben Othman Soufiene,
Chinmay Chakraborty, and Sakli Hedi

CONTENTS

10.1 INTRODUCTION

Since late December 2019, the world has been living a daily struggle with COVID-19. Because of its rapid spread, this virus has put the entire world in an unprecedented situation, bringing life to a halt all around the globe and killing thousands of people. Sneezing, coughing, and respiratory droplets are all common ways this infection spreads from person to person. Coughing, fever, and breathlessness are common symptoms of the virus, which can result in pneumonia, multiple organ failure, and death (see Figure 10.1).

Although many vaccines have been made that may help to slow the virus transmission and assist in the development of immunity through the production of appropriate antibodies, many problems are encountered in the administration of the vaccine, such as supply problems, convincing people of the necessity of vaccination, and satisfaction with the vaccines. But even with the availability of a vaccine, the

DOI: 10.1201/9781003315476-10

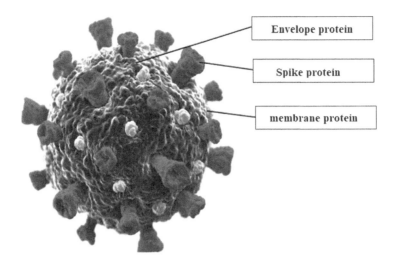

FIGURE 10.1   Modeling of COVID-19.

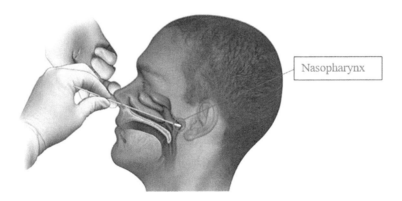

FIGURE 10.2   RT-PCR sampling.

most important factor in combating and containing the coronavirus is the effective and early detection of infected patients, so that they can obtain treatment and care right and isolate them to stop the virus from spreading and breaking the infectious cycle [1]. The RT-PCR (Figure 10.2) test is the primary screening approach used to diagnose COVID-19, which is a long, arduous, and sophisticated manual process that requires expert medical professionals. Furthermore, the sensitivity of RT-PCR testing varies greatly. As a result, there is a pressing need to develop new automated approaches for diagnosing COVID-19 that are both faster and more accurate [2].

In this context, convolutional neural networks and deep learning methods are highlighted, as well as their efficacy in computer vision and medical imaging. In this chapter, we describe a set of the most prominent recently proposed strategies for detecting COVID-19 utilizing artificial intelligence technologies.

The chapter is structured as follows: Section 10.2 presents the different technologies to combat COVID-19. In Section 10.3, deep learning algorithms and chest pictures are utilized to demonstrate a variety of COVID-19 detection approaches. Section 10.4 finishes with a conclusion and suggestions for future research.

10.2 TECHNOLOGIES TO COMBAT COVID-19

The development of information and communication technology is one of the most prominent manifestations of the last quarter of the last century and the beginning of this century. Scientists specialized in this field believe that the development of the information technology industry is the most important technological achievement that has been achieved. Before the start of the COVID-19 pandemic, the fields of communication and the information revolution of all kinds were racing against time in providing solutions and initiatives in the field of healthcare, so it was necessary to offer what it had in the battle with the pandemic and to employ its enormous potential to seize the historical moment.

- The skin temperature, heart and respiratory rates, and the level of activity and sleep in order to allow self-diagnosis of the first symptoms of the coronavirus.
- Connected "smart" mask: It is a reusable mask that connects via Bluetooth to a smartphone and monitor breathing and air and enables you to know when the filter needs to be replaced.
- Portable air purifier: This battery-powered device absorbs particles to clean the air and eliminate the "coronavirus."
- Disinfecting robot: It is a UV lamp, which can move around the room on its own to completely clean surfaces and eliminate pathogens, including the coronavirus.
- Mobile application: It is imposed by some countries to monitor and track comprehensive quarantine.
- Drones: Many developed countries have adopted drones to deliver vaccines.

These new technologies have also contributed in the following ways:

- Providing healthcare to the right people at the right time.
- Making the best choices and reducing time and effort.
- Facilitating access to available medical information at the global and local levels.

10.3 DETECTION OF COVID-19 BY CHEST IMAGES

Over several decades, CXR (chest radiography) and CT (computed tomography) have proven effective in diagnosing many diseases, including pneumonia. It has recently been used to detect and diagnose COVID-19 [3]. However, the major issue here, is that each image's reading and extracting manually the crucial information takes time and requires the expertise of a radiologist. With the advent of data science and artificial intelligence algorithms, CAD (computer-aided diagnostic) systems that integrate image processing technology can benefit doctors in the diagnosis of COVID-19, and help deliver a best knowledge of sickness development, thanks to the introduction of data science and artificial intelligence algorithms [4]. We can now analyze medical data and classify lung images in record time, without the need for radiologists. Recently, several researchers have introduced COVID-19 disclosure methods, based on convolutional neural networks (CNN), which are characterized by automatic feature extraction from the data themselves, without human intervention [5]. The next section presents some of this work.

10.3.1 The Solution of Panwar et al.

Panwar et al. [6] presented a method to find out COVID-19 patients by analyzing chest images of lungs and determining whether a person is a carrier of the virus or not. The suggested model is based on the nCOVnet network, a multilayered artificial neural network, and is expert in processing large data volume with high accuracy and lower computational cost. The fundamental framework of this network consists of the convolution, aggregation, flattening and layers that are entirely connected, as illustrated in Figure 10.3.

In this method, VGG16 is adopted as the basic model to extract the features of the database, and which consists of five layers, as shown in Figure 10.4. Despite

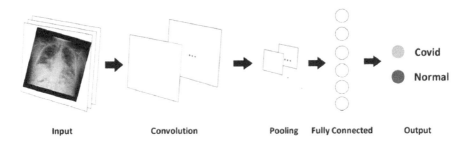

FIGURE 10.3   Basic architecture of the proposed network.

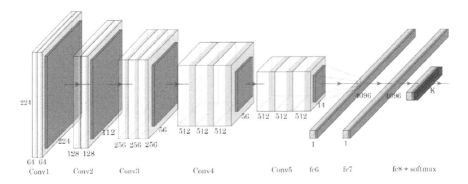

FIGURE 10.4   The architecture of the VGG-16 networks.

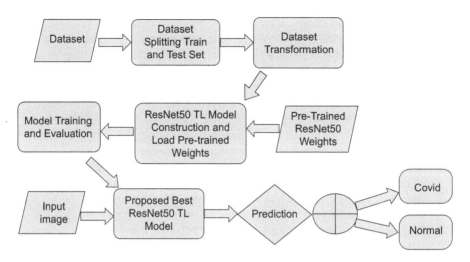

FIGURE 10.5   The diagram of the proposed methodology.

the power of the VGG16 network, this study achieved a limited overall accuracy of 88.10%.

10.3.2   THE SOLUTION OF HOSSAIN ET AL.

In Ref. [7], Hossain et al. present a method to determine whether COVID-19 is present in X-ray images, using transfer learning (TL) on a ResNet50 model. The first time, Hussein et al. used ten different weights pretrained on ResNet50, using many approaches like supervised learning, self-supervised learning, and other techniques. The ten pretrained models are ChestX-ray14, ChexPert, ImageNet, ImageNet_ChestX-ray14, ImageNet_ChxPert, iNat2021_Supervised, iNat2021_Supervised_from_Scratch, rvis2021_Mini_SwAV_v1k, MoCo_v1, and MoCo_v2 (see Figure 10.5).

Then, after suggesting the best TL model, they add two fully connected layers to the default ResNet50 model to apply fine adjustment.

10.3.3   THE SOLUTION OF SAKSHI ET AL.

Sakshi et al. [8] introduced a novel method COVID-19 virus detection, using computed tomography. This proposed model is mainly based on three main steps. Figure 10.6 shows the proposed methodology's hierarchical representation.

- **First Phase (Data Augmentation):** The data type of the image input is changed, the images are resized before being used, and the input images are normalized to ensure that the CT pictures are compatible with the selected transmission models. As we explained earlier, four different transfer learning models were chosen (ResNets18, ResNets50, ResNets101, and Squeezenet), each with different requirements for the input size. Thus, the sizes of the input images must correspond to each of them; to keep every-thing the same, the supplied images are reduced in size to $256 \times 256 \times 3$ pixels. Hence amidst the learning transfer process, the image dimensions are adjusted one more time. The data was split into two categories: 90% for train and 10% for test, and then applied augmentation of the training data using random rotation, translation, and reflection.

- **Second Phase (Learning Models):** The training-augmented images are resized based on compatibility with several pretrained CNN models. At this stage, the performance of all models is compared. For training, the authors used the SGDM optimizer (see Figure 10.6).

- **Third Phase (Localization of the Anomaly Using a Deeper Layer):** In the third phase of the suggested framework, the most effective model is chosen and implemented for the localization of the anomaly in computed tomography slides of positive cases of COVID-19. The results prove that ResNet18 consisting of 71 convolutional layers is the best compared to the rest of the models. Figure 10.6 shows the structure of ResNet18. The results proved that ResNet18 had the highest classification accuracy compared to the rest with an accuracy of 99.82% for training and 97.32% for verification.

10.3.4 THE SOLUTION OF IBRAHIM ET AL.

Another method introduced by Ibrahim et al. [9], under the name of "Deep-chest," is a deep learning model with many classifications that enables detection of COVID-19,

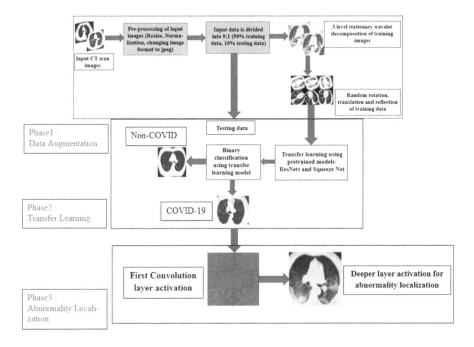

FIGURE 10.6   The architecture of proposed solution.

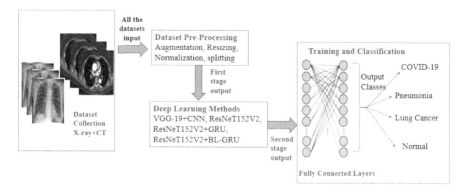

FIGURE 10.7   The proposed multi-classification deep-chest model.

normal pneumonia, and lung cancer through a blend of radiography and tomography. It is a new way to combine two types of photos at once. The model block architecture is shown in Figure 10.7. The model is divided into three stages: dataset preprocessing, feature extraction deep learning models, and classification. In the first stage, the number of images is increased and then resized and divided into two groups at random, 70% for training and 30% for validation.

In the second stage, features are extracted using four designs of deep learning approaches: ResNet152-V2, VGG19+CNN, ResNet152-V2+GRU, ResNet152-V2+Bi-GRU, and are compared. The final stage entails categorizing photographs into four groups: COVID-19, pneumonia, lung cancer, and normal cases. The VGG19+CNN model outperforms the three other models that have been offered; according to the results of the experiments, it achieved 98.05% accuracy.

10.3.5   THE SOLUTION OF JAIN ET AL.

Jain et al. [10] suggested a two-step strategy to distinguish COVID-19 cases from bacterial pneumonia, viral pneumonia, and normal persons, using chest radiography images and deep learning networks ResNet50 and ResNet101. The proposed methodology is implemented in four phases, as indicated in Figure 10.8.

- **Image Preprocessing:** This consists of two stages: determining the smallest height and width of the dataset images and then resizing them according to the ImageNet database.
- **Data Augmentation:** Due to data limitations, the authors increased the number of images using rotation and Gaussian blur.
- **The Formation of the ResNet50 Network:** This model has been trained to distinguish between viral pneumonia, bacterial pneumonia, and normal cases.
- **The Formation of the ResNet101 network:** Here COVID-19 cases are identified from the pool of pneumonia positive cases. With a dataset consisting of 1,832 images, this solution achieved an accuracy of 93.01%.

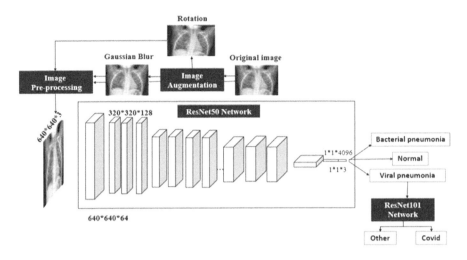

FIGURE 10.8   Architecture proposed by Jain et al.

10.3.6 THE SOLUTION OF HEMDAN ET AL.

In Ref. [11], Hemdan et al. developed a COVIDX-Net model to aid radiologists in detecting COVID-19 from a chest X-ray. This method can be summarized in three main steps:

- **Step 1:** Preprocessing
- **Step 2:** Training model and validation
- **Step 3:** Classification

VGG19, DenseNet201, InceptionV3, ResNetV2, InceptionResNetV2, Xception, and MobileNetV2 are the seven CNN architectures used in the model, as depicted in Figure 10.9. For a classification in two classes (COVID-19+ and COVID-19–), and with a database of 50 images, the accuracy of this model was 90.0%. The results show that their system is effective in terms of detection rate and detection time. However, a vast amount of data is required to prove the effectiveness of this method.

10.3.7 THE SOLUTION OF OZTURK ET AL.

Ozturk et al. [12] constructed a network based on deep learning to detect and categorize COVID-19 cases using X-ray pictures. It is one of the first solutions based on the DarkNet model, which has been named DarkCovidNet. This solution intends to deliver reliable diagnostics for paired and multiclass categorization (COVID-19, normal, and pneumonia). In the DarkCovidNet solution, there are 17 convolution layers with different filtering on each layer, as illustrated in Figure 10.10. The authors consider this solution to be perfect for COVID-19 detection; with precision of 87.02% for multiclass scenarios and 98.08% for binary classes, it offers a complete architecture that eliminates the need for human feature extraction.

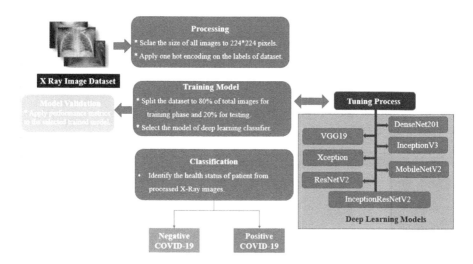

FIGURE 10.9   The COVIDX-Net model.

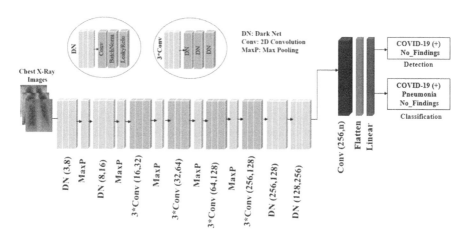

FIGURE 10.10   The proposed model's architecture (DarkCovidNet).

10.3.8   THE SOLUTION OF LIN ET AL.

A 3D deep modeling frame is proposed by Li et al. [13]. This model was dubbed COVNet; it reveals COVID-19, and distinguishes it from pneumonia cases and other lung illnesses acquired. Figure 10.11 presents the COVNet architecture. This model is based on the architecture of RestNet50, which takes a sequence of tomography slices as input and output features for each slice.

Initially, ResNet50 is taken as input to a set of computed tomography (CT) slices and generates a forecast for classifying CT images. Each CT slice's CNN features are integrated, and the generated feature map is put into the algorithm to generate

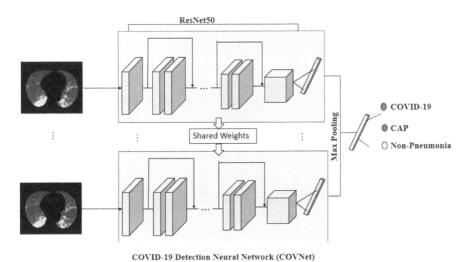

FIGURE 10.11   The COVNet architecture.

a probability score for each class. COVID-ID identification was shown to be 96% accurate.

10.3.9   THE SOLUTION OF WANG ET AL.

Wang et al. [14] presented a modern CNN architecture dubbed COVID-Net for a classification of chest X-ray images into two categories: COVID-19 infection and non-COVID-19 infection. Figure 10.12 presents the architecture of this solution. This solution uses a projection extension lightweight design pattern (PEPX), which is composed of five steps:

- *First stage dropping:* To project the input characteristics to a lower dimension.
- *Expand:* To expand features to a greater dimension than those in the input.
- *Efficient deep representation:* For spatial feature learning to minimize the complexity of computation, while preserving representation capability.
- *Second stage dropping:* To project features into a lower dimension.
- *Extension:* To obtain the final features, convolutions are used to increase the dimensionality of the channel to a higher level. This solution consists of a big number of densely connected long-span connections, as shown in Figure 10.12, and it achieved an overall accuracy of 93.3%.

10.3.10   THE SOLUTION OF ASIF ET AL.

Asif Iqbal et al. [15] proposed the CoroNet paradigm, established on the deep convolutional neural network Xception. Figure 10.13 presents the architecture of this

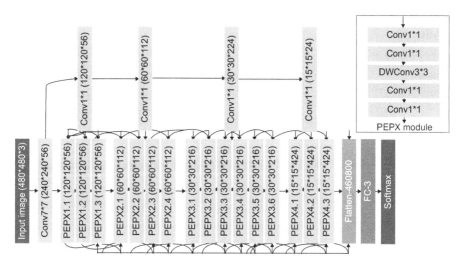

FIGURE 10.12   The architecture of COVID-Net.

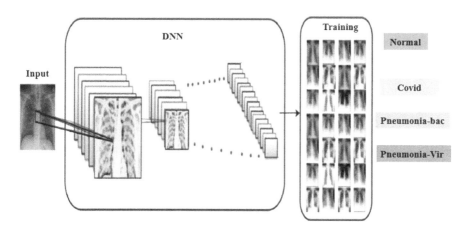

FIGURE 10.13   CoroNet model.

solution. The importance of this solution stems from the fact that the Xception is pretrained on the largest "ImageNet" dataset. CoroNet uses 71 layers to classify four cases: COVID-19, bacterial pneumonia, viral pneumonia, and healthy cases. The authors claim that this solution obtains a total accuracy rate of 89.6% and might be a really beneficial tool for clinicians and radiologists to assist in the diagnosis and follow-up of COVID-19 cases.

Table 10.1 summarizes the solutions studied previously.

TABLE 10.1

A Summary of Previous Studies on COVID-19 Detection

Authors	Technique	Image Type	No. of Images	Accuracy %
Panwar et al. [6]	nCOVnet	X-ray images	6,005	88.10
Houssain et al. [7]	Transfer learning (ResNet50)	X-ray images	21,165	99.17
Sakshi et al. [8]	Transfer learning (ResNet18)	CT-scan images	746	99.82
Ibrahim et al. [9]	Deep chest (VGG19+CNN)	CT-scan + X-ray images	5,828	98.05
Jain et al. [10]	ResNet50 + ResNet101	X-ray images	1,832	93.01
Hemdan et al. [11]	COVIDX-Net	X-ray images	50	90.0
Ozturk et al. [12]	DarkCovidNet	X-ray images	1,125	87.02
Lin et al. [13]	COVNet	CT-scan images	4,356	96
Wang et al. [14]	COVID-Net	X-ray images	13,975	93.3
Asif et al. [15]	CoroNet	X-ray images	1,215	89.6

10.4   CONCLUSION

Mass COVID-19 testing and early diagnosis are key to stopping the spread of this recent global outbreak. The three most important aspects of any disease detection method, especially COVID-19, are time, cost, and accuracy. Although RT-PCR is the most extensively utilized test, it is however slow, expensive, and not readily available. Our contribution consists in proposing a solution to solve these problems. In this chapter, we have highlighted some research works, the aim of which is to uncover from chest radiography the COVID-19, thanks to artificial intelligence algorithms.

REFERENCES

1. Manpreet, K., Mohammad, Z.K., Shikha, G., Abdulfattah, N., Chinmay, C., Subhendu, K.P., MBCP: Performance analysis of large-scale mainstream blockchain consensus protocols. *IEEE Access*, 9, 1–14, 2021. https://doi.org/10.1109/ACCESS.2021.3085187
2. Attar, H.H., Solyman, A.A.A., Alrosan, A., Chinmay, C., Mohammad, R.K., Deterministic cooperative hybrid ring-mesh network coding for big data transmission over lossy channels in 5G networks. *EURASIP Journal on Wireless Communications and Networking*, 1–18, 159, 2021. https://doi.org/10.1186/s13638-021-02032-z

3. Sravanth, K.R., Anudeep, P., Sudha, S., Chinmay, C., Comparison of attention and meditation based mobile applications by using EEG signals. *IEEE: Global Wireless Summit (GWS-SS)*, 260–265, 25–28 November 2018. https://doi.org/10.1109/GWS.2018.8686634

4. Chinmay, C., Gupta, B., Ghosh, S.K., Tele-wound monitoring through smartphone. *IEEE: International Conference on Medical Imaging, m-Health and Emerging Communication Systems (MedCom)*, 197–201, November 2014.

5. Yogesh, S., Chinmay, C., Augmented reality and virtual reality transforming spinal imaging landscape: A feasibility study. *IEEE Computer Graphics and Applications*, 41(3), 124–138, 2021. http://doi.org/10.1109/MCG.2020.3000359

6. Panwar, H., Gupta, P.K., Siddiqui, M.K., Morales-Menendez, R., Singh, V., Application of deep learning for fast detection of COVID-19 in X-Rays using nCOVnet. *Chaos, Solitons & Fractals*, 138, 109944, 2020, ISSN 0960–0779. https://doi.org/10.1016/j.chaos.2020.109944

7. Hossain, Md. Belal, Iqbal, S.M. Hasan Sazzad, Islam, Md. Monirul, Akhtar, Md. Nasim, Sarker, Iqbal H., Transfer learning with fine-tuned deep CNN ResNet50 model for classifying COVID-19 from chest X-ray images. *Informatics in Medicine Unlocked*, 30, 100916, 2022, ISSN 2352–9148, https://doi.org/10.1016/j.imu.2022.100916

8. Ahuja, S., Panigrahi, B.K., Dey, N., Rajinikanth, V., Gandhi, T.K., Deep transfer learning-based automated detection of COVID-19 from lung CT scan slices. *Applied Intelligence*, 51(1), 571–585, 2021.

9. Ibrahim, Dina M., Elshennawy, Nada M., Sarhan, Amany M., Deep-chest: Multi-classification deep learning model for diagnosing COVID-19, pneumonia, and lung cancer chest diseases. *Computers in Biology and Medicine*, 132, 104348, 2021, ISSN 0010–4825. https://doi.org/10.1016/j.compbiomed.2021.104348

10. Jain, Govardhan, Mittal, Deepti, Thakur, Daksh, Mittal, Madhup K., A deep learning approach to detect COVID-19 coronavirus with X-ray images. *Biocybernetics and Biomedical Engineering*, 40(4), 1391–1405, 2020, ISSN 0208–5216. https://doi.org/10.1016/j.bbe.2020.08.008

11. Hemdan, E.E.-D., Shouman, M.A., Karar, M.E., COVIDX-Net: A framework of deep learning classifiers to diagnose COVID-19 in X-ray images. *arXiv preprint arXiv:2003.11055*, 2020.

12. Ozturk, Tulin, Talo, Muhammed, Yildirim, Eylul Azra, Baloglu, Ulas Baran, Yildirim, Ozal, Acharya, U. Rajendra, Automated detection of COVID-19 cases using deep neural networks with X-ray images. *Computers in Biology and Medicine*, 121, 103792, 2020, ISSN 0010–4825. https://doi.org/10.1016/j.compbiomed.2020.103792

13. Li, L., Qin, L., Xu, Z., Yin, Y., Wang, X., Kong, B., Bai, J., Lu, Y., Fang, Z., Song, Q., Cao, K., Liu, D., Wang, G., Xu, Q., Fang, X., Zhang, S., Xia, J., Xia, J., Using artificial intelligence to detect COVID-19 and community-acquired pneumonia based on pulmonary CT: Evaluation of the diagnostic accuracy. *Radiology*, 296(2), E65–E71, 2020. https://doi.org/10.1148/radiol.2020200905

14. Wang, L., Lin, Z.Q., Wong, A., COVID-Net: A tailored deep convolutional neural network design for detection of COVID-19 cases from chest X-ray images. *Scientific Reports*, 10, 19549, 2020. https://doi.org/10.1038/s41598-020-76550-z

15. Khan, Asif Iqbal, Shah, Junaid Latief, Bhat, Mohammad Mudasir, "CoroNet: A deep neural network for detection and diagnosis of COVID-19 from chest x-ray images. *Computer Methods and Programs in Biomedicine*, 196, 105581, 2020, ISSN 0169–2607. https://doi.org/10.1016/j.cmpb.2020.105581

11 Monitoring ECG Signals Using e-Health Sensors and Filtering Methods for Noises

Chokri Baccouch, Nizar Sakli,
Ben Othman Soufiene,
Chinmay Chakraborty, and Sakli Hedi

CONTENTS

11.1 INTRODUCTION

The medical field has evolved considerably in recent years by merging with that of information and communication technologies (ICT), giving rise to what is now called medical informatics. In the first place, the purpose of medical informatics is to process and memorize health information relating to a patient [1–2]. It has materialized, for example, with the establishment of the electronic medical record and efforts are underway to standardize this information so that it is accessible by all the actors

DOI: 10.1201/9781003315476-11

concerned with health, under conditions respecting the integrity of the data, their confidentiality, and ethics related to medical practices.

In the examples of telehealth that we have just presented, monitoring the state of health of patients mainly remains an activity carried out occasionally in well-identified spaces (doctor's office, clinic, hospital, operating room, etc.). Pathologies requiring very frequent or even almost continuous monitoring of the state of health of certain patients require that they remain in places where such monitoring can be provided [3].

Today, with to improvements in microelectronics and telecommunications, it is possible to implant patients with complicated digital equipment that is both energy self-sufficient and capable of wireless communication. In addition, this digital equipment can be connected to sensor platforms [4]. These are used to acquire the medical data itself, to perform a calculation using an onboard microcontroller, and finally to store the data using memories. In addition, these platforms often come with short-range wireless transmission means based on protocols like ANT, ZigBee, Bluetooth, etc.

Sensor platforms generally have only limited resources. They are therefore not able to perform complex data processing, or to transmit this data over great distances [5]. To respond to medical applications expressing a strong need for resources, it is therefore not uncommon to combine sensors with more efficient mobile equipment such as smartphones or even touch tablets when the context of the application allows it. This equipment, which is now used more and more in the daily life of individuals, is equipped with numerous material resources: processors with a computing power much greater than that of microcontrollers, substantial memory capacity, access to long-term telecommunications networks range such as ADSL (Wi-Fi), GPRS, UMTS, LTE, etc.

11.2 ECG SIGNALS

Cardiovascular disease is a major public health issue in the United States. Although the heart is the major organ of the circulatory system, it is susceptible to a variety of ailments. Currently, the medical field requires new techniques and technologies, to evaluate information in an objective manner. The development of electronics and computers and their joint use in the medical field has made it possible to have more efficient devices [6]. One of the medical devices is the electrocardiograph (ECG). Its role is to collect variations in electrical potential, amplify them, and then record them in an electrical form called an electrocardiogram (ECG) signal. You can record this signal on a millimeter sheet or view it on a monitor (oscilloscope or computer), and then save it on a storage medium. The acquisition of the ECG signal is done by electrodes (2, 3, or 10 electrodes) placed on the patient's surface at a location that defines the type of leads, to convert the acquired signal into a vibration [7]. The analysis of the ECG allows a detailed study which helps in the diagnosis of dysfunctions of the heart. The heartbeat is the consequence of the contraction of the ventricles of the heart. Its measurement is expressed in number of beats per minute (bpm) [8]. We also talk about heart rate. Heart rate measurement can be performed in two different ways: either invasively, i.e., directly into the artery, or noninvasively.

• **Invasive Method**

The continuous measurement of arterial pressure by catheterization is known as invasive arterial pressure. The arterial catheter is attached to a transducer that allows a mechanical impulse to be converted into an electrical signal. The invasive heart rate measurement is performed by inserting an arterial catheter into a peripheral artery (aorta, radial, humeral, femoral, etc.) and taking the measurement directly, this is the hemodynamic method. The catheter is a medical device that consists of a flexible tube that is designed to be put into the lumen of a bodily cavity or a blood artery and facilitates fluid drainage or infusion (Figure 11.1).

Hemodynamics or "blood dynamics" is the science of physical properties generally based on the introduction of a thin catheter connected to a pressure sensor filled with an anticoagulant solution (saline/heparin) into the artery, the catheter has an access port to the pressure to be measured and another which is connected to a processing unit, the cyclic variation of the pressures thus measured makes it possible to calculate the heart rate in real time (Figure 11.2).

• **Noninvasive Method**

Noninvasive heart rate measurement can be performed by different methods depending on the needs and the tools available. The easiest way to check your heart rate is to take the pulse. This consists of pressing with one or more fingers through the skin on an artery against a bone, the pulp of the fingers allows you to feel the swelling of the artery due to the increase in blood pressure by the contraction of the heart (systole) count for a minute. Sometimes it is recommended to measure the

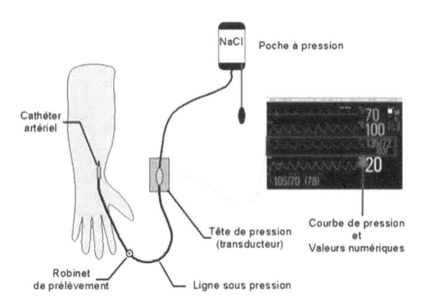

FIGURE 11.1 Continuous and invasive arterial pressure measurement technique.

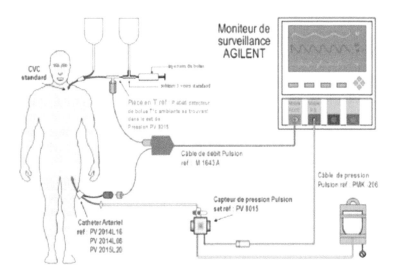

FIGURE 11.2   Invasive heart rate measurement system.

pulse with fingers other than the thumb. However, the thumb enjoys greater sensitivity than other fingers, so it is better suited to measuring the pulse [9]. It can also be taken from the carotid arteries (neck), femoral arteries (groin fold), humeral arteries (elbow fold), ulnar and radial arteries (wrist), and tibial arteries (ankle). It gives valuable insight into the state of blood flow, but the result may not be precise.

A stethoscope is an acoustic instrument, used primarily for listening to internal body sounds and sound waves emanating from the heart. It is captured using a membrane and then transmitted through a microphone and speaker system a short distance to the user's ears. Currently, stethoscopes have one or two pavilions, metal parts provided with a membrane that is applied to the patient's skin. This membrane, put into vibration by body sounds, is connected by one or two flexible rubber tubes to the tips that the operator places in these ears. The rigidity of the system at the ear level, thanks to a metal frame, the lyre constitutes an acoustic amplifier (large horn, small headphones) [10, 11]. The sensors can filter certain frequencies, to collect more specifically high-pitched or low-pitched sounds, depending on the diagnostics to be carried out.

The stethoscope has the advantage of listening to heart sounds which may lead to the calculation of the heart rate, has no side effect, but its use is limited to users who have received theoretical training. The pulse oximeter is a medical device intended to measure in a simple, noninvasive, and continuous way the pulsed saturation of hemoglobin with oxygen (SpO_2), the pulse rate, or what is called, the heart rate. This device has many applications in pulmonology, anesthesia, and especially in emergency medicine. The pulse oximeter consists of the following three components:

- The monitor which records and displays the measurements.
- The SpO_2 sensor (pulsed oxygen saturation).
- The cable that connects the monitor to the sensor.

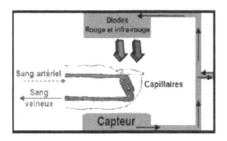
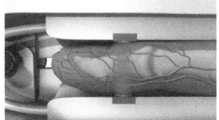

FIGURE 11.3 Principle of transmission/reception.

The principle of operation of this device is based on the emission of two lights (red and infrared), respectively, with a wavelength of 660 and 940 nm, and the measurement of their absorption by the pulsatile flow of blood [12]. The absorption of red and infrared light will vary depending on its oxygenation, in other words, its saturation. Thanks to this property that these sensors will be able to determine SpO_2. The device determines the saturation according to the color of the blood which will be deduced from the absorption of the light emitted [13]. It will therefore provide an SpO_2, but also a heart rate (Figure 11.3).

The pulse oximeter is a simple and low-risk technique. However, it has limitations that can influence the measurement [14]. Among them we find the following:

- The cold.
- Decreased cardiac output and hypotension tending to drop the values of saturation. When cardiac output drops, the readings are considered unreliable. Reading is less and less reliable.
- The artifact secondary to patient movement: Patient movement can lead to incorrect positioning of the probe on the finger.
- Colorimetric interference: The operating principle of the saturometer is based on the absorption of two wavelengths of emitted light. Anything that can interfere with signal absorption will be a source of error (angle varnish, methylene blue).

A blood pressure monitor or sphygmomanometer is a medical device used for measuring blood pressure; it is based on the principle of detecting arterial pressure waves and heart rate which is carried out by several methods, but the most used is the method oscillometric. It is performed on the limbs of the patient.

The measurement steps are as follows:

- The cuff inflates to the tension predetermined by the user above the pressure to be measured, i.e., 180 mmHg for an adult, cutting off the blood circulation in the artery of the controlled limb (here the sensor does not pick up any impulses).
- The cuff gradually deflates.

- When the cuff pressure reaches that of the systolic peak, the blood pressure monitor registers the systolic blood pressure, the sound begins to be audible (if a stethoscope is used).
- The cuff pressure decreases further until it reaches the diastolic peak. The sound or movement is no longer picked up (there is no longer a pulsation in the area of the cuff). The blood pressure monitor then records the diastolic blood pressure.

- **The Heart Rate Monitor**

For certain pathologies, the heart rate and the rate of oxygenation of the blood are warning indicators, and to prevent these pathologies properly, the cardiotachometer is used to accomplish the same mission as the methods and tools mentioned earlier, which is the detection of the heartbeat. The heart rate monitor is a device for recording the rate of the heartbeat (heart rate), it is in the form of a sensor in the fingers that is based on the opacity of the blood in the capillaries. The principle of the cardiotachometer is to take cardiac impulses, thanks to a sensor which is based on the emission of infrared light on one side of the finger and the reception of the light transmitted on the other side by a phototransistor sensitive to this light. However, some isolation from ambient light must be ensured. The movement of blood in the finger changes its opacity. The variation in light is very small; therefore, it introduces a small variation in voltage. This small variation will therefore be processed and amplified. This will calculate and display the heart rate (a number proportional to the heart rate in number of beats per minute).

11.3 THE ELECTROCARDIOGRAM

The ECG has shown good accuracy of the initial diagnosis and of the final diagnosis in treated cardiac patients [15]. The theoretical and sensible foundation for recording the electric interest of the coronary heart is proposed by Einthoven in 1901. Even though the proposed hypothesis is controversial, it is still used in the ECG [16]. In the following paragraphs, we describe in brief the state of being inactive of the heart, the scheme for recording this electric activity, and the primary frequency traits supplied by means of the ECG. ECG can diagnose a massive number of heart (or extracardiac) sicknesses associated with clinical, laboratory, or echocardiographic record. The analysis of the electrocardiogram ought to be methodical and rigorous. The standard and ordinary variant of a normal ECG must be well-known. Abnormalities in rhythm, conduction, persistent, or acute pathology can also be detected [17]. You ought to first inquire about the scientific state of affairs/symptoms motivating the overall performance of the ECG, age, intercourse and sometimes ethnicity, exam conditions (half-seated, lying down, and so forth), the morphology of the rib cage, pathologies or taking medication(s) with feasible repercussions on the heart, and the life of a pacemaker. All this statistic is useful, although it can from time to time bias the translation (expectation bias). The demand for transportable and accurate ECG tracking has multiplied dramatically. The devices electrocardiographic is in use in more than 8,000 hospitals worldwide to better diagnose and treat stroke to ultimately improve mortality and quality of life for patients. Despite the tiny length of those portable merchandise, ECG gadgets still require precision filtering and high-performance processing power, and it included high-resolution pics control that spoil away the maximum microcontroller core [18] because the medical surveillance of patients will become far-flung; the need for physical potential has emerged as strategic. Microchip-connected body and ECG demonstration board are frequently applied within the planning of superior health tracking gadgets and may also coincide with remote affected person monitoring and diagnostic device design. The primary goal of this work is to collect or get information on the electrical activity of the patient's heart and to utilize telecommunication tools to convey that information to the doctor after a well-studied optimal filtering. We are talking about an act of telemedicine called telesurveillance or remote monitoring. In the first part of this work, we describe a generality on ECG signals as well as the difficulties of monitoring these signals. The second part of this work will focus on our contribution to monitoring ECG signals via IoT system as well as the interpretation of real measurement results performed on three patients. In the last part of the work, we describe the different types of noises that can generate ECG signals as well as the different digital techniques to remove them before sending them to the doctor for good medical treatment [19–22].

11.3.1   ECG WAVES AND INTERVALS

The ECG can be analyzed by way of inspecting the waveform element. Those international components suggest the body of the energetic electrical board. The primary growing line of the ECG path is the P wave. It shows atrial contraction. The activation wave permits the repolarization and depolarization of cardiac cells which can be received by means of electrodes placed in sure places. Figure 11.4 shows the global waveform known as normal ECG because of these procedures.

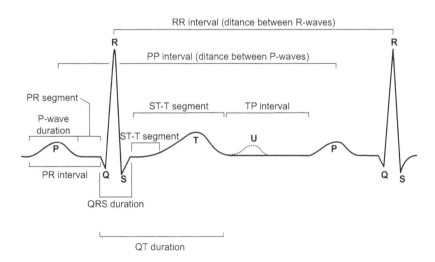

FIGURE 11.4   ECG signal.

You must read the entire ECG trace like a book, from top to bottom and then from left to start with the frontal leads and then the precordial leads and end right, with the long trace of one or more leads (generally 10 seconds provided at the bottom of the page by the manufacturers). Each deflection described by Einthoven must be analyzed. The waveforms that make up the ECG are described as follows: a P wave is a deviation to the depolarization of the left and right atria, and T wave is generally a less ascending waveform; the deviation represents the QRS complex that starts with Q and ventricular repolarization, and then a small downward deviation after which a greater upward deviation, a peak R, than a falling S wave occurs. This QRS complex display off ventricular and depolarization contraction. The QRS complex is equal to a sequence of decreases due to the depolarization of the ventricles. Regular values for declination times are Q-wave ≤ 0, 04 seconds, P-wave ≤ 0, 11 seconds, QRS complex at 0, 1 second; typically 0, 06 and 0, 08 seconds and the period of the QT wave vary relying on the heart price. It gets longer because the charge down as it will increase.

11.3.2 Leads for ECG Measurement

Frontal leads are often used to measure coronary heart rate. They use three measuring factors which are placed on the wrists and ankles. However, it is possible to convey the dimension again to the problem's trunk, in which case this dimension needs to be taken as near the extremity (Figure 11.5). There are two forms of measurements: bipolar and unipolar measurements. Within the context of bipolar measurements, they may be made with three measurements between points:

- The DI lead between the left and right arms (+) (−).
- Between the left leg (+) and the right arm (−) is the lead II.
- Between the left leg (+) and the left arm (−), there is a shunt III.

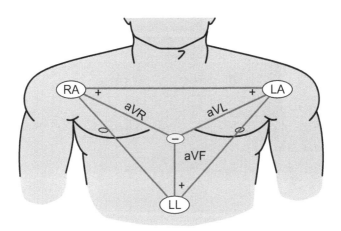

FIGURE 11.5   Unipolar lead.

11.4 ECG SIGNAL MONITORING

11.4.1 PROBLEM AND APPROACH

The wireless sensor network (WSN) is used to screen the surroundings or bodily phenomena, inclusive of noise, strain, motion, or temperature, and to transmit records to the destination. Nowadays, with the explosive boom of IoT technology, an increasing number of sensible programs may be observed in lots of fields, along with safety, smart metering, agriculture, clever towns, and greater domestic intelligence. There are different packages, in particular military, domestic automation, industrial, sanitary, and above all clinical and sanitary. This chapter proposes and explores domestic fitness care [23]. The Arduino may be used to perform a transportable ECG with the heart condition analyzing function. The main aspect of this machine is the AD8232 sensor that can examine the coronary heart charge and process the voltage of the electrodes related to the frame. By means of combining the Arduino UNO and HC 05 FC-114 microprocessor like Bluetooth or Wi-Fi, ZigBee antenna, GSM/GPRS or even XBee, the ECG display is displayed in real time on a phone. We used an ECG simulator as a synthetic corrective agent that is used as a device to justify the performance of a portable ECG based totally on the results acquired from the check. The EGC can be sent via the simulator to the cell phone or to the Matlab interface through a Wi-Fi communique module (ZigBee, Bluetooth, Wi-Fi, GSM/GPRS, or XBee) [24–26]. The precise result shows the affected person's situation in real time. In this chapter, ECG results are published through the Matlab interface. Currently, with the improvement of electronic media, especially with the advent of the Arduino module, thanks to the advantages it gives, the belief of any task has emerged as a clean challenge (Figure 11.6). On this painting, we can use the Arduino module, XBee module, and other approaches to monitor an ECG sign and its far-off emission.

Step 1 of our challenges is to collect the ECG sign. This step is assured by way of the electrodes positioned at the affected person's frame to explore and transmit the signal to an e-Health. Step 2 is zero acquisition card. This ensures the layout and processing of the electrode signal [27–29]. In turn, the e-Health acquisition board

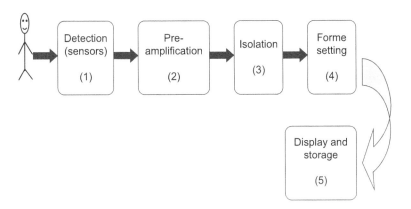

FIGURE 11.6   Block diagram of an ECG.

is attached to an Arduino board to offer analog-to-virtual (ADC) conversion of the ECG sign. Consequently, the received digital signal may be transmitted remotely to any other point through an XBee transmission module [30–32]. At the reception point, any other XBee reception module on an FTDI card will permit reception of the transmitted sign. This XBee reception module is hooked up to a microcomputer to view and process the acquired signal (Figure 11.7).

The synthesis (or end) is intended to answer the question posed through the medical situation. As an example:

- *Normal or variant ECG:* atrial repolarization, early repolarization, wandering pacemaker, etc.
- *Nonspecific QRS or repolarization abnormality:* microvoltage, intraventricular block, fragmented QRS complexes, ST depression, Chatterjee effect, secondary repolarization disorder, etc.
- *Specific anomaly:* sinus dysfunction, sinus bradycardia, sinus tachycardia, atrial fibrillation, etc.; atrial or ventricular hypertrophy, preexcitation, sequelae of necrosis, amyloidosis, etc.; bundle branch block, bifascicular block, AV block, etc.; Brugada repolarization, long QT interval, etc.
- *ECG in favor of an acute pathology:* infarction, coronary ischemia, acute pericarditis, pericardial effusion, pulmonary embolism, hyperkalemia, hypothermia, and intoxication.
- In the first phase of this work, we performed a generation of ECG signals with their spectral concentration in Matlab. Three patients with the criteria listed in Table 11.1 have their ECG signals studied.

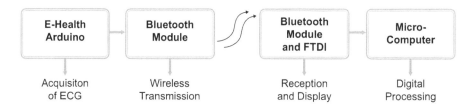

FIGURE 11.7   Block diagram of our remote ECG signal monitoring application.

TABLE 11.1
Patient Diagnosis

Patient	Patient 1	Patient 2	Patient 3
Sex	Female	Male	Male
Age	35	48	81
Diabetic	No	No	Yes
Smoking	No	No	No

Our application displays the results of ECG testing (Figure 11.8), as well as a healthy cardiac waveform (normal sinus rhythm).

11.4.2   TEST FOR ACQUIRING DATA ON THE HUMAN BODY WITH ECG

The Bluetooth-enabled wearable ECG was then tested on a real human body with heart problems. The results are provided, followed by an explanation based on medical logic and a conclusion. These signals have a 10-second period and a 1,000 Hz sample frequency. Each patient underwent 15 tests, each of which is an ECG signal, with the results shown in Figure 11.9. The two key values obtained from the data were the form of the PQRST wave and the heart's BPM. An ECG wave was recorded and visualized using a Matlab interface in this example. The P wave, the QRS complex, and the T wave are all clearly split into three components in this ECG wave. A P-type wave is caused by the register of the SA node, which was a heart-stimulating node. The QRS complex is formed when the ventricular muscle relaxes and contracts

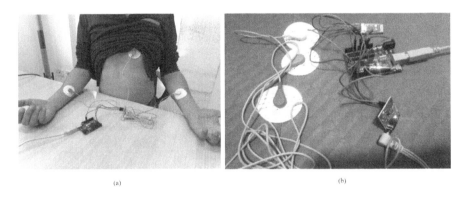

FIGURE 11.8 Reading results of ECG. (a) Actual experimental setup. (b) Data collection with Bluetooth module.

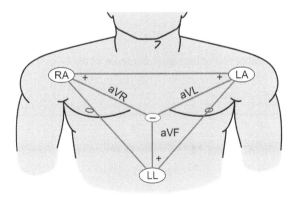

FIGURE 11.9 ECG signals for three patients.

at the same time. A recording is made as the ventricular muscles repolarize to prepare for the next heartbeat; this is the T wave (see Figure 11.9).

11.4.3 DETECTION OF THE NUMBER OF BEATS

In an ECG signal, the R-wave represents the affected person's heartbeat. For each patient, we determine the dominant "R" peaks for the given ECG sign and standard duration of the signal amplitude of the ECG signal (Figure 11.10).

The heart rate is measured in beats per minute (BPM) over a 60-second period. A healthy heart rate is 60–100 beats per minute at rest, but it increases to around 110–150 beats per minute during exercise and 40–60 beats per minute during sleep. When collecting data about a patient's heart, it's best to put them to sleep. The patient is affected by bradycardia if the heart rate is below 60 BPM or tachycardia if the rate is beyond 100 BPM for a heart rate externally ranging between 60 and 100 BPM (Table 11.2).

11.4.4 ECG SIGNAL SPECTRAL ANALYSIS

For each patient, we determined the spectrum of the ECG signal (Figure 11.11) and Nyquist frequency (Table 11.3).

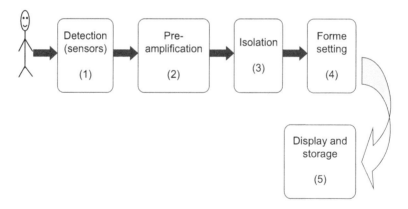

FIGURE 11.10 Typical period of the signal amplitude of the ECG signal for three patients.

TABLE 11.2
Number of Dominant Peaks "R"

Patient	Patient 1	Patient 2	Patient 3
Number of dominant peaks "R"	8	33	13
Number of beats (BPM)	12	49	20

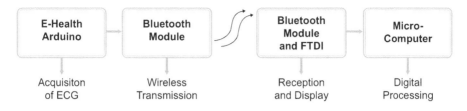

FIGURE 11.11 ECG signal spectral of patients.

TABLE 11.3
Patient Diagnosis

Patient	Patient 1	Patient 2	Patient 3
Nyquist frequency (Hz)	2.9511	6.5968	4.2440

11.5 ECG ARTIFACTS

Numerous noises occur inside the ordinary ECG. The most essential ones are the flow of the baseline (frequency much less than 5Hz), artifacts because of moves (frequency 1–10 Hz), the arena and its harmonics (essentially 50 or 60 Hz), and EMG (electromyogram) with frequency between 25 and 100 Hz.

11.5.1 BASELINE WANDER

The isoelectric line of the heart is called the baseline; it is the trace that could be visible on an ECG if the coronary heart had no electric activity. When the ECG is executed in a workplace, or all through durations of nighttime Holter recording, this line is most often horizontal due to the fact the patient does not make any movement and the signal is little disturbed via outside noise. However, during the day, the movements of the patient alter the relative positions of the electrodes, so this line provides a wavy sample (Figure 11.12).

For the analysis of an ECG recording, a skilled eye ignores this line: it is taken as a reference to have a look at the form and peak of the distinctive heart waves; but, with the intention to routinely procure this type of signal, it is imperative to find it exactly so that one can set the "zero." Within the universal ECG signal processing set of rules, baseline evaluation is performed after single-tune detection of QRS complexes and before multitrack synthesis (Figure 11.13).

Certainly, thanks to seeking out this line on each of the ECG tracks, one of a kind reliability indices may be acquired for each of them; in addition, we will outline reliability indices from the estimation of high-frequency (HF) and low-frequency (LF) noises, indices which can be vital for multitrack synthesis.

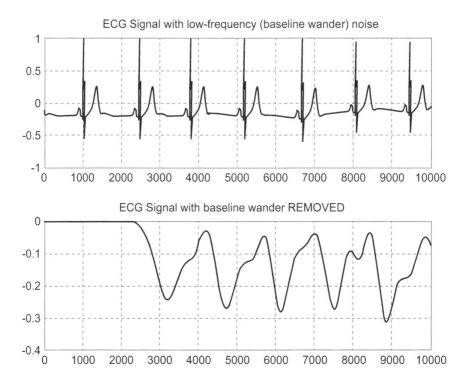

FIGURE 11.12 ECG signal with baseline deviation (above) and without baseline deviation (below) after removing it using a high-pass filter.

11.5.2 POWERLINE INTERFERENCE

It is a simultaneous activation of a region of the myocardium by two simultaneous influxes. The effect is, for instance, a fusion complicated, an aberration, or a pseudoblock. This phenomenon also explains the precise factor of QRS during atrial traumatic inflammation led with the aid of an accent package (see atrial fibrillation/ flutter and accessory package deal) (Figure 11.14).

11.5.3 ARTIFACTS OF ELECTRODE MOTION

Movement artifacts are similar to the sign features of baseline wander, but they are more difficult to fight because their spectral content spans the PQRST complex. Electrode motion artifacts are caused by skin stretching, which changes the skin's impedance around the electrode. They are most common in the 1–10 Hz range. These abnormalities appear inside the ECG as large-amplitude waveforms that are occasionally mistaken for QRS complexes. Electrode movement artifacts are particularly difficult to detect in ambulatory ECG monitoring, where they are the most common cause of incorrectly reported heartbeats (Figure 11.15).

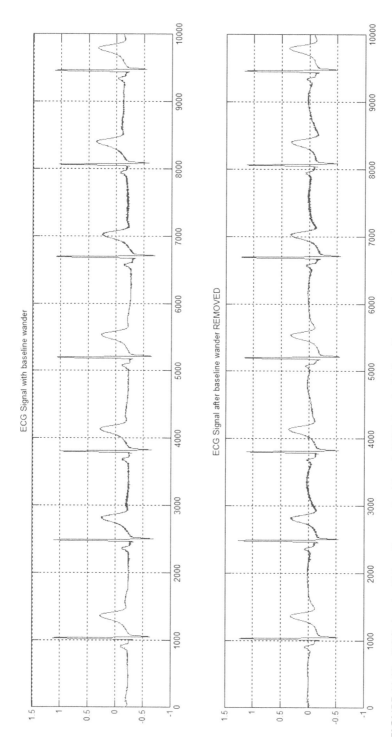

FIGURE 11.13 ECG signal with baseline wander (above); ECG signal with baseline wander reduced using DWT (below) (discrete wavelet transform).

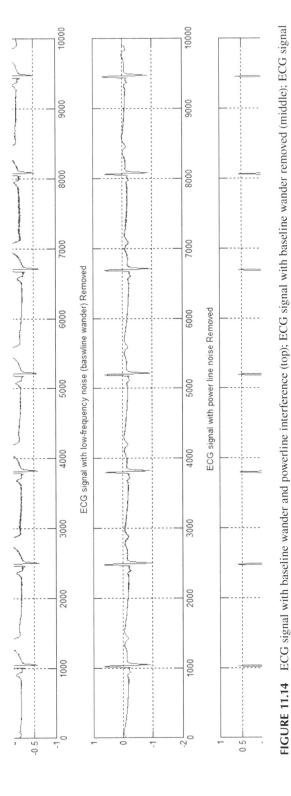

FIGURE 11.14 ECG signal with baseline wander and powerline interference (top); ECG signal with baseline wander removed (middle); ECG signal with powerline interference removed (bottom).

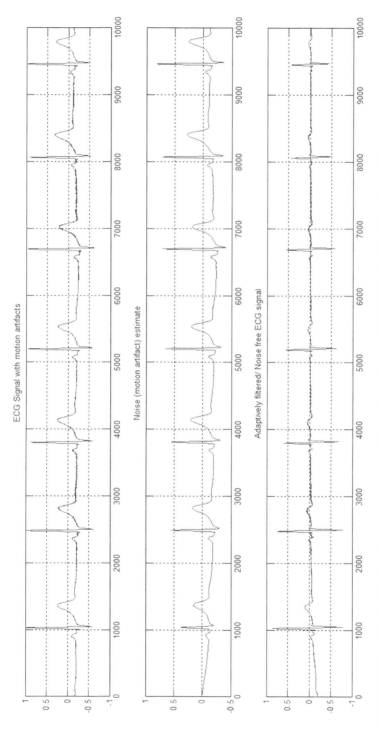

FIGURE 11.15 Adaptive filtering is used to remove motion artifacts from an ECG. ECG signal with motion artifacts (top), noise/motion artifact (middle), and noise-free ECG signal (bottom).

11.6   TECHNIQUES TO REMOVE ARTIFACTS FROM ECG SIGNAL

These techniques are simple but effective. Several signal processing strategies for removing artifacts from ECG signals have been detailed in this segment. The outcomes for the described procedures are also included in this section. ECG signal filtering is a way for eliminating noise around the sign produced by way of an ECG system. Excessive frequency noises are because of extracardiac muscle pastime and interference from electrical gadgets, and low-frequency noises because of body moves related to breathing, physicochemical modifications brought about through the electrode located at the skin and microversions in blood float.

To reduce these noises, the affected person must breathe calmly and keep away from motion or touching metal. The pores and skin must be nicely prepared (shaving the hair, simple washing and rubbing to improve the capillary glide for the peripheral electrodes, no alcohol) earlier than putting an electrode. It is also vital to keep away from overlapping recording threads (loops). Several types of filters can be used in the event of interference:

- To remove interference from electric current (removal of 50 or 60 Hz depending on the country) [33].
- To cast off very low-frequency noise, we use a conventional excessive-pass filter which gets rid of in actual mode noises below the threshold of 0.05 Hz [34]. A 0.5 Hz, actual time high pass clears out data/generates ST section distortions. This threshold can simulate an anteroseptal ST + infarction or a Brugada ECG.

Alternatively, in computerized mode (analog recording than virtual signal processing, typical mode of modern-day ECGs), a virtual linear filter out is appropriate up to the threshold of zero. At 67 Hz, it eliminates the deviations from the baseline. A traditional low-pass filter out is employed to reduce high-frequency noise, which suppresses noise over 150 Hz in actual mode [37]. A low-pass clear out calibrated to 75 Hz or much less slightly reduces the amplitude of QRSs and the ability to detect small deflections (Q microwave, fragmented QRS complexes, J wave, and epsilon wave). In addition, it smooths the direction and gets rid of many fast artifacts [35–37]. A low-skip clear out calibrated at 35 Hz or even 20 Hz significantly reduces the amplitude of QRS and can reduce signs of ventricular hypertrophy. After applying filtering steps to each patient's ECG signals, we transfer those signals to the right doctors and physicians to make the right decisions about the patient's health (Figures 11.16 and 11.17).

11.7   CONCLUSION

The use of ECG monitoring equipment has been extensively studied in the literature. We have provided an in-depth overview of the literature related to ECG monitoring systems in this chapter, focusing on a variety of factors such as application, technologies used, architecture, life cycle, categorization, and defiance. The Internet of Things (IoT) delivers remote, infinite connection and services that harness data

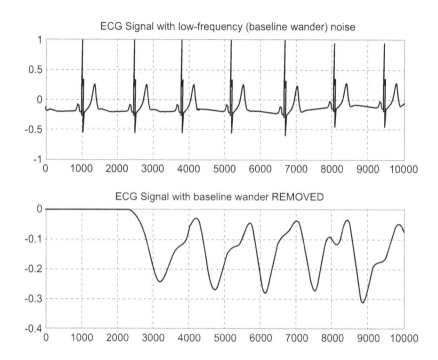

FIGURE 11.16 Filtered ECG signal.

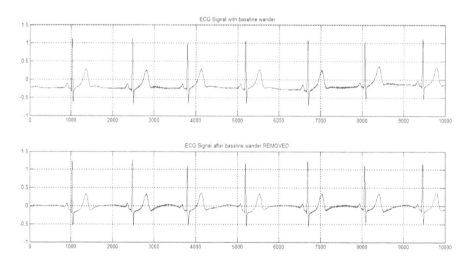

FIGURE 11.17 Filtered and shifted ECG signal.

and enable fast, relevant, and vital lifestyle decisions. We proposed a new compact IoT system for remotely monitoring ECG signals in patients. The data are shown via the Matlab interface for reading by Matlab after converting the data gathered by the electrodes and the AD8232 sensor built into the Arduino board into a "csv" or ".m" extension file. Following that, we used various digital filtering methods to remove any noise that could have caused these ECG readings. To that purpose, we support this work, as well as a detailed assessment of other related research projects that provide a comprehensive overview of the state of the art in ECG monitoring systems. It can serve as a resource for various researchers and field participants to compare, assess, and evaluate the functionality of ECG monitoring systems. It also highlights the main defiance that occurs with these systems. Finally, it discusses how next-generation ECG monitoring devices for healthcare will be perceived in the future.

REFERENCES

1. Kishor, A., Chakraborty, C. Artificial intelligence and Internet of Things based health-care 4.0 monitoring system. *Wirel Pers Commun* 119(2):617–627:July 2021. https://doi.org/10.1007/s11277-021-08708-5

2. Kishor, A., Chakraborty, C. Early and accurate prediction of diabetics based on FCBF feature selection and SMOTE. *Int J Syst Assur Eng Manag* 12(3):587–607:June 2021. https://doi.org/10.1007/s13198-021-01174-z

3. Kishor, A., Chakraborty, C., Jeberson, W. Intelligent healthcare data segregation using fog computing with internet of things and machine learning. *Int J Eng Syst Model Simul (IJESMS)*, 12;2/3:2021.

4. Kishor, A., Jeberson, W. Diagnosis of heart disease using Internet of Things and machine learning algorithms. In: Singh, P.K., Wierzchoń, S.T., Tanwar, S., Ganzha, M., Rodrigues, J.J.P.C. (eds.), *Proceedings of Second International Conference on Computing, Communications, and Cyber-Security*. Lecture Notes in Networks and Systems, vol. 203. Springer, Singapore, 2021.

5. Kishor, A., Chakraborty, C., Jeberson, W. Reinforcement learning for medical infor-mation processing over heterogeneous networks. *Multimed Tools Appl* 80:23983–24004:2021. https://doi.org/10.1007/s11042-021-108400

6. Balestrieri, E., De Vito, L., Picariello, F., Tudosa, I. A novel method for compressed sensing based sampling of ECG signals in medical-IoT era. *Proceeding of the IEEE International Symposium on Medical Measurements and Applications (MeMeA)*, 2019, Istanbul, Turkey, pp. 1–6.

7. Kamble, P., Birajdar, A. IoT based portable ECG monitoring device for smart healthcare. *Proceeding of the 5th International Conference on Science Technology Engineering and Mathematics (ICONSTEM)*, 2019, Chennai, India, pp. 471–474.

8. Miao, F., Cheng, Y., He, Y., et al. A wearable context-aware ECG monitoring system inte-grated with built-in kinematic sensors of the smartphone. *Sensors* 15;11465–11484:2015.

9. Span, E., Di Pascoli, S., Iannaccone, G. Low-power wearable ECG monitoring sys-tem for multiple-patient remote monitoring. *IEEE Sens J* 16(3):5452–5462:July 1, 2016. https://doi.org/10.1109/JSEN.2016.2564995

10. Amit, S., Lalit, G., Chinmay, C. Improvement of system performance in an IT pro-duction support environment. *Int J Syst Assur Eng Manag* 1–19:2021. https://doi.org/10.1007/s13198-021-01092-0

11. Tejedor, J., García, C.A., Márquez, D.G., Raya, R., Otero, A. Multiple physiological signals fusion techniques for improving heartbeat detection: A review. *Sensors* 19:2019.

12. Page, A., Kocabas, O., Soyata, T., Aktas, M., Couderc, J.P. Cloud-based privacy-pre-serving remote ECG monitoring and surveillance. *Ann Noninvasive Electrocardiol* 2015;20:328–337.

13. Mustafa, S., Akash, G., Chinmay, C., Bharat, G. RoC analysis for detection of epi-leptical seizures using Haralick features of Gamma band. *National Conference on Communications (NCC)*, IIT Kharagpur, February 21–23, 2020, 978-1-7281-5120-5, http://doi.org/10.1109/NCC48643.2020.9056027

14. Gusev, M., Stojmenski, A., Guseva, A. ECGalert: A heart attack alerting system. *Proceedings of the 9th International Conference*, 18–23 September 2017, Skopje, Macedonia.

15. Oresko, J.J., Jin, Z., Cheng, J., Huang, S., Sun, Y., Duschl, H., Cheng, A.C. A wearable smartphone-based platform for real-time cardiovascular disease detection via electro-cardiogram processing. *IEEE Trans Inf Technol Biomed* 2010;14:734–740.

16. Bansal, M., Gandhi, B. IoT big data in smart healthcare (ECG monitoring). *Proceedings of the International Conference on Machine Learning, Big Data, Cloud and Parallel Computing: Trends, Perspectives and Prospects, COMITCon*. Faridabad, India, February 14–16, 2019.

17. Taher, N.C., Mallat, I., Agoulmine, N., El-Mawass, N. An IoT-Cloud based solution for real-time and batch processing of big data: Application in healthcare. *Proceedings of the 2019 3rd International Conference on Bio-engineering for Smart Technologies BioSMART*. Paris, France, April 22–26, 2019, pp. 1–8.

18. Chinmay, C., Amit, B., Mahesh, H.K., Lalit, G., Basabi, C. *Internet of Things for Healthcare Technologies*, Springer—Studies in Big Data, 73, 2020. ISBN 978-981-15-4111-7

19. Mustafa, S., Akash, G., Chinmay, C., Bharat, G., Epileptical seizure detection: Performance analysis of gamma band in EEG signal using short-time Fourier trans-form, WPMC-19. *22nd Int. Symposium on Wireless Personal Multimedia Comm*. 204–09, 2019, ISBN: 978-1-7281-5419-0/19

20. Mustafa, S., Akash, G., Chinmay, C., Bharat, G. RoC analysis for detection of epi-leptical seizures using Haralick features of gamma band. *National Conference on Communications (NCC)*, IIT Kharagpur, February 21–23, 2020, 978-1-7281-5120-5, http://doi.org/10.1109/NCC48643.2020.9056027

21. Hemanta, K.B., Chinmay, C., Subhendu, K.P., Vinayak, K.R. Feature and sub-feature selection for classification using correlation coefficient and fuzzy model. *IEEE Trans Eng Manag* 1–15:2021. http://doi.org/10.1109/TEM.2021.3065699

22. Joseph, B.A., Chinmay, C., Abidemi, E.A. Intrusion detection in industrial internet of things network-based on deep learning model with rule-based features selection. *Wirel Commun Mob Comput* 1–17:2021.

23. Joseph, B.A., Chinmay, C., Abidemi, E.A, Intrusion detection in industrial inter-net of things network-based on deep learning model with rule-based feature selec-tion. *Wirel Commun Mob Comput* 2021: Article ID 7154587, 17 pages:2021. https://doi.org/10.1155/2021/7154587

24. Mohaar, G., Maleque, M., Singh, R. Framework for stochastic modelling of multi-dimensional real-time sensor data. *Proceedings of the 2015 10th International Conference on Intelligent Systems and Knowledge Engineering (ISKE)*, Taipei, Taiwan, November 24–27, 2015, pp. 244–251.

25. Xia, H., Asif, I., Zhao, X. Cloud-ECG for real time ECG monitoring and analysis. *Comput Methods Programs Biomed* 10:253–259:2013.

26. Ghosh, S., Feng, M., Nguyen, H., Li, J. Predicting heart beats using co-occurring constrained sequential patterns. *Proceedings of the Computing in Cardiology 2014*, Cambridge, MA, September 7–10, 2014, pp. 265–268.

27. Mora, F.A., Passariello, G., Carrault, G., Le Pichon, J.-P. Intelligent patient monitoring and management systems: A review. *IEEE Eng Med Biol Mag* 12;23–33:1993.

28. Ding, Q., Bai, Y., Erol, Y.B., Salas-Boni, R., Zhang, X., Li, L., Hu, X. Multimodal information fusion for robust heart beat detection. *Proceedings of the Computing in Cardiology 2014*. Cambridge, MA, September 7–10, 2014, pp. 261–264.

29. Vernekar, S., Vijaysenan, D., Ranjan, R. A novel approach for robust detection of heart beats in multimodal data using neural networks and boosted trees. *Proceedings of the 2016 Computing in Cardiology Conference (CinC)*. Vancouver, BC, Canada, September 11–14, 2016, pp. 1137–1140.

30. Chauhan, S., Banerjee, Richa, Chinmay, C., Mittal, M., Shiva, A., Ravi, V. A self-congruence and impulse buying effect on user's shopping behaviour over social networking sites: An empirical study. *Int J Pervas Comp Comm* 17(4);404–425:2021, https://doi.org/10.1108/IJPCC-01-2021-0013

31. Li, Z., Derksen, H., Gryak, J., Ghanbari, H., Gunaratne, P., Najarian, K. A novel atrial fibrillation prediction algorithm applicable to recordings from portable devices. *Proceedings of the 2018 40th Annual International Conference of the IEEE Engineering in Medicine and Biology Society (EMBC)*, Honolulu, HA, July 18–21, 2018, pp. 4034–4037.

32. Pal, S. ECG monitoring: present status and future trend, in: *Reference Module in Biomedical Sciences Encyclopedia of Biomedical Engineering, Roger Narayan.* Elsevier, 2019, pp. 363–379, ISBN 9780128051443.

33. Louis, L. Working principle of Arduino and using it as a tool for study and research. *Int J Control Autom Comm Syst (IJCACS)* 1(2):21–29:April 2016.

34. Bravo-Zanoguera, Miguel, Gonzalez, Daniel Cuevas, García-Vazquez, Juan Pablo, Avitia, Roberto Lopez. Portable ECG system design using the AD8232 microchip and open-source platform. *6th International Electronic Conference on Sensors and Applications*, November 2019.

35. Othman, Soufiene Ben, Bahattab, Abdullah Ali, Trad, Abdelbasset, Youssef, Habib. PEERP: A priority-based energy-efficient routing protocol for reliable data transmission in healthcare using the IoT. *The 15th International Conference on Future Networks and Communications (FNC)*, August 9–12, 2020, Leuven, Belgium, 2020.

36. Othman, Soufiene Ben, Bahattab, Abdullah Ali, Trad, Abdelbasset, Youssef, Habib. LSDA: Lightweight secure data aggregation scheme in healthcare using IoT. *ACM — 10th International Conference on Information Systems and Technologies*, Lecce, Italy, June 2020.

37. Othman, Soufiene Ben, Bahattab, Abdullah Ali, Trad, Abdelbasset, Youssef, Habib. RESDA: Robust and efficient secure data aggregation scheme in healthcare using the IoT. *The International Conference on Internet of Things, Embedded Systems and Communications (IINTEC 2019)*, HAMMAMET, Tunisia from December 20–22, 2019.

12 Artificial Intelligence– Enabled Wearable ECG for Elderly Patients

Nizar Sakli, Chokri Baccouch,
Ben Othman Soufiene, Chinmay Chakraborty,
Sakli Hedi, and Mustapha Najjari

CONTENTS

12.1 INTRODUCTION

While we are talking about a completely digitally transformed health system, it is interesting to wonder about the new practices resulting from telemedicine in the era of artificial intelligence (IAM) in health. IAM has been steadily improving for a decade. An example of this advancement is robotic surgery, which allows surgeons to have successfully completed certain complex surgical procedures in which the

DOI: 10.1201/9781003315476-12

dexterity of the human hand has proven to be insufficient or too "human-dependent." Surgical robots, powered by algorithms but still assisted by surgeons, are creating greater equality of opportunity in certain surgical practices.

With societal changes and major industrial innovations, telemedicine has gradually imposed itself over the last century. When the Internet began to be accessible to the public at the end of the 1990s, the Anglo-Saxon computer scientists who chose the term "e-Health" announced an upheaval in the medical organization (Internet Health) to describe this change. e-Health will replace telemedicine; medicine will replace in the health industry. Should medicine, and telemedicine, become a commercial activity responding to market rules, or should it maintain an ethical approach while benefiting from digital innovations in professional practices and organizations?

12.2   TELEMEDICINE AND MEDICAL AI

The utilitarian approach does not always create [1].

Mainly involving 15–20 million patients with chronic diseases, pathology most often is related to aging. Remote monitoring of the treatment of patients on dialysis or transplant patients at home, remote monitoring of patients suffering from arrhythmias or heart failure by implanted devices, remote monitoring of obstructive respiratory diseases at home (asthma, sleep apnea, etc.), remote monitoring of diabetic patients requiring insulin, etc. [2] are professional practices that aim to better monitor chronic patients at home, to prevent unnecessary hospitalizations, and to ensure their quality and safety care. IAM improves patient quality and safety by equipping remote medical monitoring devices with more efficient algorithms that trigger graduated alerts adapted to the patient's condition.

AMI is expanding into areas where physicians have long recognized its limitations in certain diagnostics. Let us take a few examples. A more refined cardiac diagnosis of atrial flutter (AF) on the ECG, which appears normal in the acute phase of a stroke, allows for more rapid establishment of preventive treatments for new recurrences and avoids the need for documentation. Time-consuming Holter heart rate monitor for patients and physicians [3]. Additionally, in addition to stroke, the algorithm may detect AF more quickly during cardiac assessments in older adults with frequent paroxysmal AF. Stroke can therefore be treated preventively. A criticism of teleconsultation by reluctant physicians is that teleconsultation is a low-quality medical activity compared to face-to-face consultations.

The criticism made of teleconsultation by doctors reluctant to practice is that teleconsultation is a medical exercise of mediocre quality compared to a face-to-face consultation. If the teleconsultation was useful during the period of confinement due to COVID-19 [4] to maintain a link with the confined patients who no longer moved to the medical office, its realization by telephone could only be considered less than a face-to-face consultation. Health insurance has always considered that a teleconsultation by telephone was not a quality medical practice [5] and that its reimbursement during the state of health emergency could only be temporary and derogatory [6, 7]. A quality teleconsultation must be carried out by video transmission to be relevant and reimbursed by health insurance [8, 9].

It is now possible to make teleconsultations more efficient than the simple exchange by video transmission between the doctor and his patient, an exchange which is sufficient when the teleconsultation is alternated with face-to-face consultations, especially in patients with chronic diseases [10]. The use of IAM in remote consultations can be considered in two ways. The first area concerns better access to patients' medical files for targeted clinical information, especially when the teleconsultant doctor is not the treating doctor. The Shared Medical Record (DMP) must become an essential service in the practice of teleconsultation. Of course, it must be opened by the patient and fed by all the health professionals, medical and paramedical personnel who surround the patient as part of the care coordinated by the attending physician. The DMP must allow direct and rapid access to teleconsulting doctors by ensuring that the health data it hosts are governed by algorithms, the information it was looking for [11]. In this respect, interactive and AI-allowed conversational systems could be employed in telemedicine to take more healthiness data contained in the lines of cases who advise telemedicine [12]. Another zone concerns the use of connected objects, which can ameliorate the clinical examination in the absence of a material examination. Some oppose teleconsultation by videotape transmission to "stoked" teleconsultation using connected objects, an added number of which have an individual algorithm [13]. There are now accoutrements of connected objects available in apothecaries [14] or on the Internet [15] to bear out teleconsultations which are decreasingly analogous to face-to-face consultations. Teleexpertise is a practice of telemedicine that is floundering to take off because the digital results that are supposed to allow these exchanges between a requesting croaker, frequently the primary care croaker, and a needed croaker, frequently the corresponding specialist croaker of the treating croaker, are not sufficiently nimble to use and ergonomic for medical time. Digital results more suited to this practice are being tested, for both coetaneous teleexpertise and asynchronous pipe moxie. Telemoxie is also a literacy and nonstop practice, both for the requesting croaker and for the requested croaker. Exchanges and expert opinions must be grounded on acquired and current data from medical wisdom [16].

IAM is for substantiated home medical telemonitoring. It is in this region that IAM is most anticipated. We must deliver, before 2030, in the metamorphosis of our health system, that is to talk, to move from the sanitarium-centric passage that has paid heed to "hospitalization at territory" (Homespital des Anglo-Saxons) because the growing number of cases with habitual conditions due to growing threatens to overwhelm current health systems [17]. The epidemic due to COVID-19 is an illustration of sanitarium overwhelm added to that of habitual conditions which have been on the elevation for 20 times. By 2050, the number of cases with habitual conditions will have tripled on utmost mainlands [18]. Healthcare establishments will be more and more technical, will have smaller long-term sanitarium beds, and the croakers who will work there will be medical masterminds, trained in the use of high-performance tools driven by algorithms for veritably technical care, the maturity of which will be done on an inpatient base [19]. Utmost medical and paramedical health professionals in the itinerant sector will concentrate on habitual complaint forestallment and home care. Their capability will be judged on their capability to keep people healthy for as long as possible and to avoid the circumstance of complications [20].

The challenge of organizing home care is immense and can only be achieved with AMI. There is need for computer technologies and software built by algorithms to monitor and help patients with chronic diseases. The aim of these technologies is to stabilize the chronic disease, prevent serious complications that justify costly hospitalizations, and allow this elderly and very elderly population to have a quality social life and, if possible, be independent at home. Real-time monitoring of these patients at home has become an important telemedicine topic for the next few years. After the many failures of telesurveillance in deferred mode [21], it becomes necessary to apprehend real-time remote surveillance solutions that are both effective and affordable. Thus, in the provision of health services in the years to come, priorities for patients must be addressed. They raise an important challenge, because medical decision-making is a complex process in which patients are directly involved. They are indeed considered as providers of massive health data, i.e., big data. This data must be processed in such a way that remote monitoring can be done in real time, 24 hours a day, 7 days a week.

The hospital is not suitable for the therapeutic management of a chronic disease. The mission of the hospital is changing. It becomes the place for in-depth and very specialized diagnostic assessments, for patients with cancer, cardiovascular, respiratory, neurological, renal, metabolic diseases, etc. Societies are facing a real challenge in the face of the demand for care linked to aging and longer life expectancy. In 2030, 13% of the world's population, or one billion people, will be aged 65 and over and therefore more or less affected by chronic diseases of aging. If the tertiary prevention of the complications of these chronic diseases is not better organized, emergency situations will only progress and divert hospital resources from their real missions. Hence the important role of telemedicine services is keeping patients in their homes for as long as possible without complications. We must get out of an erroneous logic that the complication of a chronic disease is inevitable, and that the hospital is there to deal with it. Many complications can be prevented. The specter of a health catastrophe linked to chronic diseases cannot be ruled out. This is what we have just experienced with COVID-19. Failure to control the development of chronic diseases and their management could lead to a real health catastrophe. IAM-assisted telemedicine can prevent such a catastrophe.

12.3 AI AND ECG

A new method using artificial intelligence (AI) is proposed to identify the risks of developing the cardiac arrhythmia called Torsade de Pointes. Identified on electrocardiograms (ECG) by its configuration, the origin of its name, Torsade de Pointes (TdP), is a fleeting cardiac event that can lead to cardiocirculatory arrest, and then to sudden death if it is not taken care of quickly. Asymptomatic in approximately 50% of patients, TdP is caused by prolongation of the QT interval. The risk of this disorder can be hereditary (congenital long QT syndrome, CLQTS) or acquired caused by taking a drug, including certain antiarrhythmics, antimalarials such as chloroquine, or even certain types of antidepressants and antibiotics. TdP is currently diagnosed primarily through the detection of QT interval prolongation on an ECG. However, this method remains insufficient and not very effective, especially for most doctors who prescribe these drugs, and who, not having immediate access to an expert consultation in cardiology, are unable to correctly quantify the risk of TdP in their patients.

12.3.1 Artificial Intelligence Applied to Risk Prediction

DeepECG4U is an original method that seeks, using artificial intelligence, to identify alterations in the ECG to predict the relative risk of developing TdP. By facilitating the interpretation of ECG data, the DeepECG4U improves the accuracy of risk assessment. Thanks to deep learning, an AI approach to imitate cognitive learning, the DeepECG4 algorithms are trained on anonymized data allowing them to create models. The results are encouraging in its experimental phase, the model has already shown the ability to detect, when coupled with the patient's ECG, risk parameters that can lead to a TdP event, or even to identify whether its cause is congenital or medication. Also, the tool discovers on the ECG and provides clinicians with detailed information describing the risk profile and making the prediction interpretable. Finally, the knowledge learned by AI makes it possible to propose new patient stratifications that can improve their care. Artificial intelligence models can now be used not only for the interpretation of ECGs, but also for the screening and prediction of various cardiac pathologies, thanks to their in-depth data analysis capability.

Artificial intelligence (AI) has put the ECG back on the agenda. Currently, many AI applications are developing, and some models are showing results that match the analysis done by cardiologists for basic interpretations. More broadly, AI has become the state-of-the-art method to be applied to all tasks: processing of images obtained by X-rays, scanners, and MRIs, but also for the analysis of medical records and the connection between medical databases, healthcare, and insurance organizations.

Machine learning (ML) is a branch of artificial intelligence in which the model is not explicitly trained to follow a set of instructions to complete a task. Indeed, the model will learn how to act by acquiring its own set of rules from its experiences (Table 12.1). The term "learning" is somewhat misleading however, because machines do not learn like humans: machine learning is in many cases an application of statistics. There are many relationships between statistical and ML algorithms, such as discriminant analysis, logistic regression, and other linear models. Statistical modeling assumes the existence of a probabilistic model generating the data (the culture of data modeling [21]); AI focuses on matching inputs and outputs through a model (the culture of algorithmic modeling). The first approach starts with a question and/or data, while the second corresponds to a task-centered approach

---

TABLE 12.1
Relationships between Basic AI Techniques

Artificial Intelligence	Machine Learning	Deep Learning
Human thought imitation system	Systems that learn from structured databases	Artificial neural structure learning systems

TABLE 12.2
Statistics: Population Inferences from Sample Machine Learning—Generalizable Predictive Models

Machine Learning	Statistics
Predictions	Inferences
Possible learning errors no problem with complexity	Preference for simple models even if complex models perform better
Focus on performance	Emphasis on interpretability
Generalization on new data	Inferences related to the population of interest
The concern: performance and robustness	The concern: inferences and robustness
Results through performance	Assumptions made a priori

(Table 12.2). ML offers a set of algorithms that can take a set of data as input, and produce a result, output.

The diversity of ECG recording techniques has become plethoric and it is sometimes difficult to navigate. ML techniques can be used from routinely used 12-lead 10-second ECG recordings to single-lead ECGs for extended durations, via implantable loop recorders (ILRs). The data placed at the input of the models can be very varied, from the entire ECG signal sampled at 1,000 Hz to the RR intervals sampled at 200 Hz, or even less. We can try to obtain as an output an interpretation, a forecast, the diagnosis of an ischemia, but also of a rhythm disorder. The ECG can be recorded repeatedly (e.g., for 30 seconds twice a day) or on demand (for long periods). On the other hand, recordings of cardiac phenomena other than the ECG can also be used: photoplethysmography (PPG) or ballistography, rediscovering the techniques of yesteryear such as mechanocardiograms. It is therefore important to properly situate the framework and methodology of the results of the studies reported in the literature, so as not to attribute to AI qualities that it does not possess.

12.3.2 AI TECHNIQUES

Deep learning (DL) does not need structured data. When all aspects of the objects to be processed cannot be classified or categorized upstream, this approach is particularly suitable for complex tasks. The network itself identifies the discriminating characteristics. While ML works from a base of a controllable amount of data, DL needs a much larger volume of data (typically several hundred thousand items) to optimize its parameters.

Recurrent neural networks (RNNs) were introduced so that the model could more efficiently handle data sequences where the order of inputs matters. RNNs process the input sequence one element at a time and use feedback from previous elements in calculating subsequent elements in the sequence. They are therefore ideal for processing data of a sequential nature, such as ECG. The long-term memory model (LSTM) is a more sophisticated variant of the RNN. Convolutional neural networks (CNN) are data-processing networks that can recognize simple patterns. The more the layers there are, the more complex the model becomes. CNNs can be applied to one-dimensional (e.g., ECG), two-dimensional (e.g., images), or even three-dimensional (e.g., video) data sequences.

12.3.3 APPLICATIONS OF AI FOR ECGs

Chang et al. developed an LSTM model capable of both identifying STEMI infarcts and 12 heart rhythms from 60,537 12-lead ECGs recorded in 35,981 patients. The AUC of their model is 0.987, which is higher than that of cardiologists (0.898), emergency physicians (0.820), internists (0.765), and a commercial algorithm (0.845). They suggest that their algorithm can be used to optimize the triage process for patients with acute chest pain and expedite reperfusion therapy for STEMI patients [22].

There is certainly some appeal in doing simple interpretations a little better than cardiologists, but there is more appeal in using AI as a tool that can allow the doctor to see what he himself cannot see. Because it is unique to everyone, the ECG can be utilized as a biometric sensor in this context, akin to a fundus or a fingerprint [23]. For this reason, it is not forbidden to believe that the ECG could be used as a technique to predict susceptibility to certain cardiovascular diseases, in the same way as genomics, in the context of precision medicine.

Attia et al. developed a DNN capable of giving sex and age to within 7 years [24]. A patient whose ECG shows a difference of more than 7 years between the age estimated by the DNN and the real age would present a risk of excess mortality which could be avoided by correcting risk factors or preventive treatment. A DNN was then employed by the same Mayo Clinic team to evaluate standard 12-lead ECGs in a population of 25,144 people over the age of 30. They found that the difference between ECG and chronological age was an independent predictor of cardiovascular and all-cause death [25]. This idea is not new: the effects of age, gender, and ethnicity on the ECG have been documented, first by Simonson from manual measurements on the ECG [26]. In 1994, Mac Farlane confirmed these results on digitized ECGs [27]. Until recently, Hnatkova showed the effect of gender and ethnicity on QRS duration [28].

Even cardiac failure can be detected using an ECG. The Mayo Clinic's Attia et al. used 44,959 individuals paired 12-lead ECG and echocardiography data. They trained their CNN to identify individuals with ventricular dysfunction, defined as an ejection fraction of less than 35%, using only the ECG. The model's AUC, sensitivity, specificity, and accuracy were all 93%, 86.3%, and 85.7%, respectively, when tested on an independent collection of 52,870 patients. Patients without ventricular dysfunction who tested positive for CNN had a fourfold increased risk of developing ventricular dysfunction in the future compared to those who tested negative [29]. Using a 12-lead ECG, Joon-myoung Kwon et al. constructed a model of LD that can detect function-preserved cardiac failure [30]. These findings show that traditional ECGs could be used to predict function-preserved heart failure.

It has almost become a habit for editors and reviewers to accept, seemingly unflinchingly, the fact that algorithms outperform cardiologists and publish reported results without testing the models and without even seeing the code used. This enthusiasm must certainly be put into perspective: the algorithms are more efficient than certified cardiologists (not experts) and for routine (non-complex) ECG interpretations. One of the advantages of AI diagnostic techniques lies in the fact of relieving cardiologists of tasks considered secondary, such as the interpretation of an ECG, and allowing them to devote themselves to much more complex and rewarding tasks in the catheterization and electrophysiology rooms. Let us note from the outset that the interpretation of the ECG, the AI, even if it is already very efficient for basic diagnoses, remains however still far from optimal performance for more arrhythmias complicated. Substantial progress is likely to be made in the years to come.

A CNN was developed by Acharya and colleagues [31] to identify a raw ECG into four categories: normal sinus rhythm, atrial fibrillation, atrial flutter, and ventricular fibrillation. Over 5-second ECG segments, sensitivity was 99.13% and specificity was 81.44%.

The fact that AI can be used in AF screening has led to the development of its use in wearables. In the Apple Watch study conducted with the Apple Watch 3, 419,297 participants were recruited. A telemedicine visit was established, and an ECG patch was mailed to the participant, who was required to wear it for up to seven days if a smartwatch-based irregular pulse detection algorithm revealed suspected AF. With a 10% confidence interval width, the major goals were to determine the proportion of reported participants with AF indicated on an ECG patch and the positive predictive value of irregular pulse intervals. Only 20.8% who received an abnormal pulse report returned the ECG patches for examination, with 34% showing AF on repeated readings and 84% of reports being consistent with AF; the detection algorithm's positive predictive value was 71%. This study demonstrated the feasibility of large-scale screening with a connected watch, but it also revealed the low diagnostic profitability of this screening in a population with a low prevalence of the disease (0.5% reported irregular pulses) and the low retention of subjects recruited until the end of the study [32]. Currently, the Apple Watch 4 makes it possible to directly make an ECG recording of a derivation and which is then sent to the smartphone for interpretation by an ML algorithm, and then possibly by a doctor for validation. Of course, almost all companies such as Samsung, Huawei, Garmin, and Polar develop their own ML algorithms. Obviously, all these algorithms are patented and generally kept secret, which can affect the transparency of data and results.

Giudicessi et al. recently demonstrated that a DNN can detect clinically significant prolongation of the corrected QT interval (QTc > 500 ms) in mobile ECG device tracings, which was comparable to ECG-based QTc measurements at 12 leads, as determined by both an expert QT cardiologist and a commercial central laboratory [33]. They find that their DNN can predict QTc as well as a standard 12-lead ECG from a two-lead ECG acquired with a smartphone. We would have preferred them to utilize their DNN as a predictor of patients who will develop Torsade de Pointes, but it is not a bad start.

Hanun et al. [34] used a DNN to identify 12 distinct arrhythmias from 91,232 single-lead ECGs collected from 53,549 individuals using the Zio Patch device. They used a 34-layer neural CNN taking as input a 30-second raw ECG signal sampled at 200 Hz. The network produces a sequence of diagnostic predictions every second. They validated their model on 328 ECGs annotated by expert cardiologists, but carefully compared its performance to interpretations by "certified" cardiologists. Their DNN reached an AUC of 0.97. DNN's sensitivity outperformed cardiologists' average sensitivity for all 12 rhythm classes when specificity was set to the average specificity obtained by cardiologists.

An arrhythmia has a greater chance of being detected longer the observation period. These devices, in the format of a USB key and implantable subcutaneously, allow loop recording of the ECG with storage of detected arrhythmia episodes. They are programmable so that their detection thresholds and recording duration can be adapted to each patient. The monitoring period is several years. Initially developed to allow the recording of conduction disorders at the origin of syncopal episodes, the ILRs saw their diagnostic capacities increased, thanks to AF detection algorithms. The algorithms used are relatively simple given that the implementation must consider a reduced memory capacity.

Sensitivity should be considered the most important performance metric for a device designed to detect and monitor AF, as undersensing might lead to underdiagnosis, placing the patient at risk for clinical complications connected to AF. Syncope or stroke can occur because of AF. The parameters most considered in all these studies are therefore sensitivity and positive predictive value (PPV).

Through a downloadable app, photoplethysmography (PPG) technologies can detect arrhythmias utilizing hardware already present on most consumer devices (smartwatches and other smartphones). The sensors of most of these wearables use the technology used by oximeters to measure heart rate by monitoring variations in the light spectrum reflected by the skin, following the capillary pulse. This pulsatile signal is interpreted as equivalent to the R wave of the ECG. An algorithm, based mainly on the irregularity of the signal, makes the diagnosis of AF. The algorithms used to analyze these PPG signals were shown to function similarly to ECG R waves [34,35]. It is also possible to use the smartphone to measure the kinetic energy transmitted by the peak shock from the G ventricle to the rib cage and to derive information concerning myocardial function, reproducing in digital mode the good old apexograms [36].

12.4   THE BIG DATA OF CONNECTED MEDICINE

The growth in computer power and the amount of data accessible are the only two factors that make DL genuinely optimal. It is in this context that the interest of connected devices in cardiology must be understood. The number of smartphone users is constantly increasing. In 2021, there were 6.4 billion worldwide, an annual increase of 5.3%. Smartphones can either collect data directly through variations in skin color detected by the camera, or collect information sent by wearables. In just three years, the number of connected wearables has more than quadrupled, from 325 million in 2016 to 722 million in 2019. In 2022, the number of these devices is estimated to exceed one billion [37]. Its various aspects in cardiology have recently been the subject of a consensus [38]. An ESC working group has also just taken stock of e-cardiology [39].

Most wearables can now record ECGs limited to a single lead. Validation studies are performed by comparing the performance of single- and dual-lead ECGs to those of 12-lead ECGs. The Physio Net Challenge 2021 also aims to identify clinical diagnoses from ECG recordings with 12 leads, 6 peripheral leads, 3 leads (I, II, and V2), and 2 leads (II and V5). Most recently, the Kardia Mobile 6L device allows a 30-second recording of the six peripheral leads, which has the advantage of allowing QT measurement in addition to AF detection. The impact of these technologies on clinical decision-making has just been evaluated in order to define the integration of data from these devices.

12.4.1 FORECAST STUDIES

Several studies have investigated the ECG signal in sinus rhythm to determine if a network can distinguish patients who will later present with a rhythm disorder. In this case, the use of AI would allow the adoption of personalized preventive medicine, which is a step further than preventive medicine based on risk factors. It remains to be determined at what precise moment this arrhythmia will manifest itself. Galloway et al. demonstrated that a smartphone-enabled device could detect an AF signature from a 20-second lead ECG with normal sinus rhythm using a deep neural network. They divided the patients with AF into two groups, depending on whether they had more or less 30% AF. Their LD model was able to determine whether an ECG was from a patient without AF or one with 30% or more AF based on normal sinus rhythm ECGs obtained before AF. The model's sensitivity and specificity were 73.1% when compared to a benchmark with equal sensitivity and specificity. Using typical 10-second, 12-lead ECGs, Attia et al. used CNN to identify an AF signature in patients with paroxysmal AF in normal sinus rhythm. For patients with paroxysmal AF, the window of interest began 31 days before the first documented ECG of AF. With an AUC of 0.87, sensitivity of 79.0%, specificity of 79.5%, F1 score of 39.2%, and overall accuracy of 79.4%, their model correctly diagnoses AF.

In a retrospective multicenter study carried out on 12,955 patients, Yong-Yeo Jo et al. developed a model of LD capable of identifying patients who will present an episode of supraventricular tachycardia while still in sinus rhythm. Their model was developed from 31,147 ECGs and presented an AUC of 0.966. Precision, sensitivity, specificity, positive predictive value, and negative predictive value were 0.970, 0.868, 0.972, 0.255, and 0.998, respectively, for precision, sensitivity, specificity, positive predictive value, and negative predictive value. Important elements for prediction included the QT interval and whether a delta wave existed.

12.5 AI APPLICATION FOR ECG

The electrocardiogram (ECG) signal is commonly used to determine a patient's heart state. It depicts changes in the heart's electrical activity as a function of time. Cardiologists must recognize and classify cardiovascular disorders based on ECG signals, which is a difficult undertaking. The ResNet50 deep learning model was constructed in this research to help cardiologists diagnose ECG data with 27 classes, including normal sinus rhythm and 26 forms of illnesses. In terms of precision and accuracy, our proposed model obtains 99.99%. These experimental results show that our proposed model is more effective than other existing methods in the literature.

Cardiac problems can be a severe warning sign for human health; in most situations, certain illnesses can result in serious harm or death. The World Health Organization (WHO) estimates that 17 million people die each year as a result of cardiovascular disease (CVD). Early diagnosis is crucial for patient care due to the high mortality rate. As a result, researchers are exploring novel ways for disease prevention, diagnosis, and treatment.

The electrocardiogram (ECG) is a real-time, noninvasive diagnostic that monitors the electrical activity of the human heart. ECG is one of the most essential techniques for diagnosing cardiac problems. It includes a wealth of information not just about the heartbeat but also about the electrical conduction system's operation. Different ECG waveforms are used to indicate different types of arrhythmias. These tracings reveal information about the heart's function and health. As a result, ECG signal monitoring and detection is a critical topic in medicine.

Electrocardiogram is the most effective technique for detecting arrhythmias. Abnormal heart rhythms are called arrhythmias, which occur because of changes in the normal sequence of electrical impulses in the heart. ECG arrhythmias can be classified by the difference in sinus normal rhythm (SNR); in this chapter, we focus on 26 arrhythmias and SNR.

The detection of arrhythmias from the ECG requires the presence of experts in the domain. In case of absence or lack of cardiologists in the hospitals, they have moved to detect the arrhythmias. The advances in technology, artificial intelligence (AI) helps cardiologists make accurate diagnoses, make optimal decisions, select the right treatment, and make predictions based on models learned from thousands of ECG signals. A number of researchers have indicated interest in AI's potential in medicine, as listed herein:

- Provide research for monitoring, associating, demonstrating, and classifying medical data.
- New technologies to aid medical decision-making, training, and research are being developed.
- Participate in events of different disciplines.
- To give the future scientific medical area a content-rich specialty.

Manual analysis of ECG signals by doctors is a tedious job, the presence of a system that helps cardiologists for the detection of cardiovascular problems is necessary. The main objective of this chapter is to propose system that can effectively distinguish patients and help specialists determine the appropriate treatment. The remainder of this document is structured in the following manner. One section reviews related literature, while the other section discusses the proposed model and our recommended approach. The training and parameters of the model are presented next. Finally, results of the proposed ECG classification model are treated as well as the conclusion and future works.

12.6   RELATED WORKS

AI refers to intelligent systems that mimic human intellect and behavior in general. Machine learning is a branch of artificial intelligence that deals with techniques that allow computers to learn from their mistakes. Artificial neural networks that learn through a hierarchy of ideas and are applied to big datasets are referred to as deep learning (DL). The main disadvantages of ML are the use of manual features extraction that requires an expert in the domain. Although ML algorithms with handcrafted features have performed well for ECG analysis, neural network methods with the power of automatic feature extraction and representation learning have demonstrated human-level performance in biomedical signal analysis.

The recent studies in DL models are powerful analytical models, although computationally expensive. Several studies have used a deep learning approach to classify ECG signals. Antonio and colleagues created a deep neural network (DNN) model to classify six different types of ECG using a private dataset of 2,322,513 recordings. The model proposed achieve a precision of 92.36%. Ahsanuzzman et al. classified a single arrhythmia, atrial fibrillation (AF), using a combination of long short-term memory (LSTM) and recurrent neural network (RNN) deep learning models and algorithms. These deep learning models and algorithms contribute to an overall accuracy of 97.57% in arrhythmia prediction. Adedinsewo et al. developed a CNN model that correctly classified left ventricular systolic dysfunction (LVSD) arrhythmias with an accuracy of 85.9%. Different studies used deep learning models to classify only one arrhythmia which is insufficient to aid cardiologists in their diagnosis. Xiong et al. used ResNet16 to train 8,528 ECG recordings from CPSC data to classify AF arrhythmias, SNR, or another arrhythmia, the model obtained an accuracy of 82%. Dongdong Zhang et al. [7] train a 34-layer ResNet 1D model to detect nine different arrhythmias in 12-lead ECG signals using the CPSC2018 database, which includes 6,877 ECG recordings. For ECG signals, this model has a classification accuracy of 96.6%.

We can observe that the number of records used to train a DL model is little, implying that DL requires a substantially higher volume of data. In this investigation, we integrated four public databases to confirm the efficacy of the provided methodology.

12.7   PROPOSED APPROACH

Our study technique is as follows: initially, our input data is ECG singles, which are then preprocessed. The following step is model training, in which a ResNet50 deep learning was proposed to train the data to predict as a result of 27 classes (see Figure 12.1).

12.7.1   Dataset Description

Public databases around the world were combined for this study on ECG signal diagnosis: CPSC 2018 and CPSC 2018 Extra from China, PTB-XL from Germany, and

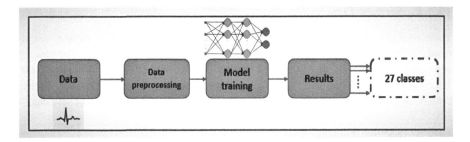

FIGURE 12.1 Our study's architecture.

TABLE 12.3
Features of Databases

Database	CPSC 2018 [8]	CPSC 2018 EXTRA [8]	PTB-XL [9]	Georgia [8]
Number of ECG recordings	6,877 M: 3,699 F: 3,178	3,453 M: 1,843 F: 1,610	21,837 M: 11,379 F: 10,458	10,344 M: 5,551 F: 4,793
Length of ECG recordings	6–60 seconds	6–60 seconds	10 seconds	10 seconds

Georgia from the United States. This combined database includes 42,511 12-lead ECG recordings at a frequency of 500 Hz for SNR and 26 arrhythmias. Table 12.3 describes the features of each database. This dataset comprises 26 types of CVDs and a normal heart state. In sum, it contains 27 classes.

12.7.2 Preprocessing of Data

The dataset includes an ECG with different durations between 6 and 60 seconds. In deep learning, the inputs must be of the same length. For this reason, and after multiple tests, the decision was to set nsteps equal to 5,000 (frequency = 500 Hz, duration = 10 seconds). Only the first 10 seconds of an ECG will be saved if it is longer than 10 seconds. Otherwise, until they have 10 seconds of recording time, they will be filled with zeros.

12.7.3 Augmentation of Data

As noted in Section 12.7.1, the problem of imbalance and insufficient data was solved using data augmentation. Amplitude scaling is used to complete the data during the training phase. It multiplies the ECG signals by a random factor from a normal distribution to extend or compress the amplitude. Although data augmentation adds noise to the model, it can assist it avoid overfitting.

12.7.4 SPLIT OF DATA

There are 42,511 ECG recordings in the dataset used in this study. First, the dataset is separated into two sets with a ratio of 0.75:0.25: training and validation and test. The training and validation sets were then subjected to a tenfold stratified cross-validation approach. This will produce ten stratified folds. These folds will be created by trying to keep the percentage of samples for each class equal. Figure 12.2 illustrates an overview of split data.

12.7.5 MODEL ARCHITECTURE

Figure 12.3 illustrates our ResNet50 model architecture.

DATA SPLIT (42 511)		
train & validation set (31 884)		Test set (10 627)
Train (25 507)	Validation (6 377)	

FIGURE 12.2 Data split.

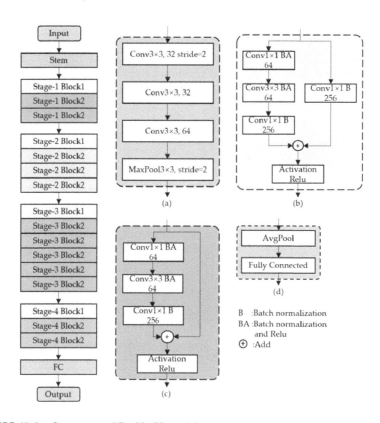

FIGURE 12.3 Our proposed ResNet50 model.

ResNet50 has 48 convolution layers, a maximum pooling layer (MaxPooling), and an overall average pooling layer (AVGPooling). The raw ECG signals $\mathbb{R}^{5000 \times 12}$ (5,000 = nsteps, 12 = number of leads) are considered as model input. The result is the multilabel classification $\mathbb{R}^{1 \times 27}$. To extract the deep features, 16 residual blocks are used. Two different residual blocks are distinguished:

- Res_Block_1 has three 1D convolutional layers (Conv1d), three batch normalization layers (BatchNorm1d), and two rectified linear unit (ReLU) activation layers on one side, and one 1D convolutional layer (Conv1d) and one batch normalization layer (BatchNorm1d) on the other.
- Three 1D convolutional layers (Conv1d), three batch normalization layers (BatchNorm1d), and two rectified linear unit (ReLU) activation layers make up Res_Block_2.

The Conv1d layers are used to automatically extract features, the BatchNorm1d layers are used to make the model faster and more stable, and the ReLU layers are used to perform nonlinear activation. Average pooling is used to pool the characteristics extracted by the residual blocks. The output layer uses the Sigmoid activation function to forecast 27 classes using the results of this pooling.

12.7.6 Model Training

A tenfold cross-validation strategy was used for model training and evaluation. The dataset was partitioned into ten folders at random. In each round, nine out of ten are used for training, one folder for validation.

To train the model, the Adam optimizer is utilized as the optimization method and the binary cross-entropy as the loss function. Table 12.4 shows the ideal values for the hyper-parameters of the deep neural network.

12.8 RESULTS AND DISCUSSION

Our proposed model was trained using OVH Cloud with NVIDIA Tesla V100 16 Go, vCore 8 and memory of 45 Go. The model was implemented on Python 3.7. Each epoch took an average of 90 seconds to complete. This section discusses and evaluates the model results.

TABLE 12.4
The Hyper-parameters Used for the Neural Network

Hyper-parameters	Optimized Value
Optimizer	Adam
Epoch	150
Batch	16
lr	0.001
Loss function	Binary cross-entropy

The accuracy acquired during the training and validation phases is 99.99% and 99.98%, respectively. In terms of precision, we obtained 99.99% and 99.87%, respectively. For loss, 78.9.10–4 and 3.83.10–4 were achieved for each phase.

The use of ten stratified folds in the data split causes the model to become disordered from fold to the next until it stabilizes in the final fold. This effect can be seen clearly in the first seven folds (epochs 01–70).

Figures 12.4 and 12.5 show model's accuracy. We note that the model gradually converges after the 70th iteration, reaching a stable accuracy and precision at the 150th iteration.

The model's loss is shown in Figure 12.6, and we can see that the model gradually converges to a low loss at the 150th iteration after the 60th iteration.

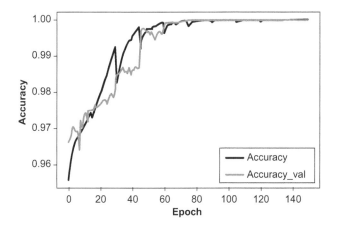

FIGURE 12.4   Training and validation accuracy utilizing our proposed model.

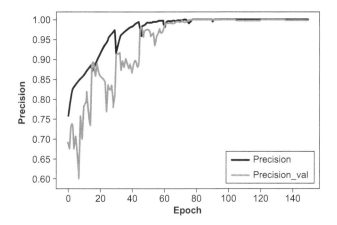

FIGURE 12.5   Precision of training and validation using our proposed model.

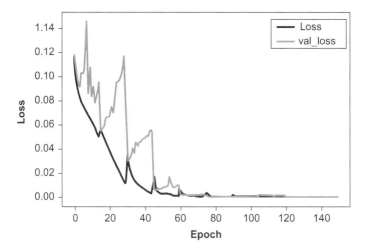

FIGURE 12.6   Precision of training and validation using our proposed model.

TABLE 12.5

Comparison of Different Literature Studies in Terms of Accuracy (Acc), Precision (Pre), and Loss

Author/Year	Number of Records	Mode I	Classes	Acc (%)	Pre (%)	Loss
Antonio et al. [3]	2,322,513	DNN	6	–	92.36	–
Ahsanuzzman et al. [4]	48	LSTM et RNN	1	97.57	–	0.01
Adedinsewo et al. [5]	6,613	CNN	1	85.9	87	–
Xiong et al. [6]	8,528	ResNet16	4	82	–	0.1
Dongdong et al. [7]	6,877	ResNet34	9	96.6	82.1	–
Our work (2021)	42,511	ResNet50	27	99.99	99.99	0.0001

A normalized confusion matrix was built to assess the suggested model's performance. Each column represents a predicted class, while each row represents an actual class. The proposed model is effective for the classes IRBBB, RAD, PVC, Brady, PR, NSR, RBBB, AF, IAVB, LBBB, and CRBBB. Indeed, their percentages of successful predictions exceed 80%. Furthermore, his performance is moderated in the classes PAC, TInv, SA, AFL, LanFB, and RAD, where their correct prediction percentages exceed 60%. The model has poor performance in the other classes, such as QAb, LAD, and LPR.

In terms of accuracy, precision, and loss, ResNet50 performed better than previous research referenced in the literature. Table 12.5 compares our results to literature studies published in the related works section.

12.9 CONCLUSION

In this chapter, we propose ResNet50, a deep learning model that uses a pooled dataset of 42,511 ECG 12-lead records to categorize 26 CVD and normal sinus rhythm. When compared to the values obtained in the literature, our proposed model reaches 99.99% accuracy and precision. This result demonstrates the efficacy of the proposed model. ResNet50 will be used as a platform for diagnosing ECG signals and assisting cardiologists in their work in the future.

REFERENCES

1. Breiman, L. Statistical modeling: the two cultures (with comments and a rejoinder by the author). *Statist Sci*, 2001, 16 (3), 199–231.
2. Chang, K.-C., Hsieh, P.-H., Wu, M.-Y., Wang, Y.-C., Wei, J.-T., Shih, E.S. et al. Usefulness of multi-labelling artificial intelligence in detecting rhythm disorders and acute ST-elevation myocardial infarction on 12-lead electrocardiogram. *Eur Heart J—Digital Health*, 2021, 2 (2), 299–310.
3. Ajay, K., Kumar, A., Chinmay, C., Natalia, K. Deep learning and Internet of Things based lung ailment recognition through coughing spectrograms. *IEEE Access*, 2021, 1–11. http://doi.org/10.1109/ACCESS.2021.3094132
4. Attia, Z.I., Friedman, P.A., Noseworthy, P.A., Lopez-Jimenez, F., Ladewig, D.J., Satam, G. et al. Age and sex estimation using artificial intelligence from standard 12-lead ECGs. *Circ Arrhythm Electrophysiol*, 2019, 12 (9), e007284.
5. Ladejobi, A.O., Medina-Inojosa, J.R., Shelly Cohen, M., Attia, Z.I., Scott, C.G., LeBrasseur, N.K. et al. The 12-lead electrocardiogram as a biomarker of biological age. *Eur Heart J—Digital Health*, 2021, 2 (3), 379–389. http://doi.org/10.1093/ehjdh/ztab043
6. Chinmay, C., Gupta, B., Ghosh, S.K., Mobile telemedicine systems for remote patient's chronic wound monitoring. In *IGI: M-Health Innovations for Patient-Centered Care*, Ch. 11, 217–243, 2016. http://doi.org/10.4018/978-1-4666-9861-1, ISBN: 9781466698611.
7. Hnatkova, K., Smetana, P., Toman, O., Schmidt, G., Malik, M. Sex and race differences in QRS duration. *Ep Europace*, 2016, 18 (12), 1842–1849.
8. Attia, Z.I., Kapa, S., Lopez-Jimenez, F., McKie, P.M., Ladewig, D.J., Satam, G. et al. Screening for cardiac contractile dysfunction using an artificial intelligence-enabled electrocardiogram. *Nat Med*, 2019, 25 (1), 70–74.
9. Kwon, J.-M., Kim, K.-H., Eisen, H.J., Cho, Y., Jeon, K.-H., Lee, S.Y. et al. Oh, Artificial intelligence assessment for early detection of heart failure with preserved ejection fraction based on electrocardiographic features. *Eur Heart J—Digital Health*, 2021, 2 (1), 106–116.
10. Acharya, U.R., Fujita, H., Lih, O.S., Hagiwara, Y., Tan, J.H., Adam, M. Automated detection of arrhythmias using different intervals of tachycardia ECG segments with convolutional neural network. *Inf Sci*, 2017, 405, 81–90.
11. Perez, M.V., Mahaffey, K.W., Hedlin, H., Rumsfeld, J.S., Garcia, A., Ferris, T. et al. Large-scale assessment of a smartwatch to identify atrial fibrillation. *N Engl J Med*, 2019, 381 (20), 1909–1917.
12. Giudicessi, J.R., Schram, M., Bos, J.M., Galloway, C.D., Shreibati, J.B., Johnson, P.W. et al. Artificial intelligence-enabled assessment of the heart rate corrected qt interval using a mobile electrocardiogram device. *Circulation*, 2021, 143 (13), 1274–1286.
13. Hannun, A.Y., Rajpurkar, P., Haghpanahi, M., Tison, G.H., Bourn, C., Turakhia, M.P. et al. Cardiologist-level arrhythmia detection and classification in ambulatory electrocardiograms using a deep neural network. *Nat Med*, 2019, 25 (1), 65–69.

14. Chinmay, C., Gupta, B., Ghosh, S.K. Chronic wound characterization using Bayesian classifier under telemedicine framework. *Int J E-Health Med Comm*, 2016, 7 (1), 78–96. http://doi.org/10.4018/IJEHMC.2016010105

15. Ciconte, G., Saviano, M., Giannelli, L., Calovic, Z., Baldi, M., Ciaccio, C. et al. Atrial fibrillation detection using a novel three-vector cardiac implantable monitor: the atrial fibrillation detect study. *EP Europace*, 2017, 19 (7), 1101–1108.

16. Noelker, G., Mayer, J., Boldt, L-H., Seidl, K., Van Driel, V., Massa, T. et al. Performance of an implantable cardiac monitor to detect atrial fibrillation: results of the DETECT AF study. *J Cardiovasc Electrophysiol*, 2016, 27 (12), 1403–1410.

17. Sanders, P., Pürerfellner, H., Pokushalov, E., Sarkar, S., Di Bacco, M., Maus, B. et al. Performance of a new atrial fibrillation detection algorithm in a miniaturized insertable cardiac monitor: results from the reveal LINQ usability study. *Heart Rhythm*, 2016, 13 (7), 1425–1430.

18. Piorkowski, C., Busch, M., Nölker, G., Schmitt, J., Roithinger, F.X., Young, G. et al. Clinical evaluation of a small implantable cardiac monitor with a long sensing vector. *Pacing Clin Electrophysiol*, 2019, 42 (7), 1038–1046.

19. Sujata D, Chinmay C, Sourav K. G, Subhendu KP, Intelligent computing on time-series data analysis and prediction of COVID-19 pandemics. *Pattern Recognit Lett*, 2021, 151, 69–75. https://doi.org/10.1016/j.patrec.2021.07.027

20. Bisignani, A., De Bonis, S., Mancuso, L., Ceravolo, G., Giacopelli, D., Pelargonio, G. et al. Are implantable cardiac monitors reliable tools for cardiac arrhythmias detection? An intra-patient comparison with permanent pacemakers. *J Electrocardiol*, 2020, 59, 147–150.

21. McManus, D.D., Chong, J.W., Soni, A., Saczynski, J.S., Esa, N., Napolitano, C. et al. Pulse-smart: pulse-based arrhythmia discrimination using a novel smartphone application. *J Cardiovasc Electrophysiol*, 2016, 27 (1), 51–57.

22. Proesmans, T., Mortelmans, C., Van Haelst, R., Verbrugge, F., Vandervoort, P., Vaes, B. Mobile phone-based use of the photoplethysmography technique to detect atrial fibrillation in primary care: diagnostic accuracy study of the FibriCheck app. *JMIR mHealth and uHealth*, 2019, 7 (3), e12284.

23. Oberlo. *How Many People Have Smartphones in 2021*? URL: www.oberlo.com/statistics (accessed: 22/07/2021).

24. Kumar, A., Kumar, A., Bharat, B., Chinmay, C. Secure access control for manufacturing sector with application of ethereum blockchain. *Peer-to-Peer Netw Appl*, 2021, 1–17. https://doi.org/10.1007/s12083-021-01108-3

25. Varma, N., Cygankiewicz, I., Turakhia, M.P., Heidbuchel, H., Hu, Y-F., Chen, L.Y. et al. 2021 ISHNE/HRS/EHRA/APHRS expert collaborative statement on mHealth in arrhythmia management: digital medical tools for heart rhythm professionals: from the International Society for Holter and Noninvasive Electrocardiology/Heart Rhythm Society/European Heart Rhythm Association/Asia Pacific Heart Rhythm Society. *Circ Arrhythm Electrophysiol*, 2021, 14 (2), e009204.

26. Jensen, M.T., Treskes, R.W., Caiani, E.G., Casado-Arroyo, R., Cowie, M.R., Dilaveris, P. et al. Esc working group on e-cardiology position paper: use of commercially available wearable technology for heart rate and activity tracking in primary and secondary cardiovascular prevention—in collaboration with the European Heart Rhythm Association, European Association of Preventive Cardiology, Association of Cardiovascular Nursing and Allied Professionals, Patient Forum, and the Digital Health Committee. *Eur Heart J—Digital Health*, 2021, 2 (1), 49–59.

27. Vinayakumar, R., Harini, N., Chinmay, C., Tuan, D.P. Deep learning based meta-classifier approach for COVID-19 classification using CT scan and chest X-ray images. *Multimedia Systems*, 2021, 1–15. https://doi.org/10.1007/s00530-021-00826-1

28. Manninger, M., Zweiker, D., Svennberg, E., Chatzikyriakou, S., Pavlovic, N., Zaman, J.A. et al. Current perspectives on wearable rhythm recordings for clinical decision-making: the wEHRAbles 2 survey. *EP Europace*, 2021, 23 (7), 1106–1113.

29. Galloway, C., Treiman, D., Schreibati, J., Schram, M., Karbaschi, Z., Valys, A. et al. 5105 a deep neural network predicts atrial fibrillation from normal ECGs recorded on a smartphone-enabled device. *Eur Heart J*, 2019, 40 (suppl 1), ehz746–0041.

30. Attia, Z.I., Noseworthy, P.A., Lopez-Jimenez, F., Asirvatham, S.J., Deshmukh, A.J., Gersh, B.J. et al. An artificial intelligence-enabled ECG algorithm for the identification of patients with atrial fibrillation during sinus rhythm: a retrospective analysis of outcome prediction. *The Lancet*, 2019, 394 (10201), 861–867.

31. Jo, Y.-Y., Kwon, J.-M., Jeon, K.-H., Cho, Y.-H., Shin, J.-H., Lee, Y.-J. et al. Artificial intelligence to diagnose paroxysmal supraventricular tachycardia using electrocardiography during normal sinus rhythm. *Eur Heart J—Digital Health*, 2021, 2 (2), 290–298.

32. Rudin, C. Stop explaining black box machine learning models for high stakes decisions and use interpretable models instead. *Nature Machine Intelligence*, 2019, 1 (5), 206–215.

33. Hoong, N.K. Medical information science—framework and potential. *International Seminar and Exhibition Computerization for Development-the Research Challenge*, Universiti Pertanian Malaysia, Kuala Lumpur, pp. 191–198, 1988.

34. Ribeiroa, Antonio H., Ribeiroa, Manoel Horta, Paixaoa, Gabriela M.M., Oliveiraa, Derick M., Gomesa, Paulo R., Canazarta, Jessica, Ferreiraa, Milton P.S., Anderssonb, Carl R., Macfarlaned, Peter W., Meira Jr., Wagner, Schonb, Thomas B. and Ribeiro, Antonio Luiz P. Automatic diagnosis of the 12-lead ECG using a deep neural network. *Nature Comm*, 2020, 11, 1–9. https://doi.org/10.1038/s41467-020-15432-4

35. Ahsanuzzaman, S.M., Ahmed, Toufiq, Rahman, Atiqur. Low cost, portable ECG monitoring and alarming system based on deep learning, *IEEE, IEEE Region 10 Symposium (TENSYMP)*, Dhaka, Bangladesh, 5–7 June 2020, pp. 316–319.

36. Zhang, Dongdong, Yuan, Xiaohui, Zhang, Ping. Interpretable deep learning for automatic diagnosis of 12-lead electrocardiogram. *iScience*, Elsevier, 2021, 24, 102373. https://doi.org/10.1016/j.isci.2021.102373

37. Othman, Soufiene Ben, Bahattab, Abdullah Ali, Trad, Abdelbasset, Youssef, Habib. PEERP: a priority-based energy-efficient routing protocol for reliable data transmission in healthcare using the IoT. *The 15th International Conference on Future Networks and Communications (FNC) August 9–12, 2020*, Leuven, Belgium, 2020.

38. Othman, Soufiene Ben, Bahattab, Abdullah Ali, Trad, Abdelbasset, Youssef, Habib. LSDA: lightweight secure data aggregation scheme in healthcare using IoT. *ACM — 10th International Conference on Information Systems and Technologies*, Lecce, Italy, June 2020.

39. Othman, Soufiene Ben, Bahattab, Abdullah Ali, Trad, Abdelbasset, Youssef, Habib. RESDA: robust and efficient secure data aggregation scheme in healthcare using the IoT. *The International Conference on Internet of Things, Embedded Systems and Communications (IINTEC 2019)*, HAMMAMET, Tunisia from 20–22 December 2019.

13 Diagnosing of Disease Using Machine Learning in Internet of Healthcare Things

Abhinay Thakur and Ashish Kumar

CONTENTS

13.1 INTRODUCTION

The aging demographic has emerged a slew of unforeseen problems for healthcare professionals. Medical rehabilitation is a comparatively recent discipline, having been established in the mid-twentieth century, and has been viewed as a novel area of therapy aimed at reducing or treating physical or mental disruptions through the remediation or restoration of defects [1–4]. Several patients have found it to be a beneficial way to improve their physical functions. Nevertheless, there are a few roadblocks in the way of expanding the spectrum of medical rehabilitation. To begin with, the majority of rehabilitation treatments are of longer duration besides being laborious. Second, more supportive services are needed to make rehabilitation treatments more accessible to patients. Third, attributed to the growing population of senior individuals in today's society, rehabilitation resources are increasingly limited. The healthcare sector could grow smarter by incorporating artificial intelligence (AI) into its operations. Disease diagnosis utilizing machine learning (ML) in smart healthcare could help medical workers save time. ML systems could be utilized for diagnosis, prediction, and providing the appropriate treatment regimen for the discovered condition to analyze and evaluate the efficacy of treatment in the healthcare field. The healthcare profession has issues in electronic data processing, electronic ailment detection, and data aggregation with the healthcare network in order to minimize healthcare costs and promote individualized health. ML offers a wide range of strategies, techniques, and resources for addressing the issues. In the field of ML, data is a valuable resource [5–9]. ML could increase its efficacy and forecast ability by increasing the quantity and quality of data. ML has been widely used to address healthcare challenges. It could be utilized to more accurately determine a patient's treatment regimen, offer advice to the patient, make forecasts, and create a disease profile depending on the symptoms detected. An ML system may give patients behavioral suggestions relying on their current health condition and background. ML algorithms could be developed to anticipate consequences. ML is often utilized in healthcare to recognize a patient's disparity and to advise a person regarding medication. In the domain of healthcare, AI and ML technologies are not simply for diagnosing diseases; they also provide therapy combinations. For instance, ML algorithms are not intended to replace physicians, but rather to assist them in making judgments and making suggestions depending on their assessment of patients. Malignancy, neurological disease, and heart disease are three major diseases where ML methods are particularly useful. Accurate diagnoses are critical in preventing patients' health issues from deteriorating. Furthermore, by improving investigative techniques on imagery, genes, Electronic Health Records, and other factors, earlier diagnosis may be possible, demonstrating the potential of AI and ML tools. Neurological, cancer and cardiac disease are all life-threatening ailments that require prompt diagnosis and treatment. ML is employed to categorize items, such as lesions, into categories like aberrant, benign, and lesions or nonlesions. Rapid identification and efficient diagnostic methods could save individuals from illnesses such as cancer, in which there is no entire reason for their development. Mammography may detect cancer up to two or three years before symptoms appear [10]. DL system, i.e., a deep learning system, also referred to as CNN (convolutional neural network) could eventually read mammograms better than a typical CAD system. CNN does have the ability to revolutionize therapeutic image analysis, particularly in the area of mammography breast cancer detection. Naive Bayes (NB), logistic regression (LR), and support vector machine (SVM) are examples of multistage classifiers. A multistage classifier comprises SVM, LDA, decision tree (DT), K-nearest neighbor (KNN), LR, and NB, and are utilized for the diagnosis, identification, and forecasting of several fatal diseases. The pattern of a particular disease can be detected with the help of the systematic examination of present medical data and also the later can assist in diagnosing several fatal diseases and its vital level. Utilizing the ML algorithms for systematic analysis can also assist in forming the prognostic models that lead to a personalized cure, inspect the detrimental remarks that appear in the patients at the time of trial run, and in addition aids the health practitioners to decide the medication for the patients. Figure 13.1 shows the various applications of ML in several healthcare fields such as smart health records, prediction and prognosis of diseases, drug discovery, etc.; ML plays a potent role in the sustainability of today's world healthcare sector.

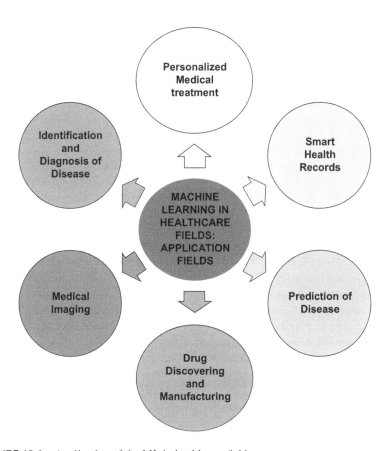

FIGURE 13.1   Application of the ML in healthcare fields.

The following major elements must be considered when selecting an ML-based framework which comprised of major characteristics of the ML framework:

- The framework must be capable of delivering optimal efficiency.
- It must be simple and user-friendly for the programmer community to use. Traditional model construction methods should be supported, as well as an easy-to-understand code approach.
- Parallelization must be completely enabled for the spread of computational activities.
- It should be backed up by a large and enthusiastic user base and network.
- It must be out rather than in a black box.
- It must be possible to simplify ML algorithms, rendering them more user-friendly and accessible to developers.

13.1.1 Machine-learning (ML) Applications in the Healthcare System

There are a variety of ML applications which have been extensively accessible in the healthcare sector, some of which are discussed in the following sections.

13.1.1.1 Recognition and Prognosis of the Disease

The healthcare sector is confronting numerous issues as a result of population increase, contemporary lifestyles, and increasing pollutants. These issues could involve poor management of large medical data and a lack of automated disease detection, diagnostic, and treatment methods. Several research facilities are collaborating with healthcare practitioners, doctors, and pharmaceutical businesses to offer essential remedies such as diagnostic equipment and therapy solutions for presymptomatic detection and treatment. Critical disorders such as malignancy, renal failure, cardiovascular disease, as well as other single-gene inheritance necessitate real-time detection and treatment so that the right cure could be administered on-site. When we examine the research efforts conducted to identify and diagnose distinct diseases, one can see how diverse enterprises have undertaken various approaches to deliver real-time treatments [11, 12]. IBM Watson for Genomics is a unified tumor sequencing and cognitive computing (genome-based) system that has been designed to expedite tumor diagnostics. Another AI-powered biotech start-up, "BERG," has established an AI-based medicinal therapy in a variety of fields, including neuroscience, rare cancer, and malignancy. Meinel et al. [13] devised a technique for semiautomated categorization. Following segmentation, 42 characteristics were calculated based on lesion size, textures, and improvement kinetics, and the 13 greatest characteristics were chosen as well as utilized as input to BNN (backpropagation neural network). The BNN was designed and evaluated on 80 BMRI lesions employing the leave-one-out technique (37 benign, 43 malignant). The reference standard was the histology of lesions. The 80 lesions were classified by five human readers with and without CAD aid. Receiver operating feature slopes were employed to examine the efficiency of the computer classifier and the human readers and multi-reader multicase (MRMC) evaluation was used to evaluate the efficiency of the human readers. In the case where CAD system was employed to help the human readers, their efficiency increased dramatically ($p < 0.05$). As per MRMC assessment, the Human reader efficiency using CAD and without using CAD system aid could be extrapolated to the intensity of cases ($p < 0.001$).

13.1.1.2   Discovery and Production of Drugs

ML can be used in each phase of drug development, from the earliest phases, including drug construction (chemical composition), to the intermediate phases, including drug verification, and the end phases, like clinical studies, production, and marketplace distribution. In two aspects, ML could assist the healthcare framework: first, this could suggest relevant solutions to cut the entire price of pharmaceuticals at the time of their debut in the marketplace. Second, as contrasted to conventional procedures, this could speed up the drug development and production procedure, rendering it extremely efficient and cost-effective [14–18]. Using molecular diagnostics and next-generation genomic tools, the clinical relevance of ML could help determine the best therapy for multiple illnesses and hereditary susceptibility. AtomNet is an "Atomwise Company" DL neural network-based system that was created specifically for the creation and development of pharmaceuticals depending on protein architecture. In comparison to existing procedures, which take months to acquire millions of possible compounds, this methodology only takes a day or two. Following the formation of protein complexes, the AtomNet simulator is used to investigate the drug's behavior in the patient. As a result, it is possible to find prospective medicines to combat a variety of ailments. Deepmind is another invention of Alphabet Incorporation, that is a division of Google, and it works in the same sector as stated earlier, with significant advancement.

13.1.1.3   Diagnosis Using Medical Imaging

In medical imaging, ML algorithms could analyze a large quantity of data at a really fast rate. Medical pictures are large datasets in health systems which could be utilized to build ML algorithms to grasp the details of MRIs and CT scans. InnerEye, a Microsoft product, was utilized to analyze photos and provide image diagnostic equipment. ML-based analytic tools have been established by organizations like Sophia and Enlitic to detect problems in medical imaging data. In contrast to medical specialists, these devices operate on all forms of medical image reports and assess them with amazing precision. LYmph Node Assistant is a technology developed by Google to assist in detecting metastasis and breast cancer promptly. This method supports pathologists and relieves their workload by producing high-quality reports. Another system was created through a collaboration between France, Germany, and the United States. This method uses a convolutional neural network (CNN) to accurately diagnose skin cancer. Ancochea et al. [2] discussed the peculiarities of COVID-19 patients at the outset of the condition, with particular emphasis on the treatment and diagnosis of female COVID-19 patients. They investigated the amorphous free text in the SESCAM Healthcare Network's electronic health records (EHRs) (Castilla La-Mancha, Spain). Between 1st January 2020 to 1st May 2020, the study samples included the whole populace with accessible EHRs (1,446,452 patients). For all COVID-19 cases, they retrieved clinical information about the patients' diagnosis, treatment, and prognosis. Finally, a maximum of 4,780 patients with a verified COVID-19 diagnosis were discovered. There were 2,443 female patients (51%), who were younger by 1.5 years on median as compared to the male patients (60.6–18.3 vs. 62.4–17.5, $p = 0.0024$). In the 15–59-year-old age group, there were significant female COVID-19 incidents, having the highest sex ratio (95%) in the 30–39-year-old group (1.58; 1.24–2.23). Females had much more headaches, anosmia, and ageusia than males when they were diagnosed. Females were less likely than males to have chest X-rays or blood tests (64.4% vs. 77.2% and 44.5% vs. 66.2%, respectively), both with $p < 0.001$. Females were less likely than men to be admitted to the hospital (44.3% vs. 62.0%) and to be divulged to the intensive care unit (ICU) (2.4% vs. 7.6%), all with $p < 0.001$. Similarly, Javed et al. [3] concentrated on enhancing the categorization of modest day-to-day activities and multipart intertwined activities. CA-SHR also performed a time-based assessment to see whether the temporal features can successfully identify handicapped people. This research identified mentally challenged people at a preliminary phase. CA-SHR assesses people's health by looking at key characteristics and improving dementia sufferers' depiction. They employed ensembles AdaBoost to classify people into various categories according to health, mild cognitive impairment (MCI), and dementia. When compared to existing methodologies, this improves the dependability of the CA-SHR by correctly assigning labels to smart home residents.

Hosseinzadeh et al. [4] used artificial neural networks (ANN) in IoMT systems to increase the diagnosis reliability of thyroid illnesses based on semantic descriptions and diagnostic data. This research proposes a collection of MMLP (multiple multi-layer perceptron) neural networks having backpropagation (BP) error capability to enhance generalization and reduce the overfitting of ANN throughout the preparation phase. In addition, to cope with the backpropagation inaccuracy, algorithm's sluggish resolution, and local minima issue, an adaptive learning rate method was utilized. The suggested MMLP significantly improved the reliability of thyroid illness classification substantially. When contrasted to a single network, MMLP has six networks improved accuracy by 0.7%. Furthermore, using an adaptive learning rate algorithm like the one used in the suggested MMLP resulted in a 4.6% in efficiency and a maximum efficiency of 99% in IoMT systems when compared to regular backpropagation. The suggested MMLP was evaluated in current thyroid illness diagnosis studies, and its efficiency was demonstrated. In this chapter, we will be discussing the impact of various forms of ML on the Internet of Healthcare Things. This will be followed by ML, various types of ML, computer-aided diagnosis (CAD), boosting algorithm, PCA, SVM, and ANN.

13.1.2 Machine Learning

In 1959, Arthur Samuel presented the term "machine learning." He was an expert in AI and electronic games. He claims that ML allows computers to understand despite having to be expressly trained. Tom Mitchell provided a structural and mathematically based description of ML in 1997, stating that a computer program uses experience "e" to understand a project "t." It uses "p" as a performance indicator on "t," which increases gradually as "e" is added. ML has emerged as the most important technology for solving many real-world issues in previous years all over the world. As a result, it is becoming a very preferred tool for issue resolution among industry and academic professionals [19, 20]. ML refers to a branch of AI which empowers machines to train from their mistakes and increase their capacity to handle problems without being given specific directions. The goal of ML is to create and use computer algorithms which can educate from a challenging region and generate improved judgments. The process of learning in ML begins with monitoring and analyzing data utilizing various strategies, including using instances, memories, depending on data pattern recognition, and so on, to enable machines to make judgments without the need for human or other interaction. To create and train a mathematical formula, machine learning algorithms use a sampling dataset as inputs, also referred to as the training dataset. Text, integer arithmetic, voice, multimodal, or video information could be gathered from a variety of sources, including sensors, programs, equipment, networking, and utilities. The mathematical framework analyzes itself to derive information from the incoming data without any active programming aid. It produces a reaction as an output following interpreting the data. The result could be in the shape of arithmetic or a floating-point number. ML algorithms, unlike traditional algorithms, can be used in a variety of domains, including pattern recognition, email filtering, e-commerce, medical systems, and many others, to give efficient and accurate responses. Figure 13.2. deliberates the input data process through the

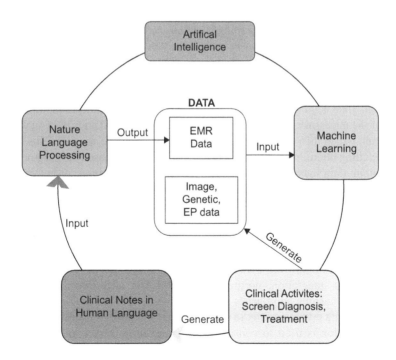

FIGURE 13.2   The workflow processing of the ML-based healthcare input and desired output.

various steps which include data transfer in the form of EMR data, genetics, EP data, and commands in natural language processing which incorporates the encompassing ML-based approaches.

13.2 ARCHITECTURE OF MACHINE LEARNING

The essential industry relevance has been built into ML framework. In conclusion, the goal is to maximize the utilization of present assets in order to attain the best possible outcome with the data given. Also, when combined with data sciences and technology, this aids in the prediction of data analytics and data forecast in wide-ranging applications. ML architecture can be developed in several phases. Each step has a distinct purpose, and all phases collaborate to improve the decision support. Data collection, data analysis, data modeling, implementation, and distribution are the five phases of the ML paradigm. The following are the specifics.

13.2.1 DATA ACQUISITION

Data collection is well-known to be problem-specific and distinct for every ML task. In addition, to gain the best value in ML tasks, precise data estimate is quite challenging. During the initial stages of data collection, it is challenging to estimate how much data will be needed to educate the model. More than two-thirds of the data generated in some research efforts is determined to be worthless. Also, until a model's training commences, it is hard to know whether the percentage of the data would be capable to deliver a meaningful and accurate outcome during the duration of data gathering. As a result, it is necessary to collect and maintain all types of data, either organized, unorganized, digital, inactive, accessible, or private [21–23]. Since the effectiveness of ML model development is dependent on the relevancy and reliability of data, this step of data collecting must be treated extremely carefully. As a result, data acquisition is the initial stage of the ML architecture, which works to gather the necessary data from various sources [22]. The data is then analyzed by the system, which then makes a judgment about how to solve an issue. This involves tasks including obtaining accurate and complete data, case-based data segmentation, and accurate data interpretation for storage and processing in accordance with the criteria. Essentially, the data is acquired in an unstructured manner from several resources, and each source has a unique form that is unsuitable for analysis.

13.2.2 DATA PROCESSING

This step receives data from a data collection level and does additional operations such as system integration, normalization, filtration, cleansing, conversion, and encoding. The learning approaches that were employed to tackle the issue also have an impact on data preprocessing. In the instance of supervised training, for instance, data segmentation is used to construct experimental data in various phases. The data collected is then used to practice the system, and the resulting sample data is commonly referred to as training data. Unlabeled data is mostly utilized for analysis in unsupervised learning. In comparison to other extant learning strategies, this learning methodology primarily works with uncertain input that is more sophisticated and requires significant processing [24–28]. In this example, data is divided into clusters, each corresponding to a distinct category. The resolution of the data determines the formation of every cluster. An additional aspect of data processing is the sort of processing that is dependent on the characteristics and actions conducted on continuous data. It also might work with discrete data. Memory constrained computation might well be required when working with datasets. As a result, the goal of this phase is to deliver a clear and well-structured dataset. This phase is often referred to as the preparation phase.

13.2.3 DATA MODELING

Data modeling entails choosing an algorithm that is most flexible for the platform in order to handle the concerns raised in the issue description. It necessitates training an ML algorithm to make forecasts dependent on accessible characteristics, variable adjustment to meet business requirements, and verification of data samples. Understanding the surroundings and implementing the training dataset utilized in the learning phase evolve the algorithms engaged in this procedure. Following effective modeling, a trained model is utilized for inferences, allowing the program to make forecasts on additional data inputs. The data scientist trains numerous models during the data modeling step. The aim of this stage is to discover the model with the best forecast reliability when compared to others. For training the model, two types of data were utilized. The initial set of data is termed training data, and it is utilized as input by the machine learning algorithm to build the model. The ML algorithm then processes the supplied data, producing a model for forecasting subsequent data. The training will proceed till the appropriate model is obtained. The model's prediction hypothesis for new data is improved, thanks to the training. To put it another way, this enables the model to anticipate the intended value given fresh data. There are two types of training data: labeled and unlabeled. The value is linked with the labeled data, whereas the unlabeled data has no preset significance. Test data is the second collection of information. The examined data is utilized to validate the model's predicted hypothesis that was developed during training. The overarching purpose of data modeling is to develop a model capable of greater forecasting and data analysis in the future.

13.2.4 EXECUTION (MODEL EVALUATION)

The algorithm (model) is applied, tested, and fine-tuned on a test dataset during the implementation phase (unseen data). The goal of this step is to get the intended result from the machine and to regulate the system's efficiency to its utmost potential. At this phase of ML design, the system's solution is competent in exploring and providing the essential data for machine decision-making.

13.2.5 DEPLOYMENT

The deployment phase determines how the model would be integrated into the platform for decision-making. At this point, the model is used in a real-world setting and is also subjected to additional analysis. In addition, the result of the functional model is sent into the system as a directive for decision-making. The ML operations' output is immediately transferred to business operations, where it leads to an improvement in allowing the machine to make informed decisions depending on output without relying on some other variables.

13.3 PERSPECTIVE OF DISEASE DIAGNOSIS USING ML

The application of ML to disease diagnosis has been demonstrated to be simple. The majority of the methods recommend using either ANN or SVM. The following is a list of diseases for which ML diagnosis has been applied.

13.3.1 ALZHEIMER'S DISEASE

There is no precise technique that could diagnose Alzheimer's disease (AD). It is diagnosed using the patient's clinical description, cognitive examinations, and electroencephalography. As a consequence, innovative methodologies are needed to allow for precise diagnosis and normative data. ML applications for detecting and classifying Alzheimer's disease have gotten a lot of interest. In the field of medical imaging assessment, ML is an expanding topic wherein researchers can utilize basic neuroimaging information to discover patterns that grab viewers. Podgorelec et al. [29] demonstrated a way of analyzing EEG waves using an ML methodology to diagnose Alzheimer's disease. They demonstrated how to collect characteristics from EEG recordings to be used in the advancement of an AD classification model incorporating ML technique. Further, it was demonstrated that using a resilient and adaptable ML approach allows for the creation of more precise (86%), well-proportioned classification models than famous synchrony metrics (83%).

Park et al. [30] used large-scale administrative healthcare information to see if ML models might forecast prospective Alzheimer's disease occurrence. They acquired the health data that was de-identified in seniors over 65 years of age group ($N = 40,736$) through the Korean National Health Insurance Service database 2002–2010, comprising 4,894 distinctive clinical characteristics such as ICD-10 digits, lab results, medication standards, the background of individual/family disease, and sociodemographics. They used two operational criteria to describe incident AD: "definite AD" ($n = 614$) with dementia medication along with diagnostic codes, and "probable AD" ($n = 2,026$) with a simple analysis. Random forest, SVM, and logistic regression were developed and verified to forecast event AD in 1–4 years. The ML models performed rather well in 1-year forecasting comprising AUCs of 0.769 and 0.772, correspondingly, depending on "certain AD" and "possible AD" results; in the two-year forecast, 0.730 and 0.693; in three-year prediction, 0.677 and 0.644; and in four-year prediction, 0.725 and 0.683. When the whole (unbalanced) specimens were utilized, the findings were comparable. Hemoglobin level, ethnicity, and urine protein level were all significant clinical variables used in logistic regression. This work demonstrated the value of a data-driven ML model built on huge organizational health data in predicting AD risk, allowing for improved identification of those at threat of AD in clinical trials or earlier identification in clinical trials.

13.3.2 THYROID DISEASE

In both men and women, the thyroid is located in the bottom part of the neck, beneath the folds of muscle and skin that could be seen. To enhance patient survival rates, it is critical to develop an accurate technique for identifying malignancy dangers. Furthermore, early detection of thyroid problem symptoms could improve survival rates by allowing therapy to begin at the earliest possible phase. As a result, ML technology must be used in the diagnostic procedure and therapy of thyroid nodules in order to obtain correct categorization. Choi et al. [31] introduced a novel economically accessible CAD system ultrasound of the thyroid which uses AI and its effectiveness was assessed in the treatment of cancerous thyroid nodules and its classification. From November 2015 to February 2016, patients having thyroid nodules having a definitive treatment, either malignant or benign, were recruited in a series of studies. Similar thyroid nodules have been investigated by another radiologist utilizing the CAD method, yielding ultrasonography features and a diagnostic of whether the nodules were harmless or cancerous. The diagnostic accuracy of the expert radiologist and the CAD system was evaluated, as well as the concordance of US features. Out of 102 thyroid nodules spotted from 89 patients enrolled in the study, 59 that turn out to be 57.8% of the total samples are benign lesions, whereas the remaining 43, i.e., 42.2% of the investigated samples, are malignant lesions. The CAD system had an identical sensitivity to the professional radiologist (91.2% vs. 87.3%, $p > 0.99$), with poorer specificity and AUROC curve (specificity: 73.5% vs. 95.1%, $p = 0.002$; AUROC: 0.83 vs. 0.92, $p = 0.021$). The radiologist and the CAD system had a high agreement on ultrasonic properties (component, direction, hypoechoic, and spongiform) ($j = 0.623, 0.732, 0.713$, and 0.643, respectively), while the margin had an acceptable agreement ($j = 0.239$). The CAD framework's sensitivities for cancerous thyroid nodules were comparable to that of a competent radiologist, but its precision and reliability were inferior. The CAD approach had high agreement with an expert radiologist in the characterization of thyroid nodules.

Similarly, Hosseinzadeh et al. [4] utilized ANN in IoMT systems to increase the diagnosis reliability of thyroid illnesses based on semantic descriptions and testing data. This research proposed a complex of MMLP neural networks having backpropagation errors capacity to increase generalization and reduce the overfitting of ANN throughout the training phase. In addition, an adaptive learning rate method was utilized to address the backpropagation error algorithm's sluggish resolution and localized minima issue. The suggested MMLP significantly improved the reliability of thyroid illness classification substantially. In comparison to a single network, MMLP employing a group of six networks improved reliability by 0.7%. Furthermore, when compared to normal backpropagation, adopting an adaptive learning rate algorithm in the suggested MMLP resulted in a 5.1% increase in efficiency and ultimate efficiency of 98.9% in IoMT systems. The suggested MMLP was evaluated in existing thyroid illness diagnosis studies, and its efficiency was demonstrated.

13.3.3 HEART DISEASE

Heart disease is also a major cause of disability, limiting the activity and eroding the quality of life of millions of older people. Manually identifying heart disease signs is tough. ML, on the other hand, is a beneficial tool for predicting the signs of cardiac disease in order to diagnose the condition and develop treatment regimens. Samhitha et al. [23] recommended using a group of classifiers to do assessments for the accuracy of prediction of cardiac disease. For preparation and validation, the Cleveland heart dataset obtained through the UCI ML repository was used. The prediction of heart disease was examined and shown to be relevant in the medical area. Regardless, the fatality rate could be effectively minimized when the disease is detected in its initial stages and thereafter, protective measures are implemented early enough. They introduced a fresh technique in this study that focuses on detecting crucial features using ML strategies, resulting in improved accuracy in the detection of cardiovascular disease. The forecast model was given several combinations of highlights as well as a few well-known grouping algorithms. Using the expectation model for heart illness with the half-breed irregular woods using a straight model, they generated an improved demonstration degree with an accuracy level of 88.7%.

Similarly, Bharti et al. [32] compared the findings and assessment of the UCI ML Heart Disease dataset using various ML and DL methods. The dataset contains 14 key attributes that were utilized in the investigation. Several encouraging outcomes have been obtained, which have been verified utilizing the reliability and ambiguity matrix. Isolation Forest was used to manage some unimportant aspects of the dataset, and the data is also standardized for improved outcomes. By utilizing a DL method, 94.2% efficiency was achieved.

13.3.4 HEPATITIS

In the recent period, ML algorithms have gotten a lot of interest in the domain of healthcare. It is feasible to find efficient classifications for extracting useful data from linked and imbalanced medical datasets. A basic instance might be a patient suffering from chest problems who visits a healthcare center. The ML algorithm can check for the top five causes of chest discomfort and declare them to be healthy. This strategy may fail for a variety of persons who are afflicted with rare disorders. We are still a long way from developing a system which could definitively diagnose all diseases, but progress is being made. A heuristic optimization approach has been used by Tang et al. [33] for optimizing the dendritic neuron model (DNM) and for computer-aided diagnostics constructed as hardware. The presented evolutionary dendritic neuron model (EDNM) is optimized by guided artificial bee colony algorithm (GABC) because the backpropagation approach is susceptible to the preliminary circumstances and could quickly collapse to the local minima. The dataset of liver disorders, Haberman's survival, Wisconsin breast cancer, hepatitis and diabetic retinopathy Debrecen were used in the experimental tests, and the efficiency of our framework was robustly affirmed in classification performance, responsivity, Cohen's kappa, selectivity, F measure, the region underneath the recipient operating characteristic curve (AUC), fast convergence, as well as statistical analgesia. Furthermore, the neural pruning mechanism allows the EDNM to streamline its neural organization following learning by deleting redundant synapses and extraneous dendrites. Ultimately, without sacrificing accuracy, the EDNM's simpler architectural morphogenesis could be substituted with a logic circuit (LC). It is worthwhile noting that, once applied by an LC, the model outperforms other classifiers in terms of performance when dealing with large amounts of data. As a result, their developed framework could be used to create a high-performing medical classifier.

Similarly, Kishor et al. [34] and his colleagues used seven ML classification algorithms to forecast nine deadly diseases, including heart disease, diabetic breast cancer, liver, hepatic issue, dermatological, surgery information, hypothyroidism, and scintigraphy cardiac. Four efficiency indicators (precision, susceptibility, precision, and region under the curve) are utilized to assess the suggested model's efficiency. For various diseases, the RF classifier records optimum precision of 97.62%, the sensibility of 99.67%, selectivity of 97.81%, and AUC of 99.32%. Physicians would be able to diagnose the condition earlier because of the established healthcare model.

13.4 ML SYSTEMS IN THE PREDICTION OF DISEASES

13.4.1 COMPUTER-AIDED DIAGNOSIS

Endoscopists are paying more emphasis to computer-aided diagnosis as it may assist them to prevent detecting and mischaracterizing polyps. The objective of CAD for colonoscopy is to identify numerous elements in a colonoscopic scans/movies and produce the projected polyp pathology or location using ML. ML is a major part of AI in which a machine could be trained to understand (in this instance, identify and categorize polyps) through repetitions and expertise. The result of CAD should preferably be displayed on the monitor in real-time, aiding the endoscopist's decision-making process. Additionally, using CAD in screening colonoscopy could assist to reduce differences in adenoma detection rates (ADR) between endoscopists or centers. Both beginner and expert endoscopists who seek to enhance their ADR may benefit from CAD training. Benzakoun et al. [35] tested the effectiveness of a commonly accessible CAD system for automated subsolid nodule identification and characterization. In 100 participants, the CAD system was tested on 50 pristine ground-glass nodules and 50 portion rigid nodules (mean size: 17 mm) found on classic CT scans. At various sensitivity parameters, genuine nodule identification and the overall number of CAD markers were assessed. Logistic regression was used to examine the impact of nodule and CT acquisition features. Spearman and Bland-Altman techniques were used to evaluate software and manually determine diameters. At a mean expense of 17 CAD marks per CT scan, 50/100 (50%) subsolid nodules were found with specificity optimized for 3-mm nodule identification. At the 5-mm level, these numbers were 26/100 (26%) and 2 correspondingly. The average number of CAD markers per CT was 41 at the maximum sensitivity setting (2-mm nodule detection), although the nodule detection performance only improved to 54%. At the 3-mm setting, portion rigid nodules were superior the identified clear ground-glass nodules: 35/50 (69%) against 16/50 (29%) ($p = 0.0001$), with no effect on the solid element thickness. No other nodule parameter affects the recognition rate save the kind. For 79 nodules, high-quality segmentation was achieved, with computerized data correlating well with manual assessments (rho = 0.90 [0.84–0.93]). Software-measured absorption levels for all part-solid nodules were more than 671 Hounsfield units (HU). This CAD system's identification rate of subsolid nodules was inadequate, but in 79% of the cases, high-quality separation was produced, enabling automated determination of size and absorption.

Choi et al. [36] contrasted the effectiveness of a CAD system in supporting radiologists in detecting cancerous solitary pulmonary nodules (SPNs) to straight personal depiction. A sum of 40 individuals enclosing SPNs were studied. An extra ten series of post-contrast scans were taken at 20-seconds increments following the pre-contrast scan. The absorbance values of the SPNs were evaluated by two researchers: a radiologist who created the ROIs and a technologist who utilized a CAD framework. The net improvement among a CAD system and straight personal sketching was compared using the Bland and Altman graphs. The diagnostic features of the cancerous SPNs were computed utilizing Fisher's exact analysis and the CAD and straight individual sketching. The net improvement differential between both the CAD system and straight personal sketching was not substantial (within two average deviations) on the Bland and Altman graph. Utilizing CAD to diagnose cancerous SPNs, the sensibility, selectivity, negative predictive value (NPV), positive predictive value (PPV), and accuracy were 91%, 85%, 75%, 96%, and 88%, correspondingly. The specificity, selectivity, positive predictive value, negative predictive value, and precision of straight drawing for diagnosing cancerous SPNs were 92%, 89%, 79%, 92%, and 88%, correspondingly.

Ha et al. [37] compared the diagnosing accuracy of abbreviated magnetic resonance imaging (MRI) and comprehensive diagnosis MRI using a CAD program in individuals having a clinical diagnosis of breast malignancy to see how kinetic features affect the efficiency of two radiologists. Between January 1, 2014, and December 31, 2017, 3,834 breast MRI examinations were performed on 2,310 individuals who had been diagnosed with breast cancer. Two radiologists examined the MRI pictures prospectively. First, two radiologists separately assessed T1- and T2-weighted pictures taken 90 seconds following the contrast media injection. The two readers used CAD to compare contrast-enhanced T1-weighted pictures with five successive postponed pictures following six months. The diagnostic accuracy of truncated and full-sequence MRI was evaluated. Breast MRI was used to detect 51 intramammary reoccurrences in 47 individuals. Thirty-six (70.6%) of the 51 tumor recurrences happened more than three years following the original cancer surgery, and seven (13.7%) occurred less than two years following the initial surgery. On the shorter sequencing, the specificity and sensitivity were 92.2–94.1% and 97.6–98.6%, respectively, while on the complete diagnostic MRI, they were 94.1–96.1% and 97.9–98.3%, respectively. Six malignant lesions out of 51 exhibited a prolonged persisting trend, three of which were non-mass enhancing and three of which were minimal boosting masses less than 1 cm in diameter. Both readers found that shortened MRI and comprehensive diagnosis MRI performed similarly in terms of comprehensive diagnostic accuracy. The reader's efficiency might be affected by CAD-generated kinetic features, and the sensitivities or precision might be enhanced depending on the reader.

13.4.2 PRINCIPAL COMPONENT ANALYSIS

Principal component analysis (PCA) is a dimensionality-reduction approach for lowering the aspect of enormous datasets by turning a vast array of components into a smaller one that maintains the significant data in the original array. Although lowering the number of components in a set of data reduces precision, the solution to dimensional minimization is to sacrifice some precision in exchange for greater transparency. ML algorithms might analyze data much more quickly and effectively without struggling with superfluous factors because compact datasets are easy to investigate and visualize.

Throughout harvesting trials, Zhang et al. [38] explored the influence of 11 canopy characteristics on mechanical harvesting for vertically trained "Scifresh" and V-trellis grown "Envy" trees. To evaluate the canopy datasets, they used a supervised ML technique using weighted k-nearest neighbors (kNN). The fruit removal condition of 2,678 ground-truth data points (apples) was divided into two binary classes: "mechanically harvested" and "mechanically unharvested" apples. The implemented approach attained an average predictive performance of 76–92% for "Scifresh" and 62–74% for "Envy" for the training dataset (85%). Overall test accuracies on "Scifresh" were 81–91%, but only 36–79% on "Envy" with the remaining 15% dataset. By computing the coefficients of principal factors, the principal components analysis was utilized to discover the important canopy characteristics (PCs). At minimum 80% of the data variance was accounted for by PC1–PC5. Fruit load per branch, branch basal diameter, and shoot length were the most relevant among all when a coefficient greater than 0.5 was assumed to be extremely relevant. These findings can help farmers enhance the effectiveness of a mechanical harvesting system by providing advice on canopy management.

Allegretta et al. [39] used a foldable energy-dispersive XRF instrument (pED-XRF), principal component analysis, as well as some ML algorithms to differentiate and provisionally classify 18 meteorite specimens of various existence and sources into three distinct macro-groups: iron meteorites, stony meteorites, and meteor-wrongs. The findings revealed that using the cubic SVM (CSVM), subspace discriminant-ensemble classifiers (SD-EC), fine kernel nearest neighbor (FKNN), and subspace discriminant KNN-EC (SKNN-EC) algorithms on the standardized spectrum, 100% accuracy in specimen classification was achieved. This technique enabled the categorization and differentiation of meteorites into macro-groups, such as irons, stony-irons, and meteor-wrongs, quickly and reliably. These preliminary findings show that using a mix of ML algorithms and XRF spectra to discriminate and categorize any actual or alleged meteorite is a very efficient and interesting method. To summarize, PCA's basic concept is to minimize the number of variables in a data collection while retaining as much knowledge as feasible.

Jo et al. [40] devised a novel method for predicting path loss using ML techniques such as dimensionality reduction, ANN-MLP, and Gaussian processes. The tests were created to see if integrating ANN-MLP and Gaussian procedure with dimensionality compression would enable a similar path loss predictive performance and offer a level of confidence in a regression challenge. The four-feature model's dimensionality was decreased utilizing the PCA technique, resulting in a more generalized model with only one component and a considerable decrease in the training phase. The effectiveness of the PCA-applied simple system is very comparable to that of the initial multifeatured training model. In comparison to a many variables model, data analysis using key variables from PCA necessitates more attention to experimental data acquisition and learning time expense. PCA could eliminate unwanted noise or unrelated independent factors, resulting in significant variables that represent the more underlying path loss qualities and improved reliability. The expense of training for using the learning technique is critical since it might be a practical aspect in the actual world. When contrasted to the four-variable model, the one variable method in ANN-MLP and the GP model consume 10% and 1% of the training time, correspondingly. As a result, in the next sections, they concentrated on a distance characteristic along with a similar frequency for ANN model training.

Polat et al.[41] used principal component analysis and the least square SVM to recognize ECG arrhythmias (LS-SVM). There are two stages to the strategy method. Utilizing principal component analysis, the dimensions of the ECG arrhythmias database, which included 279 characteristics, were limited to 15 characteristics in the initial step. The LS-SVM classifier was used to diagnose ECG arrhythmias in the second phase. They employed the ECG arrhythmias dataset from the UCI ML database in our research. The data set was then divided into two major groups: 80% of it was used for training and the remaining 20% was used for testing. The ultimate benefit might be to aid the physician in making an informed decision. This finding was for ECG arrhythmias condition, but it also indicates that this technique could be utilized with confidence to diagnose other medical diseases.

13.4.3 BOOSTING ALGORITHM

Boosting is the technique of merging weak learners to produce a robust learner, wherein a weak learner is a classifier that is only tangentially related to the real classification. A robust learner, in contrast to a weak learner, is a classifier connected with the proper classes. Sebastiani et al. [42] explain about AdaBoost.MHKR, an enhanced boosting algorithm, and how it can be used to categorize text. Boosting is a guided learning strategy which has been effectively deployed to a wide range of genres and has proved to be among the strongest producers in text categorization activities to date. Boosting is founded on the concept of depending on the aggregate judgment of a group of successively trained classifiers. Special attention is focused on the precise classification of the training documents when training the ith classifier that has proved to be more difficult for earlier taught classifiers. AdaBoost.MHKR is founded on the concept of creating a subcommittee of the K classifiers that look at the most probable at each repetition of the process of learning, rather than a single classifier. They presented the findings of a comprehensive test of this strategy using the standard Reuters-21578 benchmark. These tests revealed that AdaBoost.MHKR was more economical and efficient to train than the standard AdaBoost. Algorithm MHR.

Truong et al. [43] presented utilizing the gradient tree boosting (GTB) algorithm, among the most effective ML algorithms, an effective approach for evaluating the security of steel trusses (ML). Datasets are initially created utilizing sophisticated analysis to account for the structure's geometrical and mechanical nonlinearities. The structure's maximum load-carrying capability and distortion were then predicted using four GTB models for security assessment of durability and ease of maintenance. Input variables that were both continuous and intermittent were investigated. In order to illustrate the efficacy of the suggested approach, a comparative experiment was conducted using four popular ML methodologies: SVM, random forest (RF), decision trees (DT), and DL. The comparative analysis considers three numerical instances of steel truss constructions: a planar truss, a spatial truss, and a case study of a planar truss bridge. The quantitative findings revealed that irrespective of the volume of training data and model variables, the built GTB models deliver high accuracy (more than 90%) and have the highest efficiency in the majority of scenarios evaluated.

13.4.4 SUPPORT VECTOR MACHINE

For solving the classification as well as regression problems, a supervised learning tool, namely, SVM, has promising outcomes. However, it is primarily availed in machine learning for problems classification. The main objective of the SVM technique is to ascertain the decision boundary or best line for categorizing n-dimensional space into classes in the near future in order to place the subsequent data points into the analogous group. Further, SVM also assists in selecting the extreme points/vectors that in turn aid in building the hyperplane. The hyperplane is the optimal choice boundary. The eventual instances are support vectors, and the algorithm is known as an SVM. In the healthcare sector, Harimoorthy et al. [44] presented a generic framework for disease prediction that was tested with a diminished collection of characteristics from the kidney disease, mellitus, and cardiovascular disease datasets utilizing an enhanced SVM-radial bias kernel technique, and it was also especially likened to other ML techniques in R studio, including SVM-linear, SVM-polynomial, random forest, and decision tree. Precision, misclassification frequency, accuracy, sensitivity, and specificity were all used to assess the effectiveness of these ML methods. According to the findings of the research, the upgraded SVM-radial bias kernel method achieves reliability of 98.3%, 98.7%, and 89.9% in the kidney disease, mellitus, and cardiovascular disease datasets, correspondingly.

Chamasemani et al. [45] demonstrated a multiclass SVM classifier and how it can be used to detect and classify hypothyroidism. In the ML domain, SVM is a well-known approach for binary classification issues. MCSVMs (multiclass SVMs) are often created by mixing numerous binary SVMs. The goal of this research was to demonstrate the reliability of numerous forms of kernels for multiclass SVM classifiers, as well as a contrast of distinct multiclass SVM constructing methods, including one and one-against-all, and eventually to compare the multiclass SVM classifier's precision to AdaBoost and decision tee. One-against-all support vector machines (OAASVM) outperformed one-against-one support vector machines (OAOSVM) using polynomial kernels in simulations. On hypothyroid disorder data from the UCI ML database, OAASVM was also more accurate than AdaBoost and decision tree classifiers.

Agarap et al. [46] proposed a change to this standard by replacing the Softmax in GRU model's last output layer with a linear SVM. A margin-based function was also used instead of the cross-entropy function. While comparable research has been done, this approach was focused on the dual classification of intrusion detection utilizing 2,013 network traffic data from Kyoto University's honeypot systems.

The GRU-SVM model outperforms the conventional GRU-Softmax model, as per the conclusion. The suggested model attained a training precision of ≈79.32%, whereas a testing precision of ≈83.23%; the latter was capable to attain a training precision of ≈62.12% and a testing realism of ≈71.14%. Furthermore, the confluence of such two final output layers suggests that the SVM should exceed Softmax in terms of inference time—a logical assumption backed up by the study's actual training and testing duration.

13.4.5 ARTIFICIAL NEURAL NETWORK

ANN has performed an excellent effort in forecasting the mechanical characteristics of fiber-reinforced composites. The amount of training datasets is a critical factor in ANN prediction accuracy, according to most research. Longer training sets were shown to be more effective for more complicated nonlinear input–output relationships. The findings of various studies utilizing ANN were determined to be an effective technique in the structure–property evaluation of polymer composites, as stated by investigators. Komeda et al. [47] intended to create a one-of-a-kind CNN-CAD platform using an AI functionality which looked at endoscopic pictures retrieved from films taken with colonoscopes during normal exams. They presented the initial findings of this new CNN-CAD method for colon polyp detection. A maximum of 1,200 pictures were utilized from colonoscopy cases done at Kindai University Hospital between January 2010 and December 2016. These pictures were taken from film recordings of real endoscopic procedures. In a pilot study, supplementary video footage from ten cases of unlearned procedures was retroactively examined. They were merely labeled as adenomatous or nonadenomatous polyps. The AI utilized 1,200 photos to understand to differentiate between adenomatous and nonadenomatous tumors. These photos were culled from footage of real endoscopic procedures. Each picture was reduced to 256 × 256 pixels in size. Cross-validation of ten holds was performed. The efficiency of the tenfold cross-confirmation is 0.692, wherein efficiency is defined as the proportion of accurate responses to total answers generated by the CNN. In seven out of ten situations, CNN's decisions were accurate. A CNN-CAD method that uses routine colonoscopy to diagnose colorectal polyp categorization could be effective. To establish the efficiency of a CNN-CAD system in regular colonoscopy, more retrospective trials in an in vivo context are needed.

Choudhury et al.'s [48] particle swarm optimization (PSO) was developed as a method to increase the efficiency of ANN in the categorization of the IRIS dataset. The classifier is an ML technique for predicting data instance group membership. To make the challenge of categorization easier to understand, neural networks have been introduced. The focus of this research was on utilizing a neural network to classify IRIS plants. The issue revolves around identifying IRIS plant species based on plant attribute data. Discovering trends by evaluating the petal as well as sepal dimension of the IRIS plant and the means by which the forecast was produced by analyzing the trend to build the category of IRIS plant should be the first step in classifying the IRIS dataset. The uncertain data in upcoming decades could be anticipated more accurately utilizing this trend and categorization. Pattern categorization, linear regression, efficiency, and association recollections have all been effectively solved using ANN. The backpropagation learning approach was used to train multi-layer feed-forward networks in this study.

13.5 CONCLUSION

The globe is changing at a fast tempo right now, and people's demands changing along with it. Furthermore, we are living in the fourth industrial data revolution. As a result, effective algorithms are necessary to obtain relevant and meaningful information from massive data, as well as to understand the many approaches to machine–human interaction. Such algorithms must be capable of analyzing all elements of data and providing us with meaningful findings for a variety of applications. Machine learning has had a substantial impact on a variety of societal areas, including healthcare, production, social media sites, pharmacology, and a variety of other fields. As a result, ML has turned out to be an essential element of our day-to-day life. Owing to the rapid increase of data, simply expanding the computing capability of the machine will not be enough to receive and evaluate the data. It requires a second process to thoroughly study the data in order to offer timely and valuable data. ML has demonstrated its importance by giving data in the form that we require. YouTube, Netflix, and Amazon Prime are among the more effective ML instances. These platforms propose video, music, films, and other content depending on your streaming habits. This is possible and feasible because of the deployment of ML algorithms. Another example is the Google search engine's feature, which may offer you the most appropriate search results based on your browsing habits. In most industries, complicated redundant operations are being entirely computerized in place of manual operations in need to achieve precise and consistent outcomes. All of this is feasible owing to the strength of ML algorithms. The healthcare industry has rapidly evolved and revolutionized owing to ML. ML could aid in the immediate treatment of patients, the reduction of disease hazards in the prospective, and the streamlining of work operations. This chapter introduces a conceptual diagnostic paradigm that may be used in practice with Python. For disease diagnosis, supervised machine learning algorithms are widely utilized. The usage of a confusing matrix to evaluate the efficiency of a learning algorithm is addressed. Cancer, neurology, and cardiology are three major illness areas where ML has demonstrated its prowess. As per the case research, the SVM algorithm is more suitable for breast cancer detection. Methods based on ML are particularly effective for the diagnosis of diseases and also have the ability to improve decision-making. To summarize, it is expected that in the years ahead, ML- and AI-based diagnostic systems would provide intelligent healthcare applications. Precision medicine, automated therapy, robotic technology, and other applications of AI and ML, that will be driven by DL, are examples of the potential range of AI and ML.

REFERENCES

1. Kim TS, Sohn SY (2021) Multitask learning for health condition identification and remaining useful life prediction: deep convolutional neural network approach. *J Intell Manuf* 32:2169–2179

2. Ancochea J, Lumbreras S, Soriano JB (2021) Evidence of gender differences in the diagnosis and management of coronavirus disease 2019 patients: An analysis of electronic health records using natural language processing and machine learning. *J Women's Heal* 30:393–404

3. Javed AR, Fahad LG, Farhan AA, Abbas S, Srivastava G, Parizi RM, Khan MS (2021) Automated cognitive health assessment in smart homes using machine learning. *Sustain Cities Soc* 65:102572

4. Hosseinzadeh M, Ahmed OH, Ghafour MY, Safara F, Hama H kamaran, Ali S, Vo B, Chiang H Sen (2021) A multiple multilayer perceptron neural network with an adaptive learning algorithm for thyroid disease diagnosis in the internet of medical things. *J Supercomput* 77:3616–3637

5. Rajesh N, Maneesha T, Hafeez S, Krishna H (2018) Prediction of heart disease using machine learning algorithms. *Int J Eng Technol* 7:363–366

6. van der Schaar M, Alaa AM, Floto A, Gimson A, Scholtes S, Wood A, McKinney E, Jarrett D, Lio P, Ercole A (2021) How artificial intelligence and machine learning can help healthcare systems respond to COVID-19. *Mach Learn* 110:1–14

7. Scott I, Carter S, Coiera E (2021) Clinician checklist for assessing suitability of machine learning applications in healthcare. *BMJ Heal Care Inform* 28(1):1–8. https://doi.org/10.1136/bmjhci-2020-100251

8. Nishat MM (2021) Performance assessment of different machine learning algorithms in predicting diabetes mellitus. *Biosci Biotechnol Res Commun* 14:74–82

9. Kim J, Lee D, Park E (2021) Machine learning for mental health in social media: Bibliometric study. *J Med Internet Res* 23:1–17

10. Alizadehsani R, Roshanzamir M, Hussain S, et al. (2021) Handling of uncertainty in medical data using machine learning and probability theory techniques: a review of 30 years (1991–2020). *Ann Oper Res* 301(1–2):41–53. https://doi.org/10.1007/s10479-021-04006-2

11. Bhavsar KA, Abugabah A, Singla J, AlZubi AA, Bashir AK, Nikita (2021) A comprehensive review on medical diagnosis using machine learning. *Comput Mater Contin* 67:1997–2014

12. Mishra M (2021) Machine learning techniques for structural health monitoring of heritage buildings: A state-of-the-art review and case studies. *J Cult Herit* 47:227–245

13. Meinel LA, Stolpen AH, Berbaum KS, Fajardo LL, Reinhardt JM (2007) Breast MRI lesion classification: Improved performance of human readers with a backpropagation neural network computer-aided diagnosis (CAD) system. *J Magn Reson Imaging* 25:89–95

14. Castiglioni I, Rundo L, Codari M, Di Leo G, Salvatore C, Interlenghi M, Gallivanone F, Cozzi A, D'Amico NC, Sardanelli F (2021) AI applications to medical images: From machine learning to deep learning. *Phys Medica* 83:9–24

15. Pallathadka H, Mustafa M, Sanchez DT, Sekhar Sajja G, Gour S, Naved M (2021) Impact of machine learning on Management, healthcare and agriculture. *Mater Today Proc* 36(8):2251003. https://doi.org/10.1016/j.matpr.2021.07.042

16. Diwakar M, Tripathi A, Joshi K, Memoria M, Singh P, Kumar N (2020) Latest trends on heart disease prediction using machine learning and image fusion. *Mater Today Proc* 37:3213–3218

17. Jiang M, Li Y, Jiang C, Zhao L, Zhang X, Lipsky PE (2021) Machine Learning in Rheumatic Diseases. *Clin Rev Allergy Immunol* 60:96–110

18. Pourhomayoun M, Shakibi M (2021) Predicting mortality risk in patients with COVID-19 using machine learning to help medical decision-making. *Smart Heal* 20:100178

19. Verma C, Quraishi MA, Rhee KY (2021) Present and emerging trends in using pharmaceutically active compounds as aqueous phase corrosion inhibitors. *J Mol Liq* 328:115395

20. Tohka J, van Gils M (2021) Evaluation of machine learning algorithms for health and wellness applications: A tutorial. *Comput Biol Med* 132:104324

21. Doyle OM, Van der Laan R, Obradovic M, McMahon P, Daniels F, Pitcher A, Loebinger MR (2020) Identification of potentially undiagnosed patients with nontuberculous mycobacterial lung disease using machine learning applied to primary care data in the UK. *Eur Respir J* 56(4):1–11. https://doi.org/10.1183/13993003.00045-2020

22. Salama MS, Eltrass AS, Elkamchouchi HM (2018) An improved approach for computer-aided diagnosis of breast cancer in digital mammography. *MeMeA 2018–2018 IEEE Int Symp Med Meas Appl Proc* 3528725544:1–5

23. Keerthi Samhitha B, Sarika Priya MR, Sanjana C, Mana SC, Jose J (2020) Improving the accuracy in prediction of heart disease using machine learning algorithms. *Proc 2020 IEEE Int Conf Commun Signal Process ICCSP 2020*, 1326–1330

24. Thakur A, Kumar A, Kaya S, Vo DVN, Sharma A (2022) Suppressing inhibitory compounds by nanomaterials for highly efficient biofuel production: A review. *Fuel* 312:122934

25. Parveen G, Bashir S, Thakur A, Saha SK, Banerjee P, Kumar A (2020) Experimental and computational studies of imidazolium based ionic liquid 1-methyl- 3-propylimidazolium iodide on mild steel corrosion in acidic solution Experimental and computational studies of imidazolium based ionic liquid 1-methyl- 3-propylimidazolium. *Mater Res Express* 7:016510

26. Thakur A, Kumar A (2021) Sustainable inhibitors for corrosion mitigation in aggressive corrosive media: A comprehensive study. *J Bio- Tribo-Corrosion* 7:1–48

27. Bashir S, Thakur A, Lgaz H, Chung IM, Kumar A (2020) Corrosion inhibition efficiency of bronopol on aluminium in 0.5 M HCl solution: Insights from experimental and quantum chemical studies. *Surf Interfaces* 20:100542

28. Bashir S, Thakur A, Lgaz H, Chung I-M, Kumar A (2020) Corrosion inhibition performance of acarbose on mild steel corrosion in acidic medium: An experimental and computational study. *Arab J Sci Eng* 45:4773–4783

29. Podgorelec V (2012) Analyzing EEG signals with machine learning for diagnosing Alzheimer's disease. *Elektron ir Elektrotechnika* 18:61–64

30. Park JH, Cho HE, Kim JH, Wall MM, Stern Y, Lim H, Yoo S, Kim HS, Cha J (2020) Machine learning prediction of incidence of Alzheimer's disease using large-scale administrative health data. *NPJ Digit Med* 3:1–7. https://doi.org/10.1038/s41746-020-0256-0

31. Choi YJ, Baek JH, Park HS, Shim WH, Kim TY, Shong YK, Lee JH (2017) A Computer-aided diagnosis system using artificial intelligence for the diagnosis and characterization of thyroid nodules on ultrasound: Initial clinical assessment. *Thyroid* 27:546–552

32. Bharti R, Khamparia A, Shabaz M, Dhiman G, Pande S, Singh P (2021) Prediction of heart disease using a combination of machine learning and deep learning. *Comput Intell Neurosci* 2021:Article ID 8387680, 11 pages. https://doi.org/10.1155/2021/8387680

33. Tang C, Ji J, Tang Y, Gao S, Tang Z, Todo Y (2020) A novel machine learning technique for computer-aided diagnosis. *Eng Appl Artif Intell* 92:103627

34. Kishor A, Chakraborty C (2021) Artificial intelligence and internet of things based healthcare 4.0 monitoring system. *Wirel Pers Commun* 119(2):617–627. https://doi.org/10.1007/s11277-021-08708-5

35. Benzakoun J, Bommart S, Coste J, Chassagnon G, Lederlin M, Boussouar S, Revel MP (2016) Computer-aided diagnosis (CAD) of subsolid nodules: Evaluation of a commercial CAD system. *Eur J Radiol* 85:1728–1734

36. Eun JC, Gong YJ, Young MH, Young SL, Keun SK (2008) Solitary pulmonary nodule on helical dynamic CT scans: Analysis of the enhancement patterns using a Computer-Aided Diagnosis (CAD) system. *Korean J Radiol* 9:401–408

37. Ha T, Jung Y, Kim JY, Park SY, Kang DK, Kim TH (2019) Comparison of the diagnostic performance of abbreviated MRI and full diagnostic MRI using a computer-aided diagnosis (CAD) system in patients with a personal history of breast cancer: The effect of CAD-generated kinetic features on reader performance. *Clin Radiol* 74:817.e15–817.e21

38. Zhang X, He L, Zhang J, Whiting MD, Karkee M, Zhang Q (2020) Determination of key canopy parameters for mass mechanical apple harvesting using supervised machine learning and principal component analysis (PCA). *Biosyst Eng* 193:247–263

39. Allegretta I, Marangoni B, Manzari P, Porfido C, Terzano R, De Pascale O, Senesi GS (2020) Macro-classification of meteorites by portable energy dispersive X-ray fluorescence spectroscopy (pED-XRF), principal component analysis (PCA) and machine learning algorithms. *Talanta* 212:120785

40. Jo HS, Park C, Lee E, Choi HK, Park J (2020) Path loss prediction based on machine learning techniques: Principal component analysis, artificial neural network and gaussian process. *Sensors* (Switzerland) 7:1927. https://doi.org/10.3390/s20071927

41. Polat K, Güneş S (2007) Detection of ECG Arrhythmia using a differential expert system approach based on principal component analysis and least square support vector machine. *Appl Math Comput* 186:898–906

42. Al-Salemi B, Mohd Noah SA, Ab Aziz MJ (2016) RFBoost: An improved multi-label boosting algorithm and its application to text categorisation. *Knowledge-Based Syst* 103:104–117

43. Truong VH, Vu QV, Thai HT, Ha MH (2020) A robust method for safety evaluation of steel trusses using Gradient Tree Boosting algorithm. *Adv Eng Softw* 147:102825

44. Harimoorthy K, Thangavelu M (2021) Multi-disease prediction model using improved SVM-radial bias technique in healthcare monitoring system. *J Ambient Intell Humaniz Comput* 12:3715–3723

45. Chamasemani FF, Singh YP (2011) Multi-class Support Vector Machine (SVM) classifiers—An application in hypothyroid detection and classification. *Proc—2011 6th Int Conf Bio-Inspired Comput Theor Appl BIC-TA 2011*, 351–356

46. Agarap AFM (2018) A neural network architecture combining gated recurrent unit (GRU) and support vector machine (SVM) for intrusion detection in network traffic data. *ICMLC 2018: Proc 2018 10th Int Conf Mac Learn Comput 2018*, 26–30. https://doi.org/10.1145/3195106.3195117

47. Komeda Y, Handa H, Watanabe T, et al (2017) Computer-aided diagnosis based on convolutional neural network system for colorectal polyp classification: Preliminary experience. *Oncol* 93:30–34

48. Choudhury K, Mohd Nawi N, Muhammad Zubair Rehman Gillani S, Haruna C, Khan A, ar Hamza M (2013) Training artificial neural network using particle swarm optimization algorithm studying the effect of training Levenberg-Marquardt neural network by using hybrid meta-heuristic A . . . Hybrid learning enhancement of RBF network with particle swarm opt. *Int J Adv Res Comput Sci Softw Eng* 3:2277

14 Heart Attack Risk Predictor Using Machine Learning and Proposed IoT-Based Smart Watch Drone Healthcare System

Arun Anoop M. and Karthikeyan P.

CONTENTS

14.1 INTRODUCTION

14.1.1 HEART ANATOMY

Every day, the typical human heart beats multiple times, siphoning 2,000 gallons of blood through the body [1]. That is a ton of work for an organ no greater than a huge clench hand and gauging 8–12 ounces.[1] The "healthblog of uofmhealth" said that the heart accomplishes more actual work than some other muscle over a long period. Situated between the lungs in the chest, the heart pumps blood through the network of arteries and veins known as the cardiovascular framework. It pushes blood to the body's organs, tissues, and cells (healthblog.uofmhealth.org). The "healthblog of uofmhealth" said that blood conveys oxygen and nutrients to each cell and eliminates the carbon dioxide and other side effects made by those cells [2]. Blood is conveyed from the heart to the remainder of the body through a mind-boggling network of arteries, arterioles, and vessels. Blood got back to the heart through venules and veins (see Figure 14.1). Men in their late 40s and ladies in their late 50s are most in danger of getting a heart attack (Tables 14.1 and 14.2).[2]

DOI: 10.1201/9781003315476-14

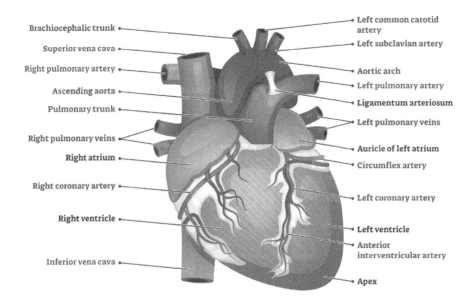

FIGURE 14.1   Heart structure.

TABLE 14.1
Study of Different Heart Parts and Its Functions

S. No.	Parts	Description/Function
1	Aorta [3]	Aorta is the body's biggest artery and takes blood to all organs [4]. One going to head and one going to lower body
2	Superior vena cava [3]	Brings deoxygenated blood from the head and upper organs
3	Right atrium [3]	• First chamber of the heart • To receive blood from all organs except lungs • Thin walls • It mixes blood from two vena cavas
4	Tricuspid valve [3]	Blood from right atrium to right ventricle
5	Right ventricle [3]	If chamber is full with blood, then pumped to pulmonary artery through pulmonary valve
6	Inferior vena cava [3]	Brings deoxygenated blood from lower organs of the body
7	Pulmonary artery [3]	Carries deoxygenated blood to the left and right lungs, where CO_2 is released into air and blood becomes oxygenated
8	Left atrium [3]	Collects blood from lungs
9	Mitral valve [3]	The valve opens when the left atrium is full and lets blood into left ventricle
10	Left ventricle [3]	Pumps out oxygenated blood to the rest of the body through aorta

TABLE 14.2

Study of Different Heart Terms

S. No.	Journal Paper	Description
1	[3]	1. Arteries convey oxygenated blood from the heart to every one of the organs [5]. When the organs have taken up the oxygen they need, the veins take the deoxygenated blood back to the heart
		2. Heart, arteries, veins make up the body's circulatory system. Oxygen goes out of the capillaries into the cells of the organ, while carbon dioxide comes into them
		3. Heart is mostly made up of muscles. And muscles require the strength to push blood with so much force that it reaches all the organs, no matter how far away they are from the heart
		4. Heart is made up of "cardiac tissue," which is laid on pericardium layer, epicardium and myocardium.
		5. Heart works without rest. Myocardium is made of cardiac muscles. When it contracts, blood is pushed out, and when it expands, new blood fills in
		6. Heart attack happens when the muscles of the heart do not get enough oxygen-rich blood. Blood clot may reduce passing oxygen-rich blood. When heart muscles stop getting oxygen and die, it may cause heart paralysis, and if it cannot pump anymore blood, it is called "heart attack"
		7. Authors mentioned the signs clearly: "chest pain," "vomiting," "sweating," "shortness of breath," "arm weakness," "speech difficulties," "severe headache," "dizziness," and "vision issues"
		8. When the heart is not able to pump blood properly, it is called heart failure
		9. The heart keeps beating as it gets signals from the brain. A problem in the nerves may cause these signals to stop. The heart stops working, and doctors call this "sudden cardiac arrest." Patients stop breathing and lose consciousness. It causes instant death if not treated in time
		10. To treat episodes of angina (chest pain) in people who have coronary artery sickness, nitroglycerine sublingual tablets are used
2	[6]	Estimates ten-year risk of heart attack. Features considered are age, gender, smoker, HDL cholesterol, systolic BP, total cholesterol, blood pressure being treated with medicines [6]
3	[7]	Demographic characteristics used here are age >65, coexisting conditions, and female, race. Coexisting conditions used are coronary artery disease, cardiac arrhythmia, diabetes mellitus, hypertension, congestive heart failure, hyperlipidemia, current smoker, former smoker, immunosuppressed condition, COPD [7]
		Risk factors noticed are >65 years of age, female, coronary artery disease, congestive heart failure, arrhythmia, current smoker, receiving ACE inhibitor, receiving ARB, COPD, receiving statin [7]
		Drugs suggested are ACE inhibitor, beta blocker, statin, ARB, insulin, another hypoglycemic agent [7]
4	[8]	Cardiotoxic effects of potential drugs or treatment of coronavirus 2019 are chloroquine, lopinavir or ritonavir, interferon alpha, favipiravir, azithromycin, monoclonal antibodies, and vitamin C [8]
5	[9, 10]	Researchers mentioned the following drugs: aspirin, angiotensin-converting enzyme (ACE) inhibitors, angiotensin receptor blockers (ARBs), beta blockers, calcium channel blockers (CCBs), diuretics, statins for cardiovascular disease prevention [9, 10]

14.1.2 Dimensionality Reduction and Test Functions

Test functions are imperative to approve and analyze the presentation of optimization calculations [11]. There have been many test or benchmark functions detailed in the writing. For any new optimization, it is fundamental to approve its exhibition and contrast other existing calculations over a decent arrangement of test functions. Two different types of functions are unimodal and multimodal which is under the categorization of test functions. Benchmark test functions mainly for testing new algorithm performance while it compares with other optimization algorithms. And the measures can use standard deviation, mean, or average which has been used recently by many researchers to check the efficiency of different optimization algorithms [12]. Dimensionality reduction is reducing redundant and irrelevant features in order to improve the system accuracy by nature or bioinspired algorithms. Moreover, objective functions play a vital role. Global optimization consists of constrained and unconstrained types [13]. Dimensionality reduction method normally plays well to reduce redundant and irrelevant features to boost the classification accuracy. Similar other terms are feature scaling and feature selection. Feature selection is the way toward diminishing the quantity of input features when fostering a predictive model [14]. Feature scaling is the interaction or sort of standardization cycle to keep the scope of free factors or features of information. Some methods we used in our previous works are max division approaches. Some may use to divide all the feature cells by max value of pixel which is presented in the input image. Optimization algorithms noticed during research are grey wolf optimization algorithm, whale-based optimization algorithm, antlion optimization algorithm, ant colony optimization algorithm, moth flame optimization algorithm, BAT ecology optimization algorithm, Dragon fly optimization algorithm, Grasshopper optimization algorithm, Salp swarm optimization algorithm, particle swarm optimization algorithm, genetic algorithm optimization algorithm, PCA, cuckoo optimization algorithm, cuttlefish optimization algorithm, chimp optimization algorithm, World Cup optimization algorithm, earthworm optimization algorithm, mayfly optimization algorithm, black widow optimization algorithm, African vultures optimization algorithm, seagull optimization algorithm, fruit fly optimization algorithm, Jaya optimization algorithm, sooty tern optimization algorithm, aquila optimization algorithm, sunflower optimization algorithm, and test functions for global optimization algorithm. At present, many modified optimization algorithms are available. Many researchers are tuning the main parameters of optimization algorithm and doing their way of improvements, while some are experimenting test functions by checking the performance of optimization algorithms. Best feature subset identifying is the key factor in all the optimization algorithms. We have processed some randomly selected test functions for identifying BAT optimization algorithm which is best for our approach previously [9]. Importance of global optimization method test functions has to be applied in the artificial neural network optimization algorithms for performance checking. *Test functions and categories:* unimodal and multimodal. *Benchmark functions:* constrained and unconstrained. Measures are standard deviation and mean value. Objective functions. *Global optimization:* constrained and unconstrained [10]. *Dimensionality reduction or feature selection or normalization:* nature-inspired and bioinspired.

Optimization algorithms: different optimization algorithms were those mentioned in Table 14.3 and Table 14.4.

Optimization algorithm mainly consists of continuous, unconstrained, discrete, constrained, and linear programming. Global optimization is the part of applied maths and mathematical investigation that endeavors to find global minima and maxima of a function. Best optimization methods are stochastic gradient

---

TABLE 14.3

Different Optimization Algorithms

Greywolf	Genetic algorithm	African vultures
Whale	PCA	Seagull
AntLion	Cuckoo	Fruit fly
Moth flame	Cuttle fish	Jaya
BAT	Chimp	Sooty tern
Dragon fly	World Cup	Aquila
Grasshopper	Earthworm	Sunflower
Salp swarm	Mayfly	Test functions
Particle swarm	Black widow	

TABLE 14.4

Different Optimization Algorithms Comparative Analysis

S. No	Optimization Algorithms	Main Idea
1	Greywolf	Is a bionic optimization algorithm which mimics the way of behaving of dark wolves to catch prey with an unmistakable division of work and common cooperation [15] and fundamental standards utilized here is the "Number of wolves"
2	Bat	Is a heuristic search algorithm, which was proposed by Yang in 2010. By reproducing the bat scrounging conduct, local and global optimality can be got through suitable iteration [16] and the fundamental measure is the "Number of Bats"
3	AntLion	Fundamental measure is the number of search agents [17]
4	Moth flame	Fundamental measure is the number of search agents (30–50) [18]
5	Whale	Fundamental measure is the number of search agents [19]
6	Dragon fly	Fundamental measure is the number of search agents [20]
7	Grasshopper	Fundamental measures is the number of search agents [21]
8	Salp swarm	Fundamental measure is the swarming mechanism of salps [22]
9	Particle swarm	Each particle moves around the solution space randomly
10	Genetic algorithm	Produce offspring of the next generation

(Continued)

TABLE 14.4 (*Continued*)
Different Optimization Algorithms Comparative Analysis

S. No	Optimization Algorithms	Main Idea
11	PCA	Minimizing information loss [23]
12	Cuckoo	Fundamental idea is inspired by the lifestyle of a family of birds called cuckoo [24]
13	Cuttle fish	Fundamental measure in cuttlefish is to solve numerical global optimization problems [25]
14	Chimp	Inspired by the sexual motivation individual intelligence of chimps in their group hunting [26]
15	World Cup	Optimization algorithm based on human society's intelligent [27]
16	Earthworm	Inspired by the earthworm in nature [28]
17	Mayfly	Inspired by the mating process flight behavior of mayflies [29]
18	Black widow	Inspired by the black widow spider's unique mating behavior [30]
19	African vultures	Inspired by the African vultures' lifestyle [31]
20	Seagull	Inspired by the migration and attacking behaviors of a seagull in nature [32]
21	Fruit fly	Based on the food finding behavior of the fruit fly [33]
22	Jaya	Changes a population of individual solutions and fit for tackling both compelled and unconstrained optimization issues [34]
23	Sooty tern	Inspired by sea bird sooty's migration and attacking behaviors [35]
24	Aquila	Inspired by the process of catching the prey of Aquila's behaviors [36]
25	Sunflower	Nature-inspired optimization method based on sunflowers' motion [37]
26	Test functions	www.sfu.ca/~ssurjano/optimization.html [38]
27	Ant colony	Number of ants in population and also it has some reward and penalty factors [39]
28	Marriage in honey bees	Social insects [40]
29	Artificial fish swarm algorithm	Social form and interactions between all fish in a group [41]
30	Termite algorithm	Inspired from intelligent behaviors of termites [42]
31	Ant bee colony	Simulates the foraging behavior of honey bees [43]
32	Wasp swarm optimization	Mimics the attribute of the wasp colony [44]
33	Monkey search	Monkey is assigned an agent that builds decision trees [45]
34	Wolf pack search algorithm	Inspired by the wolves' intelligent behaviors [46]
35	Bee collecting pollen algorithm	Lots of amounts of pollen that are easy to collect [47]
36	Dolphin partner	Mimics the hunting mechanism of dolphins [48]
37	Hunting search	Inspired by animal's group hunting [49]
38	Bird mating	Inspired by bird species' mating strategy [50]
39	Krill herd	Inspired by the tiny sea creature krill and its style of living [51]
40	Dolphin echolocation	Behavior of dolphins for their hunting process [52]
41	Boruta	Wrapper algorithm around random forest

method and the equivalent with momentum and furthermore ADAM optimizer. These best optimizers were added within convolutional neural network for better execution.

- **ADAM:** Substitution optimization calculation for SGD and utilized for preparing deep learning models. Also, it joins best properties of AdaGrad and RMSProp calculations. Another optimizer is practically the same name of ADAM, that is Nadam.
- **Genetic Algorithm:** It is a method for settling both constrained and unconstrained optimization issues in light of natural selection process that mimics biological evolution. The following are the global optimization functions, which we handled to actually look at the presentation of some optimization calculations. All the test functions codes collected from:

1. Ackley function (local minima): Multimodal [TF1]
2. Rastrigin function (local minima): Multimodal [TF2]
3. Shubert function (local minima): Multimodal [TF3]
4. De Jong function (steep ridges): Unimodal [TF4]
5. Rosenbrock function (valley-shaped): Unimodal [TF5]
6. Michalewicz function (steep ridges): Multimodal [TF6]
7. Zakharov function (plate-shaped): Multimodal [TF7]
8. Easom function (steep ridges): Unimodal [TF8]

TABLE 14.5

Test Functions

Unimodal test function

TF4	$\left(002 + \sum\limits_{i=1}^{25} \dfrac{1}{i + (x1 - a1i)^6 + (x2 - a2i)^6} \right)^{-1}$
TF5	$\sum\limits_{i=1}^{d-1} \left[100\left(xi+1 - xi^2 \right)^2 + \left(xi-1 \right)^2 \right]$
TF6	$f(x) = -\cos(x1)\cos(x2)\exp(-(x1-\pi)^2 - (x2-\pi)^2$

Multimodal test function

TF1	$-a\exp(-\dfrac{1}{d}\sum\limits_{i=1}^{d} Xi^2) - \exp\left(\dfrac{1}{d}\sum\limits_{i=1}^{d} Cos(cXi) \right) + a + \exp(1)$
TF2	$10d + \sum\limits_{i=1}^{d} \left[xi^2 - 10\cos(2\pi Xi) \right]$
TF3	$f(x) = \left(\sum\limits_{i=1}^{5} i\cos\left((i+1)X1+i\right) \right)\left(\sum\limits_{i=1}^{5} i\cos\left((i+1)X2+i\right) \right)$
TF6	$f(x) = -\sum\limits_{i=1}^{d} \sin(Xi)\sin^{2m}\left(\dfrac{iXi^2}{\pi} \right)$
TF7	$f(x) = \sum\limits_{i=1}^{d} Xi^2 + \left(\sum\limits_{i=1}^{d} 0.5iXi \right)^2 + \left(\sum\limits_{i=1}^{d} 0.5iXi \right)^4$

14.1.3 HEART FEATURES DESCRIPTION

Commonly used datasets are UCI based and Cleveland. There are generally 14 attributes to consider as features.

14.1.4 DIFFERENT CLASSIFIERS, METRICS, AND DATASETS

Classifiers used in our work are logistic regression, passive aggressive, ridge classifier, K-nearest neighbor, Gaussian NB, and Bernoulli NB.

- **Passive:** If prediction right, sit idle.
- **Aggressive:** If prediction wrong, minimally update the weights to classify accurately.
- **Ridge Classifier:** This changes over the mark data into [–1, 1] and takes care of the issue with regression strategy and is a regularization procedure, which is utilized to diminish the complexity of the model.
- **K-Nearest Neighbor Classifier:** Calculation can be utilized to tackle both classification and regression issue statements and it is to involve a database where the data focuses are isolated into a few classes to anticipate the classification of another example point [53–55].
- **Gaussian Naïve Bayes (GNB) Classifier and Bernoulli Naïve Bayes (BNB) Classifier:** Gaussian Naïve Bayes: Normal distribution, continuous data. Bernoulli Naïve Bayes: In a multivariate model, the free Boolean conditions portray the sources of info.
- **Datasets:** Used here is UCI heart disease dataset [56], another dataset is Framingham dataset [57].

Metrics are precision which is characterized as the extent of accurately anticipated positive observations to all anticipated positive observations: TP/(TP + FP). Recall is an action which measures the way the model recognizes true positives: TP/(TP + FN) F1 score is additionally an action which is used for probability that a positive prediction is right: (2*Precision * Recall)/(Precision + Recall). In this work, we propose an IoT-based smart watch drone healthcare framework and machine learning models to analyze cardiovascular diseases. To accomplish this objective, we explore different avenues regarding numerous machine learning models and thought about statewise status of diseases. In the accompanying, we sum up the fundamental commitments of this work:

- To remove noises and normalize data before main processes.
- To design IoT-based smart watch drone healthcare system.
- To design UFE 14 A Proposed System. "UFE 14 A" is nothing but it is a proposed system, and its expansion is "Utilized Feature Extraction of 14 attributes of [56] dataset."
- To evaluate UCI heart dataset with different supervised machine learning algorithms.

- To evaluate heart disease statistics based on novel attributes.
- To identify different metrics to show results.
- To classify different machine learning approaches to list best one among that.

The rest of this chapter is organized as follows: in Section 14.2, we present proposed work based on Internet of Things; Section 14.3 describes in detail the results based on machine learning and statistics. Finally, we conclude with a conclusion and future work.

14.2 IOT-BASED SMART WATCH DRONE HEALTHCARE SYSTEM

Watch to Drone Phase ("1," "2," "3" symbol)

1. Sending name and mobile number to drone.
2. Request received from drone to retrieve heart features (sex, age, chest pain, resting BPS, cholesterol, fasting blood sugar, resting electrographic, maximum heart rate, exercise-induced angina, oldpeak, slope, flourosopy, thal).
3. Extracted features sending to drone.

Drone to Cloud Phase ("1" Symbol)

1. Identity measures data forwarded to face recognition module.
2. Based on recognition, checked sentimental analysis and checked his facial expressions to decide whether he is better or serious.
3. Both data moved to cloud storage.

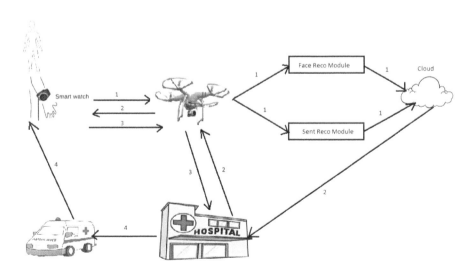

FIGURE 14.2 IoT-based smart watch drone healthcare system.

Cloud to Hospital Phase ("2" Symbol), Hospital to Ambulance ("4" Symbol), and Ambulance to Human ("4" Symbol)

1. If patient's health is better or serious, data moved to "Hospital."
2. Either better or serious message to be record for future use.
3. Serious cases will be sent to cardio experts and then those people will analyze the data based on their skills. Immediate checkups they may send "ambulance" to the tracked location.

IoT-Based Smart Watch Drone Healthcare System: An IoT-based smart healthcare system has developed for heart patients while moving from one location to another [58]. In future, anyone can monitor the same by the help of android devices. This model has developed to check the monitoring of such patient's safety [59].

14.3 EXPERIMENTAL RESULTS

Dataset used here in UCI dataset **heart.csv**

Here in the above dataset, some of the terms represented as string wise. But we required "numerical" data before processing dataset. In that 14 attributes can be seen, which is in UCI heart dataset.

1	age	sex	cp	trestbps	chol	fbs	restecg	thalach	exang	oldpeak	slope	ca	thal	target
2	63	1	3	145	233	1	0	150	0	2.3	0	0	1	1
3	37	1	2	130	250	0	1	187	0	3.5	0	0	2	1
4	41	0	1	130	204	0	0	172	0	1.4	2	0	2	1
5	56	1	1	120	236	0	1	178	0	0.8	2	0	2	1
6	57	0	0	120	354	0	1	163	1	0.6	2	0	2	1

```
df.head()
```

	Unnamed: 0	Age	Sex	ChestPain	RestBP	Chol	Fbs	RestECG	MaxHR	ExAng	Oldpeak	Slope	Ca	Thal	AHD
0	1	63	1	typical	145	233	1	2	150	0	2.3	3	0.0	fixed	No
1	2	67	1	asymptomatic	160	286	0	2	108	1	1.5	2	3.0	normal	Yes
2	3	67	1	asymptomatic	120	229	0	2	129	1	2.6	2	2.0	reversable	Yes
3	4	37	1	nonanginal	130	250	0	0	187	0	3.5	3	0.0	normal	No
4	5	41	0	nontypical	130	204	0	2	172	0	1.4	1	0.0	normal	No

```
[ ] df.tail()
```

	Unnamed: 0	Age	Sex	ChestPain	RestBP	Chol	Fbs	RestECG	MaxHR	ExAng	Oldpeak	Slope	Ca	Thal	AHD
298	299	45	1	typical	110	264	0	0	132	0	1.2	2	0.0	reversable	Yes
299	300	68	1	0	144	193	1	0	141	0	3.4	2	2.0	reversable	Yes
300	301	57	1	0	130	131	0	0	115	1	1.2	2	1.0	reversable	Yes
301	302	57	0	nontypical	130	236	0	2	174	0	0.0	2	1.0	normal	Yes
302	303	38	1	nonanginal	138	175	0	0	173	0	0.0	1	NaN	normal	No

FIGURE 14.3   Heart disease features.

- **First Column:** That is about age of a person.
- **Second Column**: Gender parameters used here. That noted as "MALE/FEMALE." It is numerical data which is either 0 or 1. And also you can process it based on any numerical values.
- **Third Column:** Next chest pain (cp) categories. Here are mainly four different types which we can identify inside of the dataset itself. That categories are {Typical, Aymptomatic, Nonanginal, Nontypical/Aptypical}, so some dataset already converts these string wise representations to numerical ones. You can denote it as {0,1,2,3} or other numerical ways. Typical angina notation "decrease blood supply to the heart." Atypical angina: "chest pain not related to heart." Non-anginal pain is non-heart related. Asymptomatic: "chest pain not showing abnormal signs."
- **Fourth Column**: "trestbps/restBP" is to denote resting blood pressure and its unit is in mm. Reason to worry range is in between 130 to 140.
- **Fifth column**: "chol" is a parameter that represented as serum cholesterol and unit is in mg/dl. Calculation of "serum = LDL + HDL + .2 * triglycerides." Reason to worry is "above 200."
- **Sixth column**: "fbs" is fasting blood sugar which is >120 mg/dl. If it is high, it is notated as 1 that is true or 0 can be used for low. Diabetes (>126) patients may face silent attacks.
- **Seventh Column**: "restecg" is "resting electrocardiographic" results and "Nothing to note" (0); "ST-T Wave abnormality" (1); "Possible or definite left ventricular hypertrophy" normally enlarged heart's main pumping chamber.
- **Eighth Column** is about "thalach" to denote maximum achieved heart rate.
- **Ninth Column** is about "exang" which is exercise-induced angina (1 can denote for "yes"; 0 for "no").
- **10th Column** is "oldpeak" which is ST depression induced and stress of heart during exercise, unhealthy heart will stress more.
- **11th Column** is "slope" which is the slope of the peak exercise ST segment. "Upsloping" can be represented as "0." "Flatsloping" can be denoted as "1" and "Downslopins" can be represented as "2" which is signs of unhealthy heart.
- **12th Column** is "ca" which is the number of major vessels (0–3) colored by flouroscopy.
- **13th Column** is "thal" which is thalium stress result. Normal can be represented as 1–3, fixed defect can be denoted as 6 (just ok), and reversible defect can be denoted as 7 (no proper blood moving during exercising).
- **14th Column** attribute is "target" that is prediction labeling. Indication of "disease affected or not." Either TRUE/FALSE or YES/No or 0/1.

Library Calling Section: Here numpy, pandas, seaborn, and matplotlib are initially used. And for comparison work, different supervised machine learning classifiers used. Classifiers used are logistic regression, passive aggressive classifier, ridge classifier, K-nearest neighbor, Gaussian Naïve Bayes, and Bernoulli Naïve Bayes. Accuracy scores calculated. Confusion matrix and ROC curve displayed. Precision and recall calculated based on cross-validation train and test splits.

TABLE 14.6
Novel Statistics Data Values

S. No.	State	Active	Mild	Severe	Cured	Death	New_Active	New_Mild	New Severe	New Cured	New Death	State Code
1	Andaman and Nicobar Islands	10	7	2	9	1	12	8	0	3	1	35
2	Andhra Pradesh	11	6	4	5	1	10	8	0	2	0	28
3	Arunachal Pradesh	15	6	7	6	2	0	0	0	0	0	12
4	Assam	9	6	3	4	0	10	8	1	3	1	18
5	Bihar	19	7	11	8	1	10	4	4	5	2	10
6	Chandigarh	20	17	2	8	1	14	4	7	5	3	4
7	Chhattisgarh	22	17	4	10	1	3	2	1	7	0	22
8	Dadra and Nagar Haveli and Daman and Diu	10	7	2	9	1	5	2	2	4	1	26
9	Delhi	13	8	5	9	0	4	2	2	4	0	7

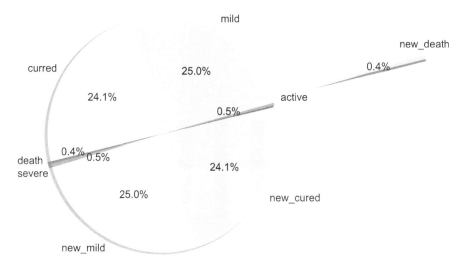

FIGURE 14.4 Active health statistics based on Table 14.6.

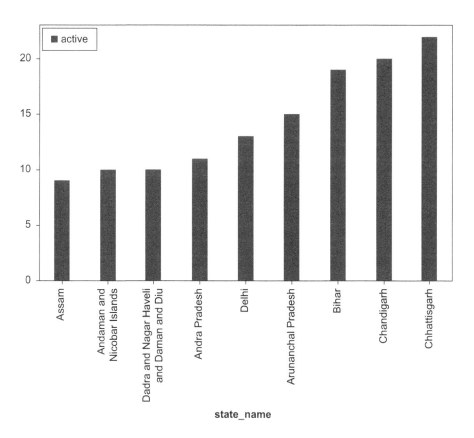

FIGURE 14.5 Death health statistics based on Table 14.6.

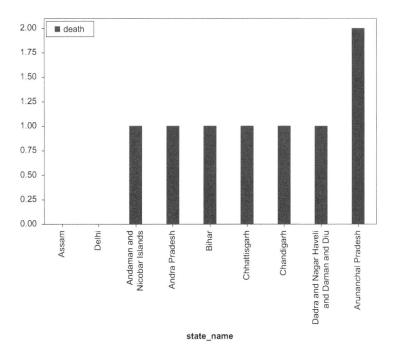

FIGURE 14.6   Severe health statistics based on Table 14.6.

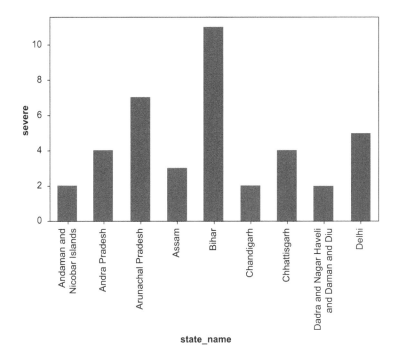

FIGURE 14.7   Cured health statistics based on Table 14.6.

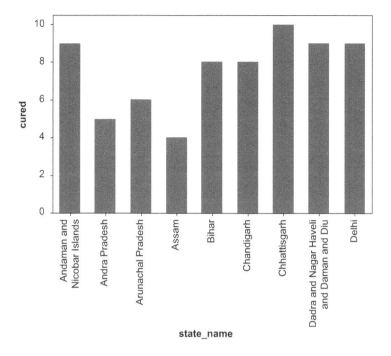

FIGURE 14.8 New cured health statistics based on Table 14.6.

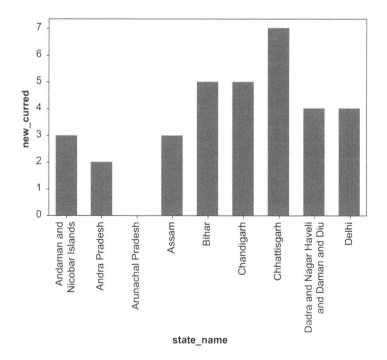

FIGURE 14.9 Cured and death health statistics based on Table 14.6.

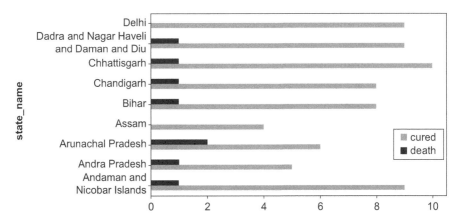

FIGURE 14.10   Severe and death health statistics based on Table 14.6: statewise.

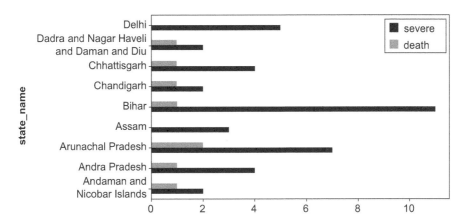

FIGURE 14.11   Cured and death health statistics based on Table 14.6: statewise.

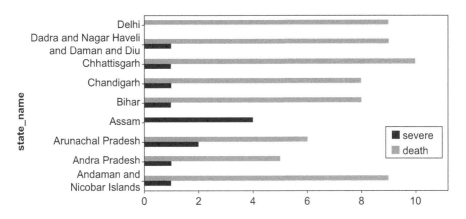

FIGURE 14.12   Active and death health statistics based on Table 14.6: statewise.

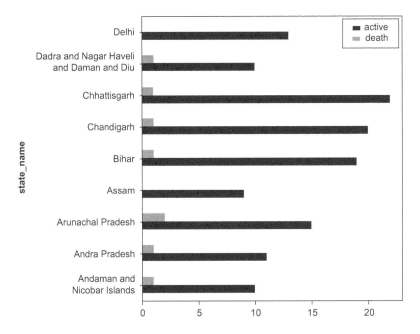

FIGURE 14.13 Health statistics based on state data (values in Table 14.6).

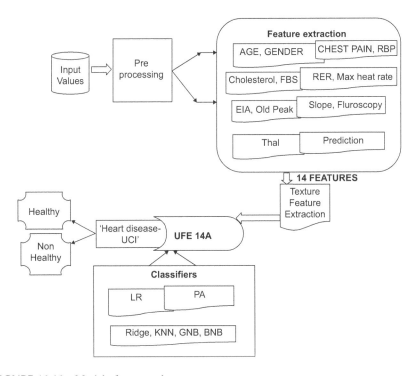

FIGURE 14.14 Model of proposed system.

In Figure 14.15, different library details for this work are clearly mentioned. Initially, numpy, pandas are added, and its name shortly mentioned by the help of "as" keyword. Seaborn is used for "statistical data visualization." Different classifiers processed and its libraries also added in Figure 14.15. Metrics and curve and cross-validation libraries added.

It is clear that Bernoulli Naïve Bayes performed well than that of other classification algorithms based on "heart disease-UCI" dataset. (No modification has been done. Predefined dataset values considered for our work.)

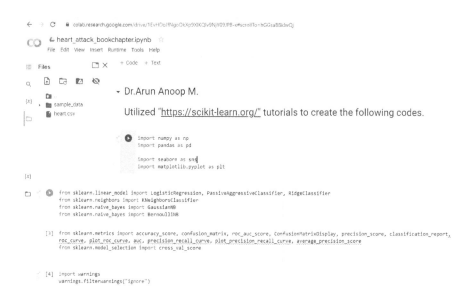

FIGURE 14.15   Libraries adding section in Colab.

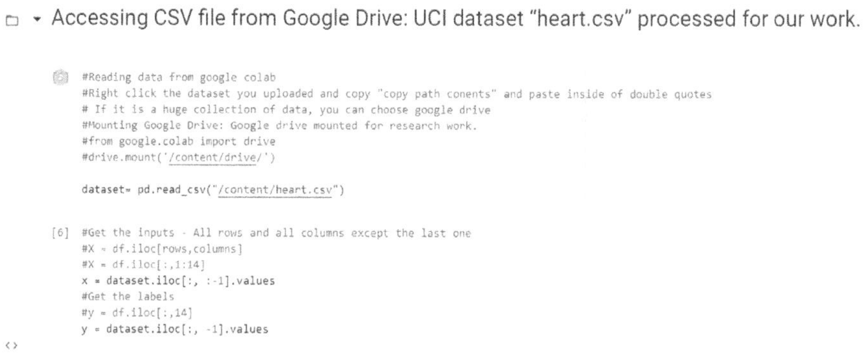

FIGURE 14.16   Dataset reading and segregation of data.

```
#https://scikit-learn.org/stable/modules/generated/sklearn.model_selection.train_test_split.html
#Splitting data: Splitting data into train and test set. "test_size=0.2" indicates test=20% and train=80%.
#If any tuning is required, can refer "scikit+train_test_split" in search engines.
from sklearn.model_selection import train_test_split
x_train, x_test, y_train, y_test = train_test_split(x, y, test_size= 0.2, random_state= 0)
```

```
#To know data count and columns/attributes count
print("Number transactions x_train dataset: ", x_train.shape)
print("Number transactions y_train dataset: ", y_train.shape)
print("Number transactions x_test dataset: ", x_test.shape)
print("Number transactions y_test dataset: ", y_test.shape)
```

```
Number transactions x_train dataset:  (242, 13)
Number transactions y_train dataset:  (242,)
Number transactions x_test dataset:  (61, 13)
Number transactions y_test dataset:  (61,)
```

FIGURE 14.17   Training and testing of data.

```
#Feature scaling: For feature scaling "standard scaler" and "min max scaler" normally use.
#Here standard scaler is used for feature scaling process.
#https://scikit-learn.org/stable/modules/generated/sklearn.preprocessing.StandardScaler.html
from sklearn.preprocessing import StandardScaler
sc = StandardScaler()
x_train = sc.fit_transform(x_train)
x_test = sc.transform(x_test)
```

```
[ ] #https://scikit-learn.org/stable/modules/generated/sklearn.preprocessing.MinMaxScaler.html
from sklearn.preprocessing import MinMaxScaler
sc = MinMaxScaler()
x_train = sc.fit_transform(x_train)
x_test = sc.transform(x_test)
```

FIGURE 14.18   Feature scaling.

```
#Logistic Regression:  "Logistic regression model" is used for classifying data.
#Individually "confusion matrix", "accuracy score" and "ROC curve" is plotted.
lr = LogisticRegression(random_state= 0)
lr.fit(x_train, y_train)
lr_pred = lr.predict(x_test)
lr_prob = lr.predict_proba(x_test)[:,1]
cm = confusion_matrix(y_test, lr_pred)
lr_acc_score = accuracy_score(y_test, lr_pred)
print(classification_report(y_test, lr_pred))
print(f'ROC AUC score: {roc_auc_score(y_test, lr_prob)}')
print('Accuracy Score: ',lr_acc_score)
```

```
              precision    recall  f1-score   support

           0       0.88      0.78      0.82        27
           1       0.84      0.91      0.87        34

    accuracy                           0.85        61
   macro avg       0.86      0.84      0.85        61
weighted avg       0.85      0.85      0.85        61

ROC AUC score: 0.9106753812636165
Accuracy Score:  0.8524590163934426
```

FIGURE 14.19   Logistic regression.

```
#Passive Aggressive Regression: "Passive Aggressive Classifier model" is used for classifying data.
#Individually "confusion matrix", "accuracy score" and "ROC curve" is plotted.
pr = PassiveAggressiveClassifier()
pr.fit(x_train, y_train)
pr_pred = pr.predict(x_test)
pr_prob = pr._predict_proba_lr(x_test)[:,1]
cm = confusion_matrix(y_test, pr_pred)
pr_acc_score = accuracy_score(y_test, pr_pred)
print(classification_report(y_test, pr_pred))
print(f'ROC AUC score: {roc_auc_score(y_test, pr_prob)}')
print('Accuracy Score: ',pr_acc_score)
```

```
              precision    recall  f1-score   support

           0       0.72      0.85      0.78        27
           1       0.86      0.74      0.79        34

    accuracy                           0.79        61
   macro avg       0.79      0.79      0.79        61
weighted avg       0.80      0.79      0.79        61

ROC AUC score: 0.883442265795207
Accuracy Score:  0.7868852459016393
```

FIGURE 14.20   Passive aggressive model.

```
[12] #Ridge Classifier: "Ridge Classifier model" is used for classifying data.
     #Individually "confusion matrix", "accuracy score" and "ROC curve" is plotted.
     rr = RidgeClassifier()
     rr.fit(x_train, y_train)
     rr_pred = rr.predict(x_test)
     rr_prob = rr._predict_proba_lr(x_test)[:,1]
     cm = confusion_matrix(y_test, rr_pred)
     rr_acc_score = accuracy_score(y_test, rr_pred)
     print(classification_report(y_test, rr_pred))
     print(f'ROC AUC score: {roc_auc_score(y_test, rr_prob)}')
     print('Accuracy Score: ',rr_acc_score)
```

```
              precision    recall  f1-score   support

           0       0.87      0.74      0.80        27
           1       0.82      0.91      0.86        34

    accuracy                           0.84        61
   macro avg       0.84      0.83      0.83        61
weighted avg       0.84      0.84      0.83        61

ROC AUC score: 0.9052287581699346
Accuracy Score:  0.8360655737704918
```

FIGURE 14.21   Ridge classifier.

```
#KNN Classifier: "KNN model" is used for classifying data.
#Individually "confusion matrix", "accuracy score" and "ROC curve" is plotted.
knn = KNeighborsClassifier()
knn.fit(x_train, y_train)
knn_pred = knn.predict(x_test)
knn_prob = knn.predict_proba(x_test)[:,1]
cm = confusion_matrix(y_test, knn_pred)
knn_acc_score = accuracy_score(y_test, knn_pred)
print(classification_report(y_test, knn_pred))
print(f'ROC AUC score: {roc_auc_score(y_test, knn_prob)}')
print('Accuracy Score: ',knn_acc_score)
```

```
              precision    recall  f1-score   support

           0       0.81      0.78      0.79        27
           1       0.83      0.85      0.84        34

    accuracy                           0.82        61
   macro avg       0.82      0.82      0.82        61
weighted avg       0.82      0.82      0.82        61

ROC AUC score: 0.9172113289760349
Accuracy Score:  0.819672131147541
```

FIGURE 14.22   K-nearest neighbor.

```
[14] #Gaussian Naïve Bayes Classifier: "Gaussian Naïve Bayes model" is used for classifying data.
     #Individually "confusion matrix", "accuracy score" and "ROC curve" is plotted.
     gr = GaussianNB()
     gr.fit(x_train, y_train)
     gr_pred = gr.predict(x_test)
     gr_prob = gr.predict_proba(x_test)[:,1]
     cm = confusion_matrix(y_test, gr_pred)
     gr_acc_score = accuracy_score(y_test, knn_pred)
     print(classification_report(y_test, gr_pred))
     print(f'ROC AUC score: {roc_auc_score(y_test, gr_prob)}')
     print('Accuracy Score: ',gr_acc_score)
```

```
              precision    recall  f1-score   support

           0       0.88      0.78      0.82        27
           1       0.84      0.91      0.87        34

    accuracy                           0.85        61
   macro avg       0.86      0.84      0.85        61
weighted avg       0.85      0.85      0.85        61

ROC AUC score: 0.9074074074074074
Accuracy Score:  0.819672131147541
```

FIGURE 14.23   Gaussian Naïve Bayes classifier.

```
#Bernoulli Naïve Bayes Classifier: "Bernoulli Naïve Bayes model" is used for classifying data.
#Individually "confusion matrix", "accuracy score" and "ROC curve" is plotted.
br = BernoulliNB()
br.fit(x_train, y_train)
br_pred = br.predict(x_test)
br_prob = br.predict_proba(x_test)[:,1]
cm = confusion_matrix(y_test, br_pred)
br_acc_score = accuracy_score(y_test, br_pred)
print(classification_report(y_test, br_pred))
print(f'ROC AUC score: {roc_auc_score(y_test, br_prob)}')
print('Accuracy Score: ',br_acc_score)
```

```
              precision    recall  f1-score   support

           0       0.85      0.85      0.85        27
           1       0.88      0.88      0.88        34

    accuracy                           0.87        61
   macro avg       0.87      0.87      0.87        61
weighted avg       0.87      0.87      0.87        61

ROC AUC score: 0.9411764705882353
Accuracy Score:  0.8688524590163934
```

FIGURE 14.24   Bernoulli Naïve Bayes classifier.

```
#'Receiver Operating Characteristic Curve': ROC curve plotted based on "Scikit" documentation notes.
#Classifiers used are Logistic Regression(lr),
#Passive Aggressive Classifier(pr), Ridge Classifier(rr), K Nearest Neighbour(knn), Gaussian Naïve Bayes(gr)
#and Bernoulli Naïve Bayes(br).
lr_false_positive_rate,lr_true_positive_rate,lr_threshold = roc_curve(y_test,lr_pred)
pr_false_positive_rate,pr_true_positive_rate,pr_threshold = roc_curve(y_test,pr_pred)
rr_false_positive_rate,rr_true_positive_rate,rr_threshold = roc_curve(y_test,rr_pred)
knn_false_positive_rate,knn_true_positive_rate,knn_threshold = roc_curve(y_test,knn_pred)
gr_false_positive_rate,gr_true_positive_rate,gr_threshold = roc_curve(y_test,gr_pred)
br_false_positive_rate,br_true_positive_rate,br_threshold = roc_curve(y_test,br_pred)

sns.set_style('whitegrid')
plt.figure(figsize=(10,5))
plt.title('Receiver Operating Characteristic Curve')
plt.plot(lr_false_positive_rate,lr_true_positive_rate,label='Logistic Regression')
plt.plot(pr_false_positive_rate,pr_true_positive_rate,label='Passive Aggressive Classifier')
plt.plot(rr_false_positive_rate,rr_true_positive_rate,label='Ridge Classifier')
plt.plot(knn_false_positive_rate,knn_true_positive_rate,label='K Nearest Neighbor')

plt.plot(gr_false_positive_rate,gr_true_positive_rate,label='Gaussian NB')
plt.plot(br_false_positive_rate,br_true_positive_rate,label='Bernoulli NB')
plt.plot([0,1],ls='--')
plt.plot([0,0],[1,0],c='.5')
plt.plot([1,1],c='.5')
plt.ylabel('True positive rate')
plt.xlabel('False positive rate')
plt.legend()
plt.show()
```

FIGURE 14.25   ROC curve evaluation and visualization.

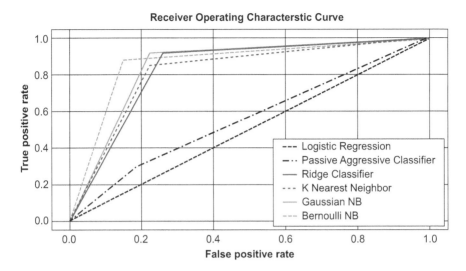

FIGURE 14.26   Receiver operating characteristics curve based on classifiers.

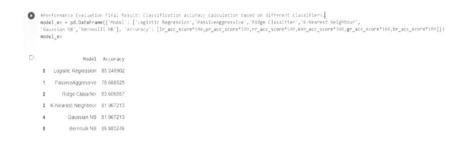

FIGURE 14.27   Different classifiers performance evaluation.

TABLE 14.7
Performance Evaluation Results

S. No.	Models	Accuracy
1	Logistic regression	85.245902
2	Passive aggressive	52.459016
3	Ridge classifier	83.606557
4	K-nearest neighbor	81.967213
5	Gaussian NB	81.967213
6	Bernoulli NB	**86.885246**

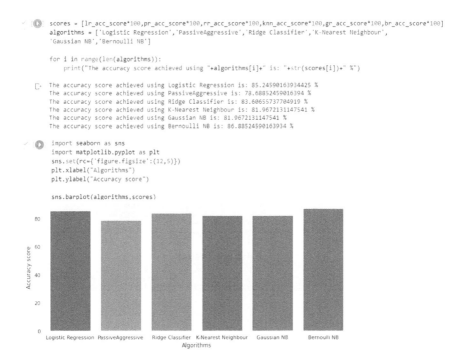

```
    scores = [lr_acc_score*100,pr_acc_score*100,rr_acc_score*100,knn_acc_score*100,gr_acc_score*100,br_acc_score*100]
    algorithms = ['Logistic Regression','PassiveAggressive','Ridge Classifier','K-Nearest Neighbour',
    'Gaussian NB','Bernoulli NB']

    for i in range(len(algorithms)):
        print("The accuracy score achieved using "+algorithms[i]+" is: "+str(scores[i])+" %")
```

```
    The accuracy score achieved using Logistic Regression is: 85.24590163934425 %
    The accuracy score achieved using PassiveAggressive is: 78.68852459016394 %
    The accuracy score achieved using Ridge Classifier is: 83.60655737704919 %
    The accuracy score achieved using K-Nearest Neighbour is: 81.9672131147541 %
    The accuracy score achieved using Gaussian NB is: 81.9672131147541 %
    The accuracy score achieved using Bernoulli NB is: 86.88524590163934 %
```

```
    import seaborn as sns
    import matplotlib.pyplot as plt
    sns.set(rc={'figure.figsize':(12,5)})
    plt.xlabel("Algorithms")
    plt.ylabel("Accuracy score")

    sns.barplot(algorithms,scores)
```

FIGURE 14.28   Different classifiers performance evaluation plot.

14.4   CONCLUSION AND FUTURE WORK

The heart and a network of veins and arteries make up the circulatory system [60]. Our heart is made up of "cardiac tissue." Left ventricle is the biggest and most grounded chamber of heart which sends blood to all parts of the body. Circulatory framework comprises the heart, endlessly blood vessels [61]. Dimensionality reduction methods, types, and test functions discussed in this chapter. Fourteen heart attack–related attributes are surveyed and clearly mentioned in this chapter. Graphs plotted are based on statewise count and UCI dataset. Heart attack–based healthcare hands on section made this chapter more informative we hope [62]. We designed a drone IoT system for healthcare division. But, because of some issues, system faced working failure (only two attributes collected by installed sensors). In future, we may focus to add more sensors to collect one or two major attributes or features. Framingham calculator is a tool designed to determine one's risk of a heart attack within next ten years (mentioned in electronic book named *Heart: A History* by Sandeep Jauhar [38]). Treadmill for stress test helps to identify coronary blockages 70% and noninvasive CT angiogram to investigate coronaries. A nitroglycerine tablet may be used to place under tongue to dilate chest arteries, injecting X-ray opaque dye into vein (mentioned in *Heart: A History* by Sandeep Jauhar [38]). In future, our work will extend to the following:

1. Developing IoT drone and smart watch system for heart patient's risk prediction and health monitoring.
2. Drug discovery for cardiovascular diseases based on computer-aided drug design.

NOTES

1. https://healthblog.uofmhealth.org/heart-health/anatomy-of-a-human-heart
2. healthblog.uofmhealth.org

REFERENCES

1. Seyedali Mirjalili (2015). The Ant Lion Optimizer. *Advances in Engineering Software* 83. http://doi.org/10.1016/j.advengsoft.2015.01.010
2. Seyedali Mirjalili (2019). Genetic Algorithm. *Evolutionary Algorithms and Neural Networks* 780. http://doi.org/10.1007/978-3-319-93025-1_4
3. Soufiene Ben Othman, Abdullah Ali Bahattab, Abdelbasset Trad, Habib Youssef (2020, June). LSDA: Lightweight Secure Data Aggregation Scheme in Healthcare using IoT. *ACM — 10th International Conference on Information Systems and Technologies*, Lecce, Italy.
4. Yassine Meraihi, Benmessaoud Gabis, Asma, Mirjalili, Seyedali, Ramdane-Cherif, Amar (2021). Grasshopper Optimization Algorithm: Theory, Variants, and Applications. *IEEE Access* 9:50001–500241. http://doi.org/10.1109/ACCESS.2021.3067597
5. S. Mirjalili, S.M. Mirjalili, A. Lewis (2014) Grey Wolf Optimizer. *Advances in Engineering Software* 69:46–61.
6. Soufiene Ben Othman, Abdullah Ali Bahattab, Abdelbasset Trad, Habib Youssef (2019). RESDA: Robust and Efficient Secure Data Aggregation Scheme in Healthcare using the IoT. *The International Conference on Internet of Things, Embedded Systems and Communications (IINTEC 2019)*, HAMMAMET, Tunisia from 20–22 December 2019.
7. Wonder House Books (2020). *Human Body—Heart and Circulatory System: Knowledge Encyclopedia for Children*. Wonder House Books, ISBN 13: 9789389931204.
8. Dr. Peter WF Wilson. *Estimates 10-Year Risk of Heart Attack*. Available: mdcalc.com/framingham-risk-score-hard-coronary-heart-disease
9. Mandeep R. Mehra, Sapan S. Desai, SreyRam Kuy, Timothy D. Henry, Amit N. Patel (2020). Cardiovascular Disease, Drug Therapy, and Mortality in COVID-19. *The New England Journal of Medicine*, 382:2582–2597. http://doi.org/10.1056/nejmoa2007621. Available: nejm.org at UNIVERSITE DE PARIS on May 1, 2020.
10. Gaurav Aggarwal, Brandon Michael Henry, Saurabh Aggarwal, Sripal Bangalore (2020). *Cardiovascular Safety of Potential Drugs for the Treatment of Coronavirus Disease 2019, 0002–9149*. Elsevier Inc, 2020. http://doi.org/10.1016/j.amjcard.2020.04.054
11. Madhusmita Panda, Bikramaditya Das (2019). Grey Wolf Optimizer and Its Applications: A Survey. *Lecture Notes in Electrical Engineering (LNEE)*, vol 556.
12. V.K. Chawla, A.K. Chanda, Surjit Angra (2019). The scheduling of automatic guided vehicles for the workload balancing and travel time minimization in the flexible manufacturing system by the nature-inspired algorithm, *Journal of Project Management* 4:19–30.
13. Bo Yang, Xiaoshun Zhang, Tao Yu, Hongchun Shu, Zihao Fang (2017). Grouped grey wolf optimizer for maximum power point tracking of doubly-fed induction generator based wind turbine. *Energy Conversion and Management* 133:427–443.

14. Binglian Zhu, Wenyong Zhu, Zijuan Liu, Qingyan Duan, Long Cao (2016). *A Novel Quantum-Behaved Bat Algorithm with Mean Best Position Directed for Numerical Optimization*. Hindawi, Computational Intelligence and Neuroscience.

15. Peifeng Niu, Songpeng Niu, Nan Liu, Lingfang Chang (2019). The Defect of the Grey Wolf Optimization Algorithm and Its Verification Method. *Elsevier, Knowledge-Based Systems* 171:37–43.

16. Ting Liu, Chao Tan, Zhongbin Wang, Jing Xu, Yiqiao Man, Tuo Wang (2019). Horizontal Bending Angle Optimization Method for Scraper Conveyor Based on Improved Bat Algorithm. *Algorithms* 12(4):84. https://doi.org/10.3390/a12040084

17. Seyedali Mirjalili (2015). The Ant Lion Optimizer. *Advances in Engineering Software* 83:80–98.

18. Mohammad Shehab, Laith Abualigah, Husam Al Hamad, Hamzeh Alabool, Mohammad Alshinwan, Ahmad M. Khasawneh (2019). Moth—Flame Optimization Algorithm: Variants and Applications. *Neural Computing and Applications* 32:9859–9884.

19. Seyedali Mirjalili, Andrew Lewis (2016). The Whale Optimization Algorithm. *Advances in Engineering Software* 95:51–67.

20. Seyedali Mirjalili (2016). Dragonfly Algorithm: A New Meta-heuristic Optimization Technique for Solving Single-objective, Discrete, and Multi-objective Problems. *Neural Computing and Applications* 27:1053–1073.

21. Shahrzad Saremi, Seyedali Mirjalili, Andrew Lewis (2017). Grasshopper Optimisation Algorithm: Theory and Application, *Advances in Engineering Software* 105:30–47.

22. S. Mirjalili, A.H. Gandomi, S.Z. Mirjalili, S. Saremi, H. Faris, S.M. Mirjalili (2017). Salp Swarm Algorithm: A Bio-inspired Optimizer for Engineering Design Problems. *Advances in Engineering Software* 114:163–191.

23. Kornel Chrominski, Magdalena Tkacz, Mariusz Boryczka (2020). Epigenetic Modification of Genetic Algorithm. In et al. *Computational Science – ICCS 2020. ICCS 2020. Lecture Notes in Computer Science*, vol 12138. Springer, Cham. https://doi.org/10.1007/978-3-030-50417-5_20

24. S. Jafari, O. Bozorg-Haddad, X. Chu (2018). Cuckoo Optimization Algorithm (COA). In Bozorg-Haddad O. (eds) *Advanced Optimization by Nature-Inspired Algorithms. Studies in Computational Intelligence*, vol 720. Springer, Singapore.

25. Amit Kishor, Chinmay Chakraborty (2021). Artificial Intelligence and Internet of Things Based Healthcare 4.0 Monitoring System. *Wireless Personal Communications*, no. 0123456789. https://doi.org/10.1007/s11277-021-08708-5

26. Mohammad Khishe, M. Mosavi (2020). Chimp Optimization Algorithm. *Expert Systems with Applications* 149:113338. http://doi.org/10.1016/j.eswa.2020.113338.

27. N. Razmjooy, M. Khalilpour, M. Ramezani (2016). A New Meta-Heuristic Optimization Algorithm Inspired by FIFA World Cup Competitions: Theory and Its Application in PID Designing for AVR System. *Journal of Control, Automation and Electrical Systems* 27:419–440.

28. Gai-Ge Wang, Suash Deb, Leandro Coelho (2015). Earthworm Optimization Algorithm: A Bio-inspired Metaheuristic Algorithm for Global Optimization Problems. *International Journal of Bio-Inspired Computation*. http://doi.org/10.1504/IJBIC.2015.10004283

29. Konstantinos Zervoudakis, Stelios Tsafarakis (2020). A Mayfly Optimization Algorithm. *Computers & Industrial Engineering* 145:106559.

30. V. Hayyolalam, A.A. Pourhaji Kazem (2020). Black Widow Optimization Algorithm: A Novel Meta-heuristic Approach for Solving Engineering Optimization Problems. *Engineering Applications of Artificial Intelligence* 87:103249.

31. H.H. Attar, A.A.A. Solyman, A. Alrosan, C. Chinmay, R.K. Mohammad (2021). Deterministic Cooperative Hybrid Ring-mesh Network Coding for Big Data Transmission Over Lossy Channels in 5G Networks. *EURASIP Journal on Wireless Communications and Networking* 159:1–18. https://doi.org/10.1186/s13638-021-02032-z

32. G. Dhiman, V. Kumar (2019). Seagull Optimization Algorithm: Theory and Its Applications for Large-scale Industrial Engineering Problems. *Knowledge-Based Systems* 165:169–196.

33. Wen-Tsao Pan (2012, February). A New Fruit Fly Optimization Algorithm: Taking the Financial Distress Model as an Example. *Knowledge-Based Systems* 26:69–74.

34. R. Venkata Rao (2016). Jaya: A Simple and New Optimization Algorithm for Solving Constrained and Unconstrained Optimization Problems. *International Journal of Industrial Engineering Computations* 7:19–34.

35. Gaurav Dhiman, Amandeep Kaur (2019). STOA: A Bio-inspired Based Optimization Algorithm for Industrial Engineering Problems. *Engineering Applications of Artificial Intelligence* 82:148–174.

36. Laith Abualigah, Dalia Yousri, Mohamed Abd Elaziz, Ahmed A. Ewees, Mohammed A.A. Al-Qaness, Amir H. Gandomi (2021). Aquila Optimizer: A Novel Meta-heuristic Optimization Algorithm. *Computers & Industrial Engineering* 157:107250.

37. G.F. Gomes, S.S. da Cunha, A.C. Ancelotti (2019). A Sunflower Optimization (SFO) Algorithm Applied to Damage Identification on Laminated Composite Plates. *Engineering with Computers* 35:619–626.

38. Soufiene Ben Othman, Abdullah Ali Bahattab, Abdelbasset Trad, Habib Youssef (2020). PEERP: A Priority-Based Energy-Efficient Routing Protocol for Reliable Data Transmission in Healthcare using the IoT. *The 15th International Conference on Future Networks and Communications (FNC) August 9–12, 2020*, Leuven, Belgium.

39. A.R. Simpson, H.R. Maier, W.K. Foong, K.Y. Phang, H.Y. Seah, C.L. Tan (2001). Selection of Parameters for Ant Colony Optimisation Applied to the Optimal Design of Water Distribution Systems. *MODSIM 2001, International Congress on Modelling and Simulation, Modelling and Simulation Society of Australia*, Canberra, Australia, 10–13 December, 1931–1936.

40. H.A. Abbass (2001). MBO: Marriage in Honey Bees Optimization—A Haplometrosis Polygynous Swarming Approach. *Proceedings of the 2001 Congress on Evolutionary Computation* (IEEE Cat. No.01TH8546), vol 1, pp. 207–214. https://doi.org/10.1109/CEC.2001.934391.

41. X. Li (2003). *A New Intelligent Optimization-artificial Fish Swarm Algorithm* [Doctor thesis]. China: Zhejiang University of Zhejiang.

42. M. Roth, W. Stephen (2006). *Termite: A Swarm Intelligent Routing Algorithm for Mobilewireless Ad-Hoc Networks.* Stigmergic Optimization, Springer, Berlin, Heidelberg, pp. 155–184.

43. B. Basturk, D. Karaboga (2006). An Artificial Bee Colony (ABC) Algorithm for Numeric Function Optimization. *Proceedings of the IEEE Swarm Intelligence Symposium*, Indianapolis, IN, May 12–14, pp. 12–14.

44. P.C. Pinto, T.A. Runkler, J.M. Sousa (2007). Wasp Swarm Algorithm for Dynamic MAXSAT Problems. Adaptive and Natural Computing Algorithms. In Beliczynski, B., Dzielinski, A., Iwanowski, M., Ribeiro, B. (eds) *Adaptive and Natural Computing Algorithms. ICANNGA 2007. Lecture Notes in Computer Science*, vol 4431. Springer, Berlin, Heidelberg, pp. 350–357.

45. A. Mucherino, O. Seref (2007). Monkey Search: A Novel Metaheuristic Search for Global Optimization. *AIP Conference Proceedings* 953:162. https://doi.org/10.1063/1.2817338

46. C. Yang, X. Tu, J. Chen (2007). Algorithm of Marriage in Honey Bees Optimization Based on the Wolf Pack Search. *Proceedings of the 2007 International Conference on Intelligent Pervasive Computing*, IPC, pp. 462–467.

47. X. Lu, Y. Zhou (2008). A Novel Global Convergence Algorithm: Bee Collecting Pollen Algorithm. Advanced Intelligent Computing Theories and Applications with Aspects of Artificial Intelligence. In Huang, D.S., Wunsch, D.C., Levine, D.S., Jo, KH. (eds) *Advanced Intelligent Computing Theories and Applications. With Aspects of Artificial Intelligence. ICIC 2008. Lecture Notes in Computer Science*, vol 5227. Springer, Berlin, Heidelberg, pp. 518–525. https://doi.org/10.1007/978-3-540-85984-0_62

48. Y. Shiqin, J. Jianjun, Y. Guangxing (2009). A dolphin partner optimization. *GCIS '09: Proceedings of the WRI Global Congress on Intelligent Systems*, vol 1, pp. 124–128. https://doi.org/10.1109/GCIS.2009.464

49. R. Oftadeh, M.J. Mahjoob, M. Shariatpanahi (2010). A Novel Meta-heuristic Optimization Algorithm Inspired by Group Hunting of Animals: Hunting Search. *Computers & Mathematics with Applications* 60:2087–2098.

50. A. Askarzadeh, A. Rezazadeh (2012). A New Heuristic Optimization Algorithm for Modeling of Proton Exchange Membrane Fuel Cell: Bird Mating Optimizer. *International Journal of Energy Research* 37:1196–1204.

51. A.H. Gandomi, A.H. Alavi (2012). Krill Herd: A New Bio-inspired Optimization Algorithm. *Communications in Nonlinear Science and Numerical Simulation* 17(12): 4831–4845.

52. A. Kaveh, N. Farhoudi (2013). A New Optimization Method: Dolphin Echolocation. *Advances in Engineering Software* 59:53–70.

53. Koby Crammer, Ofer Dekel, Joseph Keshet, Shai Shalev-Shwartz, Yoram Singer (2006). Online Passive-Aggressive Algorithms. *Journal of Machine Learning Research* 7:551–585.

54. B.V. Kiranmayee, C. Suresh, S. SreeRakshak (2022). Classification of the Suicide-Related Text Data Using Passive Aggressive Classifier. In Shakya S., Balas V.E., Kamolphiwong S., Du K.L. (eds) *Sentimental Analysis and Deep Learning. Advances in Intelligent Systems and Computing*, vol 1408. Springer, Singapore. https://doi.org/10.1007/978-981-16-5157-1_34

55. https://medium.com/@adi.bronshtein/a-quick-introduction-to-k-nearest-neighbors-al-gorithm-62214cea29c7

56. S. Yogesh, C. Chinmay (2021). Augmented Reality and Virtual Reality Transforming Spinal Imaging Landscape: A Feasibility Study. *IEEE Computer Graphics and Applications* 41(3):124–138. http://doi.org/10.1109/MCG.2020.3000359

57. *UCI Machine Learning Repository*. Available: https//archive.ics.uci.edu/ml/datasets/Heart+Disease

58. https://medium.com/@sarojthapa60_76302/what-is-overfitting-and-how-to-avoid-it-56d4b9ba0688

59. Shaica. Available: https://jovian.ai/forum/t/difference-between-logistic-regression-and-linear-regression/14649/2

60. *Framingham Dataset*. Available: www.kaggle.com/eeshanpaul/framingham

61. Logistic Regression Classifier. Available: www.shuhanyu.com/2018/07/12/Logistic RegressionInMultiClassClassificationProblems/

62. https://thevivekpandey.github.io/posts/2017-10-08-deeplearning-coursera-course-2.html

15 Thermal Face Image Reidentification Based on Variational Autoencoder, Cascade Object Detector Using Lightweight Architectures

Jafar Majidpour, Aram M. Ahmed,
Bryar A. Hassan, Mohammed H. Abdalla,
Shko M. Qader, Noor B. Tayfor, and
Tarik A. Rashid

CONTENTS

15.1 INTRODUCTION

Person reidentification (ReID) has great potential to contribute to tasks, such as surveillance [1], industry [2], security [3], and earthquake research [4]. Face recognition in thermal infrared images has become popular because of the fast development of infrared thermal sensors, particularly in some harsh conditions where a visible image is not sufficient for recognition. For example, when a full-time system fails to recognize visual faces at night, thermal infrared imaging systems can be used to obtain better accuracy. Another example is when professional makeup techniques are used to make significant changes in the appearance and hence making apparent facial recognition is more difficult. In these circumstances, a thermal infrared face recognition system can be used as an alternative because they are less affected and can capture many details of an image that color imaging cannot [5]. The techniques of feature extraction and machine learning have been extensively employed to identify thermal infrared images; for example, Ref. [6] used LPB, meaning local binary pattern and Haar wavelet transform in the area of recognition systems of the thermal image. In addition, they decreased the dimensionality of the information through the principal component analysis (PCA) method. The accuracy of their results on several classifications was greater than 90%. Reference [7] implemented discrete wavelet transform (DWT) method to extract features and diminish data dimension. They achieved a recognition rate of over 93% on the Terravic facial IR dataset. Moreover, Ref. [8] obtained texture characteristics by employing SFTA (segmentation-based fractal texture analysis) algorithm. The authors implemented two distinct dimensionality decreasing approaches; linear discriminant analysis (LDA) and principal component analysis [9, 10]. Then, they used the random linear oracle ensembles for identification purposes. They achieved an accuracy ratio of 94.12% on the (IR) dataset, which stands for Terravic facial.

Deep convolutional neural network recently has been actively employed by the scientific community. It is usually employed to train exceptionally large datasets to create a different feature representation. Cross-modal applications have been used in this strategy to find a representative embedding space [11, 12]. Furthermore, many studies were conducted on thermal image identification, first for the synthesis of visible images using generative adversarial networks (GAN) and then for identification using CNN networks. For example, Ref. [13] suggested a thermal image identification model based on the conversion of thermal images to visual pictures. First, a conditional generative adversarial networks (CGAN) model was used to produce realistic images, and then two simultaneous CNN networks were used to recognize the generated images. They applied their model to the Carl dataset, and they achieved an accuracy of 80%. Thermal infrared facial recognition is suggested by using a CNN model. Based on the properties of thermal images, the convoluted edges are considered primary features. In this regard, regional parallel construction is developed for extracting multiscale characteristics. When using different classifiers, statistical tests show that features retrieved using regional parallel structure (RPS) net attain decent accuracy [5]. VisDCNN (visible spectrum deep convolutional neural network) and polarimetric thermal DCNN or PolDCNN were used to obtain deep global features by using polarimetric information in the convolutional neural network [14]. The authors of Ref. [15] presented the ThermalGAN framework for the reidentification of cross-modality color-thermal people (ReID). They used a stack of GAN for a probe image of a single color to be transformed into a probe set of thermal or multimodal. As a signature of thermal, they also used thermal histograms and feature descriptors. In Ref. [16], MTCNN, which is called the multi-task cascaded convolutional networks model, was employed for perceiving face, whereas FaceNet has been utilized for extracting features. Using the triplet loss function, the network is trained to learn the facial features. On a public thermal face database, the suggested method achieved an impressive validation rate. Furthermore, the method has some generalization capacity under a variety of illumination circumstances while the best validation ratio of the thermal facial recognition was 88.81%, and the FAR was 50.66%.

Even though different models have been proposed to recognize thermal images, the results are not satisfying yet and more research need to be conducted. Therefore, in this study, a novel thermal image recognition scheme is proposed. To acquire high accuracy of face recognition from generated images, the VAE network is employed to produce visible images of thermal with high quality; next, the face portion from the generated pictures is extracted using cascade object detector such that only the person's face will remain. This eliminates details and similar pixels from all images and hence increases the identification accuracy. Finally, three lightweight architectures, which have lower parameters and higher speeds, are employed to recognize and classify the generated pictures. This chapter is prepared to reflect the subsequent sections; Section 15.2 provides the methodology of this work; Section 15.3 explains and addresses the realized outcomes; conclusively, Section 15.4 finishes the study and affords future recommendations.

15.2   METHODOLOGY

The design method of this chapter combines three significant techniques, namely, VAE, cascade object detector, and lightweight CNN architecture to form the proposed model. Figure 15.1 clearly confirms the general structure of the technique. The recognition procedure consists of four phases: within the first phase, the VAE model is used to create images with high quality and within the second phase, the value of the shaped images is assessed using different criteria such as structural similarity index method (SSIM), peak signal-to-noise ratio (PSNR), mean square error (MSE), and Fréchet inception distance (FID) metrics. In the third phase, cascade object detector is used to acquire the region of interest, i.e., crop the face of generated images and eliminate the unwanted pixels. Finally, three lightweight CNN architectural techniques, such as MobileNet, SqueezeNet, and ShuffleNet, are employed to identify the thermal face images. The next sections provide more details regarding the employed techniques of the model.

15.2.1   Autoencoding Variational Bayes

Autoencoder is one of the most common methods to compress data into smaller spaces and reduce its dimensionality. In a normal autoencoder, the image (in our

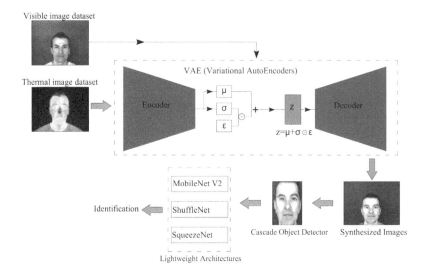

FIGURE 15.1   Proposed structure.

study, thermal face image), or the vector, which has a high dimension is fed to a model to compress the data and produce a smaller representation. This model consists of three parts; loss function, plus encoder, and decoder. The encoder is simply a neural network that can be fully connected or convolutional. It takes the data as input, produces a hidden representation as output, and possesses weights and biases. The output of this encoder is usually known as a bottleneck, which has less dimensionality compared to the input data. Furthermore, the decoder is also an artificial neural network (ANN), which takes inputs and produces parameters for the data's probability distribution and has weights and biases. The decoder tends to reconstruct the input using its layers. Then, this reconstructed version can be utilized to train the model by computing the reconstruction loss concerning the inputs [17], as presented in Figure 15.2.

In the variational autoencoder, instead of mapping the input data into a fixed vector, it will be mapped onto a distribution, as shown in Figure 15.3. So, the bottleneck is substituted by two separate vectors, which signify the standard deviation and average distribution. Therefore, a sample from the distribution is fed to the decoder to reconstruct the input data. The loss function consists of two portions: reconstruction loss, which instigates the decoder in the data reconstruction, and Kullback–Leibler divergence, which calculates how much information is lost. Finally, the reparameterization trick for the variational lower bound is required to produce a lower bound estimator that can be optimized directly using typical stochastic gradient or propagation methods [18].

15.2.2   CASCADE OBJECT DETECTOR

The cascade object detector is a Viola–Jones algorithm–based classifier that detects people's expressions, fronts, senses, etc. [19].

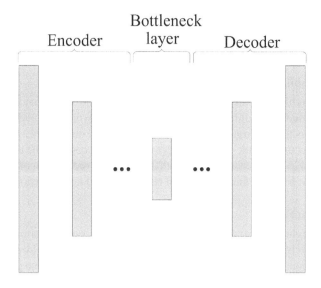

FIGURE 15.2   Normal autoencoder.

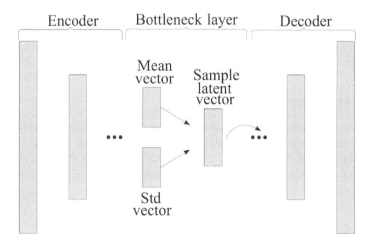

FIGURE 15.3   Variational autoencoder.

15.2.3   LIGHTWEIGHT CNN-BASED MODELS

The classification employs supervised learning to classify the generated images. Many images identification and classification methods and advancements may be traced back to CNN. An ANN is trained on local sympathetic images that create an adequate level of weight to scan a small portion of an image [20, 21]. Lightweight CNN-based models, including MobileNet, SqueezeNet, and ShuffleNet, is used to classify synthetic thermal face images to decrease model parameters, speed up computations, and achieve high performance [22]. Therefore, the next sections provide details regarding these lightweight models.

15.2.3.1 MobileNetV2

It is a CNN architecture that is suitable for portable and those vision systems that can be embedded. To build a compact deep neural network. MobileNet's precision is not as high as that of larger CNN designs. MobileNet, on the other hand, excels in the resource/accuracy trade-off. It provides excellent precision at the expense of limited resources [23]. Moreover, MobileNetV2 is an improved version of MobileNetV1, making it more accurate and powerful in terms of speed and precision [24].

15.2.3.2 ShuffleNet

It is a lightweight CNN architecture optimized for low-power mobile devices [25]. ShuffleNet's architecture makes use of two novel operations to minimize computation costs without compromising precision. These are the pointwise group convolution as well as channel shuffle operations, respectively. The channel shuffle process enables the division of each group's channels into numerous subgroups and then feeding each subgroup into the next layer's groups.

15.2.3.3 SqueezeNet

It is a compact CNN architecture to obtain a more controlled method for the design-space exploration of convolutional neural networks. Finally, it enlarges the activation maps of the convolution layers by downsampling layers in the network [26].

15.2.4 MEASUREMENTS

In our study, we evaluated classification accuracy using two distinct kinds of metrics: first, we employed observational error metrics, including accuracy, recall, F1 score, and precision. Second, using the SSIM [27], MSE [28], PSNR [29], and FID [30] metrics, compare the synthesized image quality with the original visible images [31–33].

15.2.5 CARL DATASET

Carl dataset was collected by taking images of 41 individuals using three different colors of light. The images in the Carl dataset were gathered throughout four separate sessions, each with a distinct type of lighting. The thermal images have a resolution of 60×120 pixels and can be shown in four separate chronological sessions. Images for each lighting situation, kind, and session are included for each topic. Because of this, we utilized 4,920 photos in total. It is separated into 80% training and 20% testing in this study. There are 60 pairs of images (thermal and visible) in this dataset; each subject has a total of 60 pairs of images (thermal and visible). For each person, we utilized 48 of these images to train and 12 to test [34, 35]. Some instances of the dataset for Indian scripts are shown in Figure 15.4.

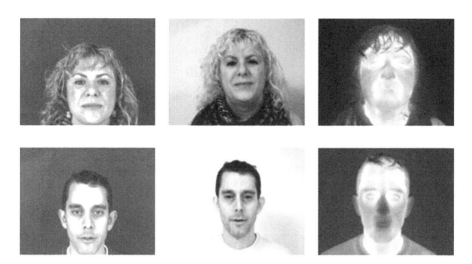

FIGURE 15.4   Samples of the Carl dataset: (a) normal (visible) images, (b) infrared images, and (c) thermal images.

15.3   RESULT AND DISCUSSION

This chapter proposes a mechanism for recognizing thermal images. As previously mentioned, detecting thermal images is impossible for computers and even humans; thus, our major aim is to overcome this challenge [36]. We were also able to considerably bridge the gap between thermal and normal photos, resulting in images that can be comprehended and recognized by both computers and people, as seen in Figure 15.5. Training and testing methods are all detailed in this section. Then it is time to discuss how to assess the quality of the picture that has been created Lastly, the study results of the suggested methodologies are shown and reviewed.

15.3.1   TRAIN AND TEST PHASES

As previously mentioned, the suggested technique for synthetic thermal face images is based on VAE, while the identification method is based on lightweight architecture. Training and testing stages were done separately in two scenarios for image creation and verification systems. Both situations were optimized using an Adam optimizer [37], in which AdaGrad and RMSProp techniques are used in Adam to give an optimization method for noisy problems with sparse gradients with 0.0001 learning rate, accuracy metric, and categorical cross-entropy. In the first scenario, the suggested VAE architecture is used to generate more realistic images by producing noticeable images from images of the thermal face. A VAE is a probabilistic version of an AE that compresses large-scale input data into a smaller demonstration. The method generates a continuous, organized latent space that may be used to generate images. The VAE takes all of the Carl dataset's thermal images, which have been separated for the training stage, as input to generate high-quality visible

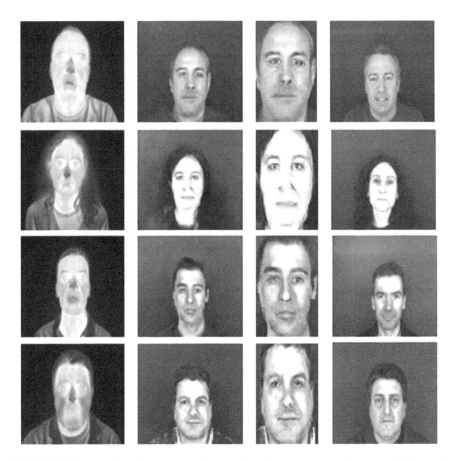

FIGURE 15.5   Samples of synthesized images based on our proposed model. (a) Thermal images as input to the VAE. (b) Synthesized image from thermal images. (c) Cascade object detector on the generated images. (d) Ground truth images.

images. In the second scenario, the proposed identification approach was trained to utilize lightweight architecture. In this work, we employed CNN models such as MobileNet, SqueezeNet, and ShuffleNet. To illustrate our system's performance, we used fivefold cross-validation (CV), which means we trained and tested our system five times with different data at any time, employing 80% for training and 20% for testing. Finally, the average of all fivefold CVs was determined. Table 15.1 summarizes the classification outcomes. Figures 15.6 and 15.7 display outcomes that are compared [13], illustrating original noticeable images and generated images for testing in the proposed model, respectively.

15.3.2   Generated Image Quality

To assess the value of created noticeable images, metrics like SSIM, MSE, FID, and PSNR are displayed (see Table 15.2)

TABLE 15.1

Results Obtained Using Our Proposed Model and Ref. [13]

	Type of Learning	CNN Model	Accuracy	Precision	Recall	F1 Score
[13]	Train = G and test = O	MobileNet	75	N/A	74	N/A
	Train = G and test = O	2-CNN	80	N/A	80	N/A
VAE	Train = G and test = O	MobileNetV2	82.808	82.49333	82.644	82.086
	Train = G and test = O	SqueezeNet	85.394	84.56	85.11	86.33
	Train = G and test = O	ShuffleNet	81.16	82.8	83.2	81.74
VAE + COD	Train = G and test = O	MobileNetV2	85.012	84.95667	85.012	84.398
	Train = G and test = O	**SqueezeNet**	**87.682**	**88.44333**	**87.682**	**87.348**
	Train = G and test = O	ShuffleNet	83.372	84.855	83.172	82.702
VAE	Train = G and test = G	MobileNetV2	93.07	93.11	92.61	92.73
	Train = G and test = G	SqueezeNet	91.45	91.31	90.41	92.65
	Train = G and test = G	ShuffleNet	89.13	89.38	88.25	88.94
VAE + COD	Train = G and test = G	**MobileNetV2**	**94.57**	**95.21**	**95.68**	**94.63**
	Train = G and test = G	SqueezeNet	93.54	93.81	92.48	93.22
	Train = G and test = G	ShuffleNet	90.25	91.11	90.57	90.46

Abbreviations: VAE: variational autoencoder; COD: cascade object detector; O: original normal image; G: generated image.

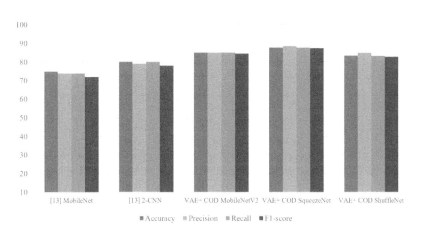

FIGURE 15.6 The obtained results when the original normal images are used for testing.

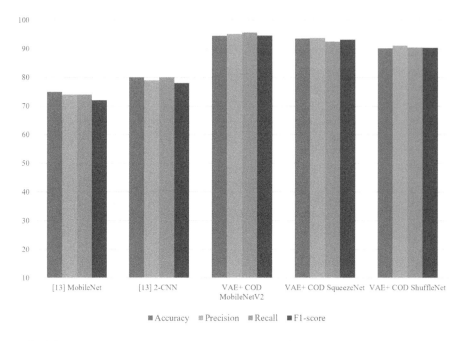

FIGURE 15.7 The obtained results when the generated images are used for testing.

TABLE 15.2
The Value of Synthesized or Created Images for Different Noises

	SSIM	MSE	PSNR	FID
Edge to visible [13]	0.681	0.039	28.453	0.034
Our proposed	0.75	0.032	33.3	0.029

15.4 RESULT

The results of tests to recognize thermal images are reported in this section and are divided into four groups, as shown in Table 15.1. First, three types of classification were conducted on images generated with the VAE but without face extraction. One of the most interesting aspects of this research is that the identification network was trained using images obtained from the VAE, and the network was tested using the visible images in the database. This makes the system's identification performance more realistic. The results for all three categories are better than the 2-CNN proposed in Ref. [13], and the SqueezeNet, with an accuracy of 85%, outperforms the other categories. The faces are taken from the VAE-generated image and passed to lightweight architecture for identification as the second result. The useful features of the face are saved when the face is extracted from the image, which improves the identification system's performance, and background pixels are eliminated from the images, which have the same values in all of the images obtained from the VAE, which reduces the accuracy of the identification system. The presented model has the highest accuracy of 87%, and the results of this stage employed images generated by the VAE for training and visible images from the database for testing.

Data generated by the VAE was utilized for training and testing the network in the third and fourth stages, resulting in the accuracy of the network in the third stage without face extraction and in the fourth stage with face extraction. The network's accuracy is over 93% in both phases. The accuracy of the results acquired in stages one and two compared to stages three and four has a small gap, indicating that the images synthesized are of excellent quality and that effective CNN network models were used. Table 15.2 shows the SSIM, MSE, PSNR, and FID metrics used for gauging the superiority of the produced images much better than those in Ref. [13].

15.5 CONCLUSION

Our proposed model was able to generate thermal face identification by synthesizing visible images with the VAE model, which preserved the original face structure and generated high-quality images from thermal images. To identify the generated images, we used three models based on lightweight architecture, which fundamentally has high accuracy in face detection by reducing parameters and executing at high speed. The suggested model could detect thermal face images when trained and tested with different data, making it applicable to new thermal face images without the need for an extra training step to identify the faces. In the future, GAN models can be introduced to the scheme to reduce the gap between the synthetic and original images and hence improve the image quality.

REFERENCES

1. Tronin, A. A., Hayakawa, M., & Molchanov, O. A. (2002). Thermal IR satellite data application for earthquake research in Japan and China. *Journal of Geodynamics*, 33(4–5), 519–534.
2. Bhowmik, M. K., Saha, K., Majumder, S., Majumder, G., Saha, A., Sarma, A. N., & Nasipuri, M. (2011). Thermal infrared face recognition a biometric identification technique for robust security system. In *Reviews, refinements and new ideas in face recognition* (Vol. 7). London: IntechOpen. https://www.intechopen.com/chapters/17173. doi: 10.5772/18986
3. Ginesu, G., Giusto, D. D., Margner, V., & Meinlschmidt, P. (2004). Detection of foreign bodies in food by thermal image processing. *IEEE Transactions on Industrial Electronics*, 51(2), 480–490.
4. Zhang, L., Xie, X., Feng, S., & Luo, M. (2018). Heuristic dual-tree wavelet thresholding for infrared thermal image denoising of underground visual surveillance system. *Optical Engineering*, 57(8), 083102.
5. Wang, P., & Bai, X. (2018). Regional parallel structure based CNN for thermal infrared face identification. *Integrated Computer-Aided Engineering*, 25(3), 247–260.
6. Bhattacharjee, D., Seal, A., Ganguly, S., Nasipuri, M., & Basu, D. K. (2012). Comparative study of human thermal face recognition based on haar wavelet transform and local binary pattern. *Computational Intelligence and Neuroscience*, 2012(6).

7. Seal, A., Ganguly, S., Bhattacharjee, D., Nasipuri, M., & Basu, D. K. (2013). Thermal human face recognition based on haar wavelet transform and series matching technique. In *Multimedia Processing, Communication and Computing Applications* (pp. 155–167). Springer.

8. Gaber, T., Tharwat, A., Ibrahim, A., Snáel, V., & Hassanien, A. E. (2015). Human thermal face recognition based on random linear oracle (RLO) ensembles. In *INCOS '15: Proceedings of the International Conference on Intelligent Networking and Collaborative Systems (INCOS)* (pp. 91–98). https://doi.org/10.1109/INCoS.2015.67

9. Tharwat, A., Gaber, T., Ibrahim, A., & Hassanien, A. E. (2017). Linear discriminant analysis: A detailed tutorial. *AI Communications (Preprint)*, 1–22.

10. Tharwat, A. (2016). Principal component analysis-a tutorial. *International Journal of Applied Pattern Recognition*, 3(3), 197–240.

11. He, Y., Xiang, S., Kang, C., Wang, J., & Pan, C. (2016). Cross-modal retrieval via deep and bidirectional representation learning. *IEEE Transactions on Multimedia*, 18(7), 1363–1377.

12. Xu, D., Ouyang, W., Ricci, E., Wang, X., & Sebe, N. (2017). Learning cross-modal deep representations for robust pedestrian detection. *arXiv preprint arXiv:1704.02431*.

13. Majidpour, J., Kais Jameel, S., & Anwar Qadir, J. (2021). Face identification system based on synthesizing realistic image using edge-aided GANs. *The Computer Journal*, 144. https://doi.org/10.1093/comjnl/bxab144

14. Iranmanesh, S. M., Dabouei, A., Kazemi, H., & Nasrabadi, N. M. (2018, February). Deep cross polarimetric thermal-to-visible face recognition. In *2018 International Conference on Biometrics (ICB)* (pp. 166–173). IEEE.

15. Mahouachi, D., & Akhloufi, M. A. (2021, April). Adaptive deep convolutional neural network for thermal face recognition. In *Proceedings of SPIE 11743, Thermosense: Thermal Infrared Applications XLIII, 1174304* (Vol. 11743). International Society for Optics and Photonics. https://doi.org/10.1117/12.2586974

16. Ghojogh, B., Ghodsi, A., Karray, F., & Crowley, M. (2021). Factor analysis, probabilistic principal component analysis, variational inference, and variational autoencoder: Tutorial and survey. *arXiv preprint arXiv:2101.00734*.

17. Viola, P., & Jones, M. J. (2004). Robust real-time face detection. *International Journal of Computer Vision*, 57(2), 137–154.

18. Howard, A. G., Zhu, M., Chen, B., Kalenichenko, D., Wang, W., Weyand, T., Andreetto, M., & Adam, H. (2017). Mobilenets: Efficient convolutional neural networks for mobile vision applications. *arXiv preprint arXiv:1704.04861*.

19. Othman, Soufiene Ben, Bahattab, Abdullah Ali, Trad, Abdelbasset, & Youssef, Habib. (2020, June). LSDA: Lightweight secure data aggregation scheme in healthcare using IoT. In *ACM — 10th International Conference on Information Systems and Technologies*, Lecce, Italy.

20. Ranjan, R., Sankaranarayanan, S., Castillo, C. D., & Chellappa, R. (2017, May). An all-in-one convolutional neural network for face analysis. In *2017 12th IEEE International Conference on Automatic Face & Gesture Recognition (FG 2017)* (pp. 17–24). IEEE.

21. El-Saadawy, H., Tantawi, M., Shedeed, H. A., & Tolba, M. F. (2020, April). A two-stage method for bone X-rays abnormality detection using MobileNet network. In *The International Conference on Artificial Intelligence and Computer Vision* (pp. 372–380). Cham: Springer.

22. Othman, Soufiene Ben, Bahattab, Abdullah Ali, Trad, Abdelbasset, & Youssef, Habib. (2020). PEERP: A priority-based energy-efficient routing protocol for reliable data transmission in healthcare using the IoT. In *The 15th International Conference on Future Networks and Communications (FNC) August 9–12, 2020*. Leuven, Belgium.

23. Othman, Soufiene Ben, Bahattab, Abdullah Ali, Trad, Abdelbasset, & Youssef, Habib. (2019). RESDA: Robust and efficient secure data aggregation scheme in healthcare using the IoT. In *The International Conference on Internet of Things, Embedded Systems and Communications (IINTEC 2019)*, HAMMAMET, Tunisia from 20–22 December 2019.

24. Howard, A., Zhmoginov, A., Chen, L. C., Sandler, M., & Zhu, M. (2018). Inverted residuals and linear bottlenecks: Mobile networks for classification, detection and segmentation. *arXiv:1801.04381v2*.

25. Zhang, X., Zhou, X., Lin, M., & Sun, J. (2018). ShuffleNet: An extremely efficient convolutional neural network for mobile devices. In *2018 IEEE/CVF Conference on Computer Vision and Pattern Recognition* (pp. 6848–6856). https://doi.org/10.1109/CVPR.2018.00716

26. Iandola, F. N., Han, S., Moskewicz, M. W., Ashraf, K., Dally, W. J., & Keutzer, K. (2016). SqueezeNet: AlexNet-level accuracy with 50x fewer parameters and< 0.5 MB model size. *arXiv preprint arXiv:1602.07360*.

27. Wang, Z., Bovik, A. C., Sheikh, H. R., & Simoncelli, E. P. (2004). Image quality assessment: From error visibility to structural similarity. *IEEE Transactions on Image Processing*, 13(4), 600–612.

28. Lehmann, E. L., & Casella, G. (2006). *Theory of Point Estimation*. Springer Science & Business Media. ISBN 0-387-98502-6.

29. Hore, A., & Ziou, D. (2010, August). Image quality metrics: PSNR vs. SSIM. In *2010 20th International Conference on Pattern Recognition* (pp. 2366–2369). IEEE.

30. Heusel, M., Ramsauer, H., Unterthiner, T., Nessler, B., & Hochreiter, S. (2017). GANs trained by a two time-scale update rule converge to a local Nash equilibrium. *Advances in Neural Information Processing Systems*, 30.

31. Cadik, M., & Slavik, P. (2004, July). Evaluation of two principal approaches to objective image quality assessment. In *Proceedings. Eighth International Conference on Information Visualisation*, IV (pp. 513–518). IEEE.

32. Nguyen, T. B., & Ziou, D. (2000). Contextual and non-contextual performance evaluation of edge detectors. *Pattern Recognition Letters*, 21(9), 805–816.

33. Elbadawy, O., El-Sakka, M. R., & Kamel, M. S. (1998, May). An information theoretic image-quality measure. In *Conference Proceedings. IEEE Canadian Conference on Electrical and Computer Engineering* (Cat. No. 98TH8341) (Vol. 1, pp. 169–172). IEEE.

34. Espinosa-Duro, V., Faundez-Zanuy, M., & Mekyska, J. (2013). A new face database simultaneously acquired in visible, nearinfrared and thermal spectrums. *Cognitive Computation*, 5(1), 119–135.

35. Sarfraz, M. S., & Stiefelhagen, R. (2017). Deep perceptual mapping for cross-modal face recognition. *International Journal of Computer Vision*, 122(3), 426–438.

36. Dosselmann, R., & Yang, X. D. (2005, May). Existing and emerging image quality metrics. In *Canadian Conference on Electrical and Computer Engineering, 2005* (pp. 1906–1913). IEEE.

37. Kingma, D. P., & Ba, J. (2014). Adam: A method for stochastic optimization. *arXiv preprint arXiv:1412.6980*.

16 IoT-Based Label Distribution Learning Mechanism for Autism Spectrum Disorder for Healthcare Application

Anurag Shrivastava, Namita Rajput,
P. Rajesh, and S.R. Swarnalatha

CONTENTS

16.1 INTRODUCTION

Recent studies have shown that autism spectrum disorders are related to abnormal brain function in patients [1–6], and resting-state functional MRI, which reflects functional changes such as brain metabolic activity in patients under resting state by using blood oxygen–dependent levels Resonance imaging has become a powerful tool to quantify brain neural activity and has gradually become one of the essential means for the study of brain diseases such as autism spectrum disorder

DOI: 10.1201/9781003315476-16

(ASD) [7–9]. Based on this diagnosis, researchers have proposed a variety of computer-aided autism diagnosis algorithms [10–15]. For example, in Ref. [14], the author proposed multivariate graph learning for additional diagnosis of autism, and also explored the relationship between brain regions through deep understanding correlation for IoT-based auxiliary diagnosis of autism [15] and so on. However, these methods can only deal with dichotomous problems. In the clinic, autism spectrum disorder includes several disorders related to developmental disorders, such as autism, Asperger's syndrome (Asperger's disease), nonspecific general developmental disorder [4, 16], and so on. Most of the existing IoT-based auxiliary diagnosis models for autism can only solve the problem of binary classification and cannot distinguish several related diseases of ASD at the same time. Furthermore, these methods also do not deal with label noise in a targeted manner. Labeling noise is a challenge in the IoT-based auxiliary diagnosis of multiclass ASD and has serious adverse effects on classifier performance [17]. Label noise refers to the deviation between the target label of the training sample and the actual label of the corresponding instance. There are many factors in the generation of labeling noise, such as the subjectivity of the labeling process, the low recognizability of the samples to be labeled, and communication/coding problems. Labeling noise is prevalent in autism diagnosis scenarios. Subjectivity in the diagnostic process, inconsistent diagnostic criteria, and blurring of the boundaries of ASD subcategories contribute to labeling noise. The class imbalance problem under high-dimensional features is another challenge in the IoT-based auxiliary diagnosis of multi-class ASD. The neuroimaging data usually used for additional diagnosis of ASD often have hundreds or thousands of parts. The number of training samples is minimal, which quickly leads to overfitting problems during classifier training. Moreover, the models used to construct the ASD classifier have the problem of class imbalance, which causes the classification prediction results to be biased toward the majority class [18]. Aiming at the above issues, this chapter proposes a cost-sensitive label distribution support vector regression learning for the IoT-based auxiliary diagnosis of ASD. First, multiclass ASD diagnosis is faced with the problem of label noise. The unique label form of label distribution can better overcome the influence of label noise on the classifier through the description of the same sample by different labels to accurately express the difference between labels degree of correlation between. This makes the learning process contain richer semantic information, can better distinguish the relative importance differences of multiple markers, and has better pertinence to the problem of marker noise in the IoT-based auxiliary diagnosis of ASD [19–20]. At the same time, the support vector regression introduces the kernel method. Through the nonlinear mapping of the kernel method, the linearly inseparable data in the original input space can be mapped into a linearly separable feature space, providing more discriminative information. Finally, to overcome the problem of category imbalance, a cost-sensitive mechanism is introduced. By introducing the imbalance of misjudgment costs of different categories, in reality, the algorithm can adapt to the needs of practical applications to a certain extent and treat a small number of people fairly class and majority class.

16.2   DEEP LABEL DISTRIBUTION LEARNING

LDL (labeled distribution learning) is a machine learning technique that has gained popularity in recent years. It explains how to use single-label and multi-label learning to distribute labels. If a sample is linked to many markers in a multi-marker situation, the significance of these markers to the model will often vary. The marker distribution is a kind of marker that represents the relevance of other variables in a model. Label distribution learning is a machine learning approach that uses label distribution as a learning objective and has a wide range of applications. Author proposed a deep label distribution learning algorithm combining convolutional neural networks and label distribution learning to estimate age through faces [19]. To automatically identify the user's emotional state from text, the author proposed a multivariate label distribution learning algorithm to achieve head pose detection (see Figure 16.1). However, it has yet to be documented for IoT-based auxiliary brain illness diagnosis.

Label distribution learning requires that the training data contain label distribution information. However, people often label samples in single-label or multi-label in real life, making it challenging to obtain label distribution information directly. Nonetheless, the labels of these data still contain relevant information about the distribution of the brands. Marker enhancement enhances the supervised information of samples through the implicit correlation between different sample markers, thereby achieving better results in marker distribution learning. For example, author proposed tag augmentation as an auxiliary algorithm for tag distribution learning, which is used to mine the implied tag importance information in the training set, promote the original logical tag to tag distribution, and assist tag distribution learning. Furthermore, the author proposed label-enhanced multi-label learning to reconstruct latent label importance information from rational brands to improve the performance of label distribution learning.

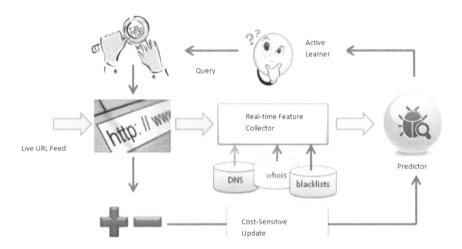

FIGURE 16.1   Support vector regression–based label distribution.

16.3   AUTISM SPECTRUM DISORDER

16.3.1   LABEL DISTRIBUTION LEARNING ALGORITHM SYMBOLS

The main symbols in this chapter are expressed as follows: use $x_i \in S^q$ to represent the ith sample, where q represents the dimension of the feature vector, $X = [x_1, x_2, \ldots, x_N] \in S^{q \times N}$; $m_i = [m_i^1, m_i^2, \ldots, m_i^k]^U$ represents the logical token corresponding to x_i, K represents the number of possible tokens, and $m_i^j \in \{0,1\}$. Similarly, $d_i = [d_i^1, d_i^2, \ldots, d_i^k]^U \in S^K$ represents the label distribution of the ith sample, where $d_i^j \in [0, 1]$ represents the jth value of the label distribution of the ith sample, satisfying $\sum_{j=1}^{k} d_i^j = 1$, $E = [e_1, e_2, \ldots, e_N] \in S^{K \times N}$.

16.3.2   LABEL DISTRIBUTION LEARNING ALGORITHM

The label distribution learning algorithm for multi-category autism IoT-based auxiliary diagnosis proposed in this chapter is shown in Figure 16.1. First, the rs-fMRI images are preprocessed, the functional connectivity matrix is constructed on this basis, and each sample's available connectivity feature vector is obtained based on the available connectivity matrix. At the same time, combining the logical marker data and useful connectivity features for marker enhancement, the marker distribution form of the sample is obtained. Finally, a cost-sensitive label distribution learning model is performed to obtain a multi-classification model for the IoT-based auxiliary diagnosis of autism.

16.3.3   LABEL DISTRIBUTION LEARNING DESCRIPTION

Label distribution learning describes the degree of correlation between each label and sample by introducing descriptive degree so that it can obtain richer semantic information from the data than multi-label, and more accurately express the relative importance difference of multiple labels of the same sample. However, the essential requirement of labeled distribution learning is to have labeled distributed datasets, which is often challenging to meet in reality. The marker distribution data can be obtained by transforming a given multi-marker form sample by a marker enhancement method. The label enhancement method is adopted based on FCM (fuzzy C-means) and vague operation. The basic idea is as follows:

- Use FCM to divide N samples into p fuzzy clusters, and find the center of each group, so that the sum of the weighted distances from all training samples to the cluster center is the smallest. Equation (16.1) lists the specific weighted distance formula:

$$m_{x_i}^k = \cfrac{1}{\sum_{j=1}^{P} \left(\cfrac{Dist\left(y_i, \mu_k\right)}{Dist\left(y_i, \mu_j\right)} \right)^{\frac{1}{\beta-1}}} \qquad (16.1)$$

Among them, $m_{x_i}^k$ represents the membership degree of the ith sample to the kth cluster center, μ_k represents the kth cluster center, β is a fuzzy factor greater than 1, *Dist*

(∗,∗) represents the distance measure. Each sample's membership degree represents the strength of the association between the model and the cluster. The clustering results of traditional FCM are greatly affected by the initial value. Therefore, they cannot ensure convergence to the optimal global solution, but in label enhancement, the clustering results of FCM are only used as a transitional bridge. Although the clustering results fluctuate, it has little effect on the results of marker enhancement. The difference between Chebyshev distance and KL divergence (Kullback–Leibler divergence) of the results of multiple marker enhancements is below 10–6.

- Construct an association matrix A between markers and clusters. The elements in the matrix represent the degree of association between traits and sets. The calculation method of the association matrix is as shown in formula (16.2):

$$B_j = B_j + n_{x_i}^k, \; if m_i^j = 1 \tag{16.2}$$

In the formula, B_j is the jth row of the matrix, and Aj is the sum of the membership degree vectors of the samples of the jth class. After the rows are normalized, the association matrix B can be regarded as a fuzzy relationship matrix of clustering and labeling.

- According to the fuzzy logic reasoning mechanism, the vague synthesis operation is performed on the association matrix and the membership degree, and the membership degree of the sample to the label is obtained. Then, after normalization, it is the label distribution.

The marker enhancement based on FCM and fuzzy operation introduces cluster analysis as a bridge. Through the compound operation between the membership degree of the sample to the cluster and the membership degree of the group to the marker, the membership degree of the model to the title is obtained, that is, the designation distributed. In this process, the topological relationship of the sample space is mined through fuzzy clustering. This relationship is projected to the label space through the association matrix. The simple logical labeling generates richer semantic information and transforms it into label distribution.

16.3.4 ANALYSIS OF ASD DATA

The following two key issues need to be considered in modeling labeled distribution learning for ASD-aided diagnosis: first, the various distributions of ASD data samples are unbalanced. Studies have shown that class imbalance can adversely affect training. It involves the convergence in the training phase and the model's generalization ability on the test set. Therefore, this chapter introduces a cost-sensitive mechanism based on the labeled distribution support vector regression to balance the influence of the majority class and the minority class on the objective function. Second, ASD datasets are mostly multi-category data, and the data guiding label distribution learning training should be label distribution data. To this end, label augmentation is introduced to transform the label of each training sample into a label distribution. The process of marking enhancement has been briefly described in Section 2.3.

Assume that the label distribution d corresponding to the sample x can be linearly represented by the projection of the sample on the feature space:

$$e = f(x) = \frac{1}{1 + \exp(-x)} \tag{16.3}$$

Among them, $z = Z\phi(x) + c$ is the dividing hyperplane of the feature space, $\phi(x)$ is the nonlinear projection of x in the feature space S^H, and $Z \in S^{K \times H}$ and $c \in S^K$ are model parameters. Activate z using the sigmoid function to obtain the predicted marker distribution $e^\wedge$. But using the Euclidean distance of e and $e^\wedge$ as the loss function is not convex, and it is not easy to find the optimal value. To this end, it is transformed, using the Euclidean distance of x and $x^\wedge$ corresponding to x and $e^\wedge$ as the loss function ($e = f(x)$), and introducing a cost-sensitive mechanism to balance the majority class and minority class on the objective function impact. The objective function of cost-sensitive label distribution support vector regression (CSLDSVR) is defined as follows:

$$U(Z,c) = \frac{1}{2} \sum_{j=1}^{k} \| z^j \|^2 + D \sum_{j=1}^{k} \frac{M(u_i)}{O_j} \tag{16.4}$$

$$M(u_i) = \begin{cases} 0, u_i < \varepsilon \\ (u_i - \varepsilon)^2, u_{i \geq \varepsilon} \end{cases} \tag{16.5}$$

$$u_i = \| e_i \| = \sqrt{e_i^T e_i} \tag{16.6}$$

$$e_i = z_i - z_i^\wedge = -I\left(\frac{1}{d_i} - 1\right) - \left(Z\phi(y_i) + c\right) \tag{16.7}$$

Among them, z^j is the transpose of the jth row of W, $L(ui)$ is the loss function value of the ith sample, D is the weight coefficient, and O_j is the number of instances of the jth class. From this, the result is determined by the ε insensitive region, that is, the part where the loss is less than ε can be ignored. Using the loss function with a sensitive area setting makes the loss function have a certain scarcity, which improves the computational efficiency of the algorithm and can better overcome the noise of the data and improve the robustness of the algorithm. However, when the threshold is set to a significant value, it is easy to cause the loss of useful information, resulting in the degradation of the algorithm performance. The introduction of $\frac{1}{O_i}$ is to balance the influence of the majority class samples on the value of the objective function so that the weight of the misjudgment cost of the minority class is greater than that of the majority class, thus balancing the algorithm's tendency to different types. Theorem 1 $M(u_i)$ is a convex function concerning z^j c^j. Prove that formula (16.5) is a convex function, that is, prove that the second derivative of $M(u_i)$ concerning z^j, c^j is always greater than or equal to 0:

$$\frac{\partial^2 M(u_i)}{\partial(z^j)^2} = 2\varphi^U(y_i)\varphi(y_i)\sqrt{G(z^j,\varphi(y_i))} \tag{16.8}$$

Here $G(z^j,\varphi(y_i))$ is a function of $z^j,\varphi(y_i)$. Formula (16.8) is always greater than or equal to 0. Similarly, it can be proved that $M(u_i)$ is nonnegative concerning c^j, and the theorem is proved. This chapter uses the iterative quasi-Newton method to optimize Equation (16.4). First, the second part of Equation (16.4) is expanded by the Taylor series, and its linear part is taken as the approximate value. In the pth iteration, the approximate value is as follows:

$$U(Z',c') \approx \frac{1}{2}\sum_{j=1}^{k}\|z^j\|^2 + D\sum_{j=1}^{K}\frac{1}{O}\sum_{i=1}^{O_i}\left[M(u_i') + \frac{dU(u_i)}{du_i}\bigg|\frac{(f_i')^U}{u_i'}(e_i - e_i')\right] \tag{16.9}$$

Among them, Z' and c' are the values corresponding to the pth iteration. Substitute Z' and c' into Equation (16.6) and Equation (16.7) and obtain u_i' and u_i' through calculation. Equation (16.9) can be a quadratic approximation:

$$\begin{aligned}U(Z',c') &\approx \frac{1}{2}\sum_{j=1}^{k}\|z^j\|^2 + D\sum_{j=1}^{K}\frac{1}{O}\sum_{i=1}^{O_i}\left[M(u_i') + \frac{dU(u_i)}{du_i}\bigg|\frac{(u_i)^2 - (u_i')^2}{u_i'}\right]\\ &= \frac{1}{2}\sum_{j=1}^{k}\|z^j\|^2 + 2\sum_{j=1}^{K}\frac{1}{O}\sum_{i=1}^{O_i}a_iu_i^2 + \gamma\end{aligned} \tag{16.10}$$

Here τ is a constant independent of Z, c. Formula (16.10) calculates the partial derivative of Z_j and c_j, respectively, and sets the value of the partial product to 0; the formula can be obtained as follows:

$$\left[\frac{1}{2}\Phi E_a T\Phi + \frac{1}{4}J\Phi^U Tb\right]\begin{bmatrix}Z^U\\c^T\end{bmatrix} = \begin{bmatrix}-\Phi^U E_a.In\left(\frac{1}{E^U} - 1\right)\\-b^U T.In\left(\frac{1}{E^U} - 1\right)\end{bmatrix} \tag{16.11}$$

Among them, $\Phi = [\phi(x_1), \phi(x_2), \ldots, \phi(x_N)]^U$, I is the identity matrix, 1 is the all-one column vector, $b = [b_1, b_2, \ldots, a_N]^U$, $E_a = \text{diag}(b_1, b_2, \ldots, b_N)$, $T = \text{diag}(t_1, t_2, \ldots, t_N)$, t_i represents the cost weight of the ith sample, which is set to $\frac{1}{M_k}$ in this chapter, and M_k included in the class to which t_i belongs is the number of samples. According to the literature, Z_j can be obtained by the linear combination of training samples in the projection space of the samples, namely $w^j = \Phi^U \beta^j$, $Z^T = \Phi^T C^T$, $C^T = [\beta^1, \beta^2, \ldots, \beta^K]$, substituting into formula (16.11):

$$\begin{bmatrix}\frac{1}{2}TK + \frac{1}{4}E_a^{-1} & E_a^{-1}Tb\\ b^T Tk & 1^T Ta\end{bmatrix}\begin{bmatrix}C^T\\c^T\end{bmatrix} = \begin{bmatrix}-T.In\left(\frac{1}{E^U} - 1\right)\\-b^T T.In\left(\frac{1}{E^U} - 1\right)\end{bmatrix} \tag{16.12}$$

Among them, $L_{ij} = l(x_i, x_j) = \phi^T(x_i)\phi(x_j)$, L_{ij} is the element value of the ith row and jth column of the matrix L, and $l(x_i, x_j)$ is the kernel function. So far, by substituting C^T and c^T into Equation (16.3), the prediction function can be updated as follows:

$$e_i = \frac{1}{1 + \exp\left(-(C\Phi\varphi(y_i) + c\right)} \qquad (16.13)$$

The corresponding label distribution can be calculated from the input feature space of the sample. The result of the label distribution is the importance of ASD and its subclasses for the same model, and the maximum possible label is taken as the result:

$$m_i^j = \begin{cases} 0, e_i^j < \max\left(e_i^{\ j}\right)\left(i = 1, 2, \ldots, N; j = 1, 2, \ldots, K\right)) \\ 1, e_i^j = \max\left(e_i^{\wedge j}\right) \end{cases} \qquad (16.14)$$

Among them, e_i^j and m_i^j are the predicted values corresponding to e_i^j and m_i^j $\max(e_i^j)$ is the maximum value in the vector. A classifier from the original input feature space to the multi-classification results is obtained from this. The algorithm is described as follows.

16.4 LABEL DISTRIBUTIONS

16.4.1 METRIC OF THE LABEL DISTRIBUTION

This chapter uses the evaluation metric of the label distribution and the evaluation metric of the multi-classification task for algorithm evaluation. All evaluation indicators and calculation formulas are shown in Table 16.1. The first six are evaluation indicators for label distribution learning, and the last two are evaluation indicators for multi-classification tasks. "↑" after the index, the name means that the larger the value, the better the algorithm effect; with "↓", the smaller the value, the better the algorithm effect.

16.4.2 ANALYSIS OF DATASET

All rs-fMRI datasets used in this chapter are from ABIDE web platform. Table 16.2 shows the composition of various samples in each dataset. Taking the NYU

TABLE 16.1
Statistics of Datasets

Dataset	No. of Samples	Normal	Autism	Asperger's Syndrome
NYU	177	103	53	21
UM	144	76	57	11
KKI	48	31	8	9
Leuven	102	62	21	19
UCLA	81	53	16	12

TABLE 16.2
Range of Parameters

Parameter Name	Parameter Range
Weight factor	0.001, 0.01, 0.1, 1, 10, 100,1 000
Type of kernel function	Linear kernel, polynomial kernel, Gaussian kernel
Insensitive area size	0.000 1, 0.001, 0.01, 0.1
The kernel bandwidth of the Gaussian kernel	0.01,0.1,1,10,100

(New York University) dataset as an example, the data collection institution of the NYU dataset is New York University. The subjects remained in a still state during the collection process and did not perform any actions. The specific parameters are shown in Table 16.1.

In Table 16.1, UM stands for University of Michigan, KKI stands for Kennedy Krieger Institute, Leuven stands for KU Leuven, and UCLA stands for University of California, Los Angeles.

Although brain regions are spatially isolated, neural activity influences each other. Therefore, this chapter uses the brain functional connectivity matrix between brain regions as a classification feature. The calculation steps of the available connectivity matrix [13] (i.e., the preprocessing step) are as follows:

- The DPARSF tool to extract the average time series signals of each brain region and calculate the Pearson coefficient between brain regions and obtain the functional connectivity matrix.
- Take each row of the functional connectivity matrix as the feature description of each brain region, take the upper triangular matrix of the available connectivity matrix, and connect the rows in series to obtain the corresponding eigenvectors.

16.4.3 TWO MULTI-CLASSIFICATION ALGORITHMS

The proposed CSLDSVR method is compared with six existing LDL algorithms and two multi-classification algorithms. Two multi-classification algorithms are decision tree and K-nearest neighbor (KNN), both of which are classic multi-classification algorithms. The six existing LDL algorithms are PT-SVM, PT-BAYES, AA-KNN, AA-BP (backpropagation), SA-IIS (improved iterative scaling), and LDSVR, where "PT" means problem transformation (problem transformation), "AA" stands for algorithm adaptation, and "SA" stands for specialized algorithm. The CSLDSVR algorithm proposed in this chapter has four parameters, namely, the weight coefficient C, the type of the kernel function, the size of the insensitive region ε, and the kernel bandwidth of the Gaussian kernel. The specific range of parameters is shown in Table 16.2. Results were calculated using tenfold cross-validation. The particular operation steps are as follows: randomly divide the dataset into ten equal parts, in each fold cross-validation; take 1 part as the test set, and the remaining nine parts as the training set. Repeat this process ten times, and take the average of the ten results as the evaluation index.

16.4.4 Distribution Learning Algorithms

Table 16.3 summarizes the experimental results of six labeled distribution learning algorithms and CSLDSVR on five different datasets, and the experimental results are recorded in the form of mean ± standard deviation. Among them, the bold is the best value of each indicator in different methods on the current dataset. Compared to

TABLE 16.3

Performance Comparison of CSLDSVR and LDL Algorithms

Evaluation Metrics	Algorithm	NYU	UM	Leuven	UCLA	KKI
Chebyshev↓	AA-BP	0.2237 ± 0.035	0.2184 ± 0.045	0.2480 ± 0.044	0.2506 ± 0.053	0.2547 ± 0.052
	AA-KNN	0.1441 ± 0.011	0.1540 ± 0.021	0.1579 ± 0.026	0.1426 ± 0.031	0.1572 ± 0.029
	LDSVR	0.1501 ± 0.024	0.1400 ± 0.012	0.1629 ± 0.034	0.1694 ± 0.053	0.1602 ± 0.057
	SA-IIS	0.1478 ± 0.011	0.1535 ± 0.023	0.1748 ± 0.021	0.1458 ± 0.032	0.1627 ± 0.049
	PT-BAYES	0.3818 ± 0.111	0.2057 ± 0.009	0.2069 ± 0.007	0.2135 ± 0.009	0.2154 ± 0.008
	PT-SVM	0.2005 ± 0.041	0.1885 ± 0.042	0.1831 ± 0.040	0.1958 ± 0.033	0.1822 ± 0.058
	CSLDSVR	0.1413 ± 0.016	0.1352 ± 0.023	0.1402 ± 0.024	0.1386 ± 0.038	0.1267 ± 0.034
Cosine↑	AA-BP	0.8731 ± 0.034	0.8818 ± 0.035	0.8622 ± 0.049	0.8399 ± 0.057	0.8437 ± 0.058
	AA-KNN	0.9354 ± 0.009	0.9286 ± 0.017	0.9274 ± 0.020	0.9297 ± 0.022	0.9130 ± 0.024
	LDSVR	0.9377 ± 0.019	0.9448 ± 0.013	0.9325 ± 0.029	0.9285 ± 0.052	0.9326 ± 0.047
	SA-IIS	0.9407 ± 0.009	0.9344 ± 0.016	0.9205 ± 0.016	0.9395 ± 0.020	0.9246 ± 0.042
	PT-Bayes	0.7985 ± 0.071	0.9156 ± 0.006	0.9151 ± 0.005	0.9104 ± 0.006	0.9092 ± 0.005
	PT-SVM	0.8987 ± 0.038	0.9043 ± 0.042	0.9145 ± 0.030	0.8974 ± 0.036	0.9068 ± 0.045
	CSLDSVR	0.9405 ± 0.012	0.9473 ± 0.018	0.9234 ± 0.025	0.9428 ± 0.036	0.9363 ± 0.029
Clark↓	AA-BP	0.4681 ± 0.064	0.4613 ± 0.099	0.5170 ± 0.083	0.5371 ± 0.110	0.5427 ± 0.104
	AA-KNN	0.2631 ± 0.020	0.2822 ± 0.036	0.2873 ± 0.047	0.2613 ± 0.053	0.2832 ± 0.053
	LDSVR	0.2729 ± 0.036	0.2557 ± 0.021	0.2872 ± 0.062	0.2956 ± 0.092	0.2819 ± 0.100
	SA-IIS	0.2663 ± 0.019	0.2788 ± 0.039	0.3113 ± 0.033	0.2623 ± 0.055	0.2939 ± 0.088

Evaluation Metrics	Algorithm	NYU	UM	Leuven	UCLA	KKI
	PT-BAYES	0.8936 ± 0.359	0.3520 ± 0.014	0.3523 ± 0.012	0.3636 ± 0.016	0.3663 ± 0.013
	PT-SVM	0.3580 ± 0.070	0.3481 ± 0.075	0.3253 ± 0.065	0.3505 ± 0.056	0.3287 ± 0.098
	CSLDSVR	0.2616 ± 0.032	0.2463 ± 0.037	0.2539 ± 0.041	0.2484 ± 0.062	0.2334 ± 0.061
Canberra↓	AA-BP	0.7176 ± 0.102	0.7104 ± 0.152	0.8108 ± 0.125	0.8118 ± 0.169	0.8319 ± 0.160
	AA-KNN	0.4066 ± 0.029	0.4296 ± 0.057	0.4475 ± 0.070	0.3984 ± 0.084	0.4380 ± 0.083
	LDSVR	0.4321 ± 0.064	0.3998 ± 0.039	0.4699 ± 0.097	0.4935 ± 0.129	0.4640 ± 0.159
	SA-IIS	0.4268 ± 0.034	0.4384 ± 0.067	0.5022 ± 0.060	0.4224 ± 0.093	0.4696 ± 0.127
	PT-BAYES	1.4721 ± 0.574	0.6022 ± 0.026	0.6048 ± 0.022	0.6245 ± 0.029	0.6299 ± 0.023
	PT-SVM	0.5736 ± 0.106	0.5411 ± 0.127	0.5227 ± 0.111	0.5510 ± 0.087	0.5115 ± 0.165
	CSLDSVR	0.3863 ± 0.047	0.3875 ± 0.061	0.3938 ± 0.069	0.4023 ± 0.109	0.3544 ± 0.093
Intersection↑	AA-BP	0.7763 ± 0.035	0.7816 ± 0.045	0.7520 ± 0.044	0.7494 ± 0.053	0.7453 ± 0.052
	AA-KNN	0.8559 ± 0.011	0.8460 ± 0.021	0.8421 ± 0.026	0.8574 ± 0.031	0.8428 ± 0.029
	LDSVR	0.8499 ± 0.024	0.8600 ± 0.012	0.8371 ± 0.034	0.8306 ± 0.053	0.8398 ± 0.057
	SA-IIS	0.8522 ± 0.011	0.8465 ± 0.023	0.8252 ± 0.021	0.8542 ± 0.032	0.8373 ± 0.049
	PT-BAYES	0.6182 ± 0.111	0.7943 ± 0.009	0.7931 ± 0.007	0.7865 ± 0.009	0.7846 ± 0.008
	PT-SVM	0.7995 ± 0.041	0.8115 ± 0.042	0.8169 ± 0.040	0.8042 ± 0.033	0.8178 ± 0.058
	CSLDSVR	0.8587 ± 0.041	0.8648 ± 0.023	0.8598 ± 0.024	0.8614 ± 0.038	0.8733 ± 0.034
KL↑	AA-BP	0.1667 ± 0.042	0.1612 ± 0.051	0.1920 ± 0.069	0.2222 ± 0.089	0.2279 ± 0.076
	AA-KNN	0.0685 ± 0.010	0.0760 ± 0.018	0.0766 ± 0.022	0.0746 ± 0.023	0.0932 ± 0.026
	LDSVR	0.0665 ± 0.019	0.0593 ± 0.014	0.0703 ± 0.032	0.0749 ± 0.062	0.0711 ± 0.049
	SA-IIS	0.0639 ± 0.009	0.0698 ± 0.017	0.0837 ± 0.016	0.0639 ± 0.021	0.0800 ± 0.044
	PT-BAYES	0.4929 ± 0.251	0.0879 ± 0.006	0.0880 ± 0.006	0.0935 ± 0.008	0.0948 ± 0.006
	PT-SVM	0.1081 ± 0.041	0.1055 ± 0.047	0.0906 ± 0.032	0.1104 ± 0.040	0.1003 ± 0.048

the label distribution learning algorithm, CSLDSVR shows excellent results in most cases, and it is more evident on the UM, UCLA, KKI datasets. Among the indicators of labeled distribution, KL divergence is an indicator describing the difference between the two distributions, and the LDL algorithm used as a comparison uses KL divergence as the objective function. The KL divergence of the prediction result of CSLDSVR can be minimized. It shows that the label distribution predicted by the new algorithm is the closest to the actual data distribution on the whole, which is better than the comparison algorithm. Figure 16.2 with Table 16.2 summarizes the results of CSLDSVR and the marker distribution algorithm multiclass metrics precision and mAP. On the two most critical multiclass metrics, CSLDSVR performs better. Some algorithms have a high accuracy rate but a low macro-average because these algorithms do not consider the class imbalance problem. The model classification is biased toward the majority class. CSLDSVR uses the kernel trick to solve the problem in a more discriminative feature space, and CSLDSVR considers the size of each type, which effectively solves the pain caused by class imbalance. To verify the performance improvement of the cost-sensitive mechanism, the algorithm in this chapter is compared with the LDSVR without the cost-sensitive mechanism. As shown in Table 16.4, in most cases, the learning effect of the algorithm CSLDSVR in

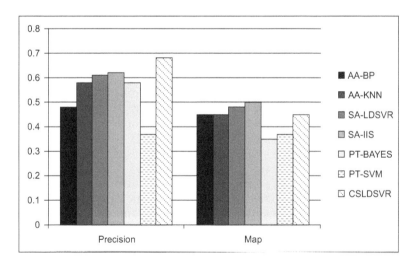

FIGURE 16.2   Evaluation with label distribution algorithms.

TABLE 16.4
Evaluation with Label Distribution Algorithms

Serial	AA-BP	AA-KNN	SA-LDSVR	SA-IIS	PT-BAYES	PT-SVM	CSLDSVR
Precision	0.48	0.58	0.61	0.62	0.58	0.37	0.68
Map	0.45	0.45	0.48	0.5	0.35	0.37	0.45
Precision	0.48	0.58	0.61	0.62	0.58	0.37	0.68
Map	0.45	0.45	0.48	0.5	0.35	0.37	0.45

this chapter is better; in addition, the standard deviation of the results is maintained at a low level. That is, the stability of the algorithm is improved. However, LDSVR does not introduce a cost-sensitive mechanism, and the standard deviation of the results obtained by the algorithm is significant and fluctuating. For example, the standard deviation of the Canberra indicators in UCLA and KKI exceeds 0.1.

16.4.5 Two Classical Multi-classification Algorithms

Table 16.5 and Figure 16.2 show the comparison results of five datasets of the precision and mAP metrics of CSLDSVR and two classical multi-classification algorithms, decision tree, and KNN. The bold is the best value of the corresponding indicator in different methods on the current dataset. Observing the experimental results of the KNN method, it can be found that the mAP of the KNN method appears 0.3333 many times. This is because KNN is too biased toward the majority class, and there is an extreme case of classifying all samples into the majority class. In the case of high-dimensional imbalance of autism neuroimaging data, traditional multi-classification algorithms are prone to fall into the dimensional trap or bias toward the majority class.

The algorithm CSLDSVR in this chapter solves the above problems using kernel techniques and cost-sensitive mechanisms and achieves better results: good classification model. The cost-sensitive mechanism reduces the overall misclassification cost by increasing the misclassification cost of the minority class, reducing the misclassification cost of the majority class, and making the model avoid leaning toward the majority class. In other words, the cost-sensitive mechanism is based on the original standard cost loss function, adding some constraints and weight constraints so that the final model is biased toward another minority class that is more concerned with practical applications. This chapter achieves the purpose of different

TABLE 16.5
Performance Evaluation of Proposed Work for Multi-classification Algorithms

	Decision Tree		KNN		CSLDSVR	
Dataset	Precision	mAP	Precision	mAP	Precision	mAP
NYU	0.548	0.409	0.614	0.364	0.655	0.451
	8 ± 0.1423	3 ± 0.0703	4 ± 0.1525	7 ± 0.0527	4 ± 0.0571	7 ± 0.038
UM	0.576	0.385	0.528	0.374	0.701	0.497
	7 ± 0.1325	9 ± 0.0872	5 ± 0.1214	0 ± 0.0861	4 ± 0.0708	1 ± 0.1250
Leuven	0.617	0.424	0.608	0.333	0.617	0.448
	1 ± 0.2261	2 ± 0.2086	5 ± 0	3 ± 0	6 ± 0.0725	2 ± 0.0861
UCLA	0.605	0.442	0.654	0.333	0.665	0.443
	2 ± 0.1833	0 ± 0.2086	3 ± 0	3 ± 0	2 ± 0.1504	4 ± 0.1659
KKI	0.559	0.395	0.646	0.333	0.687	0.447
	8 ± 0.2567	4 ± 0.2941	5 ± 0	3 ± 0	5 ± 0.1237	6 ± 0.1016

misjudgment costs for different categories by introducing $1N_j$. In theory, this can avoid the tendency of the algorithm model to the majority class and improve the prediction accuracy for the minority class [18]. The experimental results in Table 16.5 also verify this theory in the experiment. In most cases, the algorithm's stability has also been improved, and the standard deviation of the experimental results is slight.

16.4.6 ANALYSIS OF GRAPH

In this section, we study the effect of parameter changes on the algorithm CSLDSVR. Figure 16.3 shows the changes in the precision and KL divergence evaluation indicators when the parameters C and ε take different values on five different datasets. Comparing and studying two graphs of the same parameter and other indicators, such as Figure 16.3a and b with Table 16.6, it can be found that the curve trend of the same dataset is basically opposite, and the point where precision takes the maximum value is generally the same as the KL divergence. The minimum value, which also corresponds to the previous analysis of KL divergence, indicates that when the KL divergence is slight, the label distributions of the two are more similar, and the classification results are more accurate for different datasets, the parameter values for obtaining the optimal solution are not the same, which also shows that

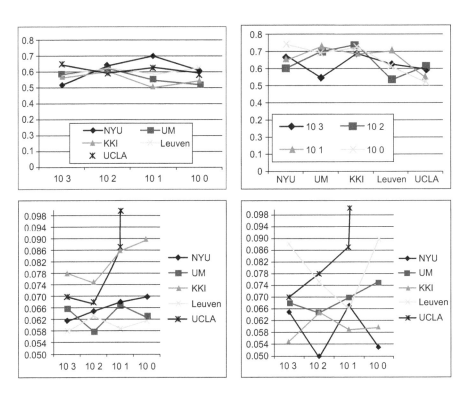

FIGURE 16.3   (a) Impact of C on precision. (b) Impact of ε on precision. (c) Impact of C on KL. (d) Impact of ε on KL.

TABLE 16.6
Impact of *C* on Precision

Serial	NYU	UM	KKI	Leuven	UCLA
10^3	0.52	0.59	0.57	0.58	0.65
10^2	0.64	0.62	0.6	0.63	0.6
10^1	0.7	0.55	0.51	0.59	0.63
10^0	0.61	0.52	0.54	0.62	0.59

in the diagnosis of autism, the data distribution of different data centers is further. Therefore, the parameters for building the model should also be other. Moreover, it is found that in the dataset with fewer samples, the result is more sensitive to the change of parameters. For example, the KKI dataset with only 48 pieces fluctuate when the parameter value changes. The parameters of the CSLDSVR algorithm should be based on the characteristics of the dataset, and the corresponding parameter values should be set to build a model. If the parameter settings are reasonable, CSLDSVR can overcome the high dimensionality and category imbalance of the autism dataset: better classification effect.

16.5 CONCLUSION

The brain function of ASD patients is different from that of ordinary people [4–6], and rs-fMRI is an effective tool to reflect brain activity. This chapter proposes a cost-sensitive marker distribution support ASD-aided diagnosis method for vector regression based on the functional connectivity features extracted from rs-fMRI. The introduction of label distribution learning overcomes the label noise problem of ASD-aided diagnosis based on multi-classification. Moreover, the new method introduces class balance based on the labeled distribution support vector regression technique. It can effectively solve the imbalanced data problem in ASD diagnosis. However, the improved model is still biased toward the majority class to a certain extent, and the imbalanced data problem should be further improved. You can try to improve the sampling method of the data or use the synthetic minority sample method, etc., which is worthy of further research; at the same time, the loss function can be changed to a more complex distance measure, and the Euclidean distance treats each feature equally so that it can reflect the individual absolute difference in the eigenvalues. But it is also necessary to introduce relatively high-level spaces, but this requires more prior knowledge. No more prior knowledge is currently used, so Euclidean distance is used. Other advanced lengths have their advantages, which will be further improved in future research.

REFERENCES

[1] J. Wang et al., "Multi-Class ASD Classification Based on Functional Connectivity and Functional Correlation Tensor via Multi-Source Domain Adaptation and Multi-View Sparse Representation," in *IEEE Transactions on Medical Imaging*, vol. 39, no. 10, pp. 3137–3147, Oct. 2020, doi:10.1109/TMI.2020.2987817.

[2] H.-C. Shin et al., "Deep Convolutional Neural Networks for Computer-Aided Detection: CNN Architectures, Dataset Characteristics and Transfer Learning," in *IEEE Transactions on Medical Imaging*, vol. 35, no. 5, pp. 1285–1298, May 2016, doi:10.1109/TMI.2016.2528162.

[3] G. Han et al., "The LISS—A Public Database of Common Imaging Signs of Lung Diseases for Computer-Aided Detection and Diagnosis Research and Medical Education," in *IEEE Transactions on Biomedical Engineering*, vol. 62, no. 2, pp. 648–656, Feb. 2015, doi:10.1109/TBME.2014.2363131.

[4] K. Drukker, C. A. Sennett and M. L. Giger, "Automated Method for Improving System Performance of Computer-Aided Diagnosis in Breast Ultrasound," in *IEEE Transactions on Medical Imaging*, vol. 28, no. 1, pp. 122–128, Jan. 2009, doi:10.1109/TMI.2008.928178.

[5] H. Jing and Y. Yang, "Image Retrieval for Computer-aided Diagnosis of Breast Cancer," in *2010 IEEE Southwest Symposium on Image Analysis & Interpretation (SSIAI)*, 2010, pp. 9–12, doi:10.1109/SSIAI.2010.5483930.

[6] S. Kato et al., "Blood Vessel Structure Analysis in Endoscopic Images for Computer-Aided Diagnosis," in *2020 9th International Congress on Advanced Applied Informatics (IIAI-AAI)*, 2020, pp. 493–498, doi:10.1109/IIAI-AAI50415.2020.00104.

[7] R. Michida et al., "A Lesion Classification Method Using Deep Learning Based on JNET Classification for Computer-Aided Diagnosis System in Colorectal Magnified NBI Endoscopy," *2021 36th International Technical Conference on Circuits/Systems, Computers and Communications (ITC-CSCC)*, 2021, pp. 1–4, doi:10.1109/ITC-CSCC52171.2021.9501420.

[8] H. R. Roth et al., "Improving Computer-Aided Detection Using Convolutional Neural Networks and Random View Aggregation," in *IEEE Transactions on Medical Imaging*, vol. 35, no. 5, pp. 1170–1181, May 2016, doi:10.1109/TMI.2015.2482920.

[9] Z. Z. Htike, W. Y. Nyein Naing, S. L. Win and S. Khan, "Computer-Aided Diagnosis of Pulmonary Nodules from Chest X-Rays Using Rotation Forest," in *2014 International Conference on Computer and Communication Engineering*, 2014, pp. 96–99, doi:10.1109/ICCCE.2014.38.

[10] R. T. Sousa et al., "Evaluation of Classifiers to a Childhood Pneumonia Computer-Aided Diagnosis System," in *2014 IEEE 27th International Symposium on Computer-Based Medical Systems*, 2014, pp. 477–478, doi:10.1109/CBMS.2014.98.

[11] J. Gutierrez-Cáceres, C. Portugal-Zambrano and C. Beltrán-Castañón, "Computer Aided Medical Diagnosis Tool to Detect Normal/Abnormal Studies in Digital MR Brain Images," in *2014 IEEE 27th International Symposium on Computer-Based Medical Systems*, 2014, pp. 501–502, doi:10.1109/CBMS.2014.110.

[12] Soufiene Ben Othman, Faris A. Almalki, Chinmay Chakraborty and Hedi Sakli, "Privacy-preserving Aware Data Aggregation for IoT-Based Healthcare with Green Computing Technologies," in *Computers and Electrical Engineering*, vol. 101, p. 108025, 2022, doi:10.1016/j.compeleceng.2022.108025.

[13] Soufiene Ben Othman, Abdullah Ali Bahattab, Abdelbasset Trad and Habib Youssef, "PEERP: A Priority-Based Energy-Efficient Routing Protocol for Reliable Data Transmission in Healthcare using the IoT," in *The 15th International Conference on Future Networks and Communications (FNC) August 9–12, 2020*, Leuven, Belgium, 2020.

[14] K. Abe, K. Shirakawa, M. Minami and K. Yoshikawa, "Automated Extraction of the Essential Region in Computer-Aided Diagnosis of Helicobacter Pylori Infection Using Gastric X-ray Images," in *2018 7th International Congress on Advanced Applied Informatics (IIAI-AAI)*, 2018, pp. 626–629, doi:10.1109/IIAI-AAI.2018.00131.

[15] Segyeong Joo, Woo Kyung Moon and Hee Chan Kim, "Computer-aided Diagnosis of Solid Breast Nodules on Ultrasound with Digital Image Processing and Artificial Neural Network," in *The 26th Annual International Conference of the IEEE Engineering in Medicine and Biology Society*, 2004, pp. 1397–1400, doi:10.1109/IEMBS.2004.1403434.

[16] S. -F. Huang, H. -Y. Chaoa, C. -C. Hsu, S. -F. Yang and P. -F. Kao, "A Computer-aided Diagnosis System for Whole Body Bone Scan Using Single Photon Emission Computed Tomography," in *2009 IEEE International Symposium on Biomedical Imaging: From Nano to Macro*, 2009, pp. 542–545, doi:10.1109/ISBI.2009.5193104.

[17] T. Okamoto et al., "Feature Extraction of Colorectal Endoscopic Images for Computer-Aided Diagnosis with CNN," in *2019 2nd International Symposium on Devices, Circuits and Systems (ISDCS)*, 2019, pp. 1–4, doi:10.1109/ISDCS.2019.8719104.

[18] T. Okamoto et al., "Implementation of Computer-Aided Diagnosis System on Customizable DSP Core for Colorectal Endoscopic Images with CNN Features and SVM," in *TENCON 2018–2018 IEEE Region 10 Conference*, 2018, pp. 1663–1666, doi:10.1109/TENCON.2018.8650331.

[19] H. Zhang, W. Zuo, Y. Chen, K. Wang and D. Zhang, "TDS and Its Application in Computer Aided TCM Diagnostics Education," in *2010 Second International Workshop on Education Technology and Computer Science*, 2010, pp. 260–263, doi:10.1109/ETCS.2010.358.

[20] Soufiene Ben Othman, Abdullah Ali Bahattab, Abdelbasset Trad and Habib Youssef, "LSDA: Lightweight Secure Data Aggregation Scheme in Healthcare using IoT," in *ACM — 10th International Conference on Information Systems and Technologies*, Lecce, Italy, June 2020.

Index

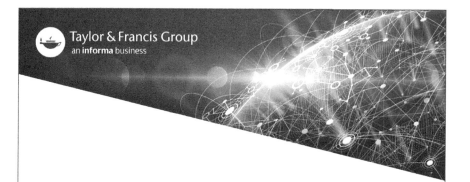